Statistics And Experimental Design
For Toxicologists

D1158694

Statistics and Experimental Design For Toxicologists

Shayne C. Gad
G.D. Searle and Company
Skokie, Illinois

and

Carrol S. Weil
C.S. Weil, Inc.
Pittsburgh, Pennsylvania

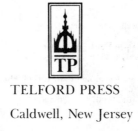

TELFORD PRESS

Caldwell, New Jersey

Copyright © by the Telford Press, Inc.
All rights reserved.
No part of this publication may be reproduced or transmitted in any form
or by any means, electronic or mechanical, including photocopy, recording,
or any information storage or retrieval system, without permission in writ-
ing from the publisher.

THE TELFORD PRESS, INC.
285 Bloomfield Avenue, Caldwell, New Jersey, 07006

Library of Congress Cataloging-in-Publication Data
Statistics and Experimental Design for Toxicologists
1. Toxicology—Statistical methods.
2. Toxicology, Experimental—Statistical methods. I. Gad, Shayne, C.,
1948— II. Weil, Carrol S.
RA1199.4.S73S73   1986   615.9'0072   86—1953
ISBN 0-936923-01-6
ISBN 0-936923-00-8 (pbk.)

DEDICATION

To my beloved Suzann, who made me real again and brought me back to the World.

SCG

CONTENTS

ACKNOWLEDGEMENTS

There are a number of people without whom this book would either never have been completed or would be much less than it is. Lorie Abraham and Nancy Bruce spent many hours struggling with translating handwritten pages into the final polished manuscript—a feat of typing, given the use of unfamiliar specialized symbols, which was certainly beyond the scope of any job requirement. And Gary Roy and Ann Smith provided exacting proofreading of the manuscript without which the final product would not be nearly as lucid as it is. We wish to thank these fine people for their support.

PREFACE

Statistics and Experimental Design for Toxicologists has been designed as a source and textbook for both practicing and student toxicologists with the central objective of equipping them for the regular statistical analysis of experimental data. Starting with the assumption of only basic mathematical skills and knowledge, it provides a complete and systematic yet practical introduction to the statistical methodologies that are available for, and utilized in, the discipline. For every technique that is presented, a worked example from toxicology is also presented.

Because toxicology is the study of the adverse responses of biological units to chemicals and physical agents, any understanding and valid analysis must originate from an understanding of the underlying biological mechanisms, and from this understanding selecting the best methods of analysis in accordance with their limitations and necessary assumptions. This book is written from the perspective of toxicologists, drawing on the authors' combined experience of more than 50 years to provide insight and philosophical underpinnings for the overall structure of analysis and for the specific usage examples. It is the purpose of this book to provide both the methodological tools necessary to analyze experimental toxicology data and the insight to know when to use them.

Statistics and Experimental Design for Toxicologists is organized to provide an ordered development of skills and yet still facilitate ease of access to the information that is desired. The first section, (Chapters I - IV) develops some basic principles, establishes (or reviews) introductory statistical concepts, presents an overview of automated computational hardware and software, and presents decision tree guidelines for selecting actual analytical techniques. The second section (Chapters V - X) presents actual techniques, organized by their functional objectives. The third section (Chapters XI - XIV) reviews all the major possible data analysis applications in toxicology (LD_{50}/LC_{50} calculation, clinical chemistry, reproduction studies, behavioral studies, risk assessment, SAR's etc.) and in each case provides examples and guidelines for analysis. The last chapter stands apart, and presents an overview of the areas of controversy in "statistical toxicology", such as the question of the existence of thresholds. Each of these chapters not only should enable a person to perform a type of analysis, but should also ensure sufficient understanding of its assumptions and limitations to prevent misuse.

CHAPTER 1

INTRODUCTION

This book has been written for both practicing and student toxicologists, as both a basic text and a practical guide to the common statistical problems encountered in toxicology and the methodologies that are available to solve them. It has been enriched by the inclusion of discussions of why a particular procedure or interpretation is suggested, by the clear enumeration of the assumptions that are necessary for a procedure to be valid, and by worked-through examples and problems drawn from the actual practice of toxicology. A set of tables has been included to make this volume complete.

Since 1960, the field of toxicology has become increasingly complex and controversial in both its theory and practice. Much of this change is due to the evolution of the field. As in all other sciences, toxicology started as a descriptive science. Living organisms, be they human or otherwise, were dosed with or exposed to chemical or physical agents and the adverse effects which followed were observed. But as a sufficient body of descriptive data was accumulated, it became possible to infer and study underlying mechanisms of action - to determine in a broader sense why adverse effects occurred. As with all sciences, toxicology has thus entered a later state of development, the mechanistic stage, where active contributions to the field encompass both descriptive and mechanistic studies. Frequently, in fact, present day studies are a combination of both approaches.

As a result of this evolution, studies are being designed and executed to generate increased amounts of data which are then utilized to address various areas of concern. The resulting problems of data analysis have then become more complex and toxicology has drawn more deeply from the well of available statistical techniques. At the same time however, the field of statistics has also been very active and growing during the last twenty-five years - to some extent, at least, because of the very growth of toxicology. These simultaneous changes have led to an increasing complexity of data and, unfortunately, to the introduction of numerous confounding factors which severely limit the utility of the resulting data in all too many cases.

One (and perhaps the major) difficulty is that there is a very real necessity to understand the biological realities and implications of a problem, as well as to understand the peculiarities of toxicological data before procedures are selected and employed for analysis. Some of these characteristics include the following.

(1) The need to work with a relatively small sample set of data collected from the members of a population (laboratory animals, cultured cells and bacterial cultures) which is not actually our population of interest (that is, people or a wildlife population).

(2) Dealing frequently with data resulting from a sample which was censored on a basis other than by the investigator's as design. By censoring, of course, we mean that not all data points were collected as might be desired. This censoring could be the result of either a biological factor (the test animal being dead or too debilitated to manipulate) or a logistic factor (equipment being inoperative or a tissue being missed in necropsy).

(3) The conditions under which our experiments are conducted are extremely varied. In pharmacology (the closest cousin to at least classical toxicology), the possible conditions of interaction of a chemical or physical agent with a person are limited to a small range of doses via a single route over a short course of treatment to a defined patient population. In toxicology however, all these variables (dose, route, time span and subject population) are determined by the investigator.

(4) The time frames available to solve our problems are limited by practical and economic factors. This frequently means that there is not time to repeat a critical study if the first attempt fails. So a true iterative approach is not possible.

Unfortunately, there are very few toxicologists who are also statisticians, or vice versa. In fact, the training of most toxicologists in statistics has been limited to a single introductory course which concentrates on some theoretical basics. As a result, the armertarium of statistical techniques of most toxicologists is limited and the tools that are usually present (t-tests, chi-square, analysis of variance, and linear regression) are neither fully developed nor well understood. It is hoped that this book will help change this situation.

As a point of departure toward this objective, it is essential that any analysis of study results be interpreted by a professional who firmly understands three concepts; the difference between biological significance and statistical significance, the nature and value of different types of data, and causality.

For the first concept, we should consider the four possible combinations of these two different types of significance, for which we find the relationship shown below.

		STATISTICAL SIGNIFICANCE	
		No	Yes
BIOLOGICAL	No	Case I	Case II
SIGNIFICANCE	Yes	Case III	Case IV

Cases I and IV give us no problems, for the answers are the same statistically and biologically. But cases II and III present problems. In Case II (the "false positive"), we have a circumstance where there is a statistical significance in the measured difference between treated and control groups, but there is no true biological significance to the finding. This is not an uncommon happening, for example, in the case of clinical chemistry parameters. This is called type I error by statisticians, and the probability of this happening is called the α(alpha) level. In Case III (the "false negative"), we have no statistical significance, but the differences between groups are biologically/toxicologically significant. This is called type II error by statisticians, and the probability of such an error happening by random chance is called the β(beta) level. An example of this second situation is when we see a few of a very rare tumor type in treated animals. In both of these latter cases, numerical analysis, no matter how well done, is no substitute for professional judgment. Here, perhaps, is the cutting edge of what really makes a practicing toxicologist. Along with this, however, must come a feeling for the different types of data and for the value or relative merit of each.

We will more fully explore the types of data (the second major concept) and their value (and the implications of value of data to such things as animal usage) in the next chapter of this book.

The reasons that biological and statistical significance are not identical are multiple, but a central one is certainly causality. Through our consideration of statistics, we should keep in mind that just because a treatment and a change in an observed organism are seemingly or actually associated with each other does not "prove" that the former caused the latter. Though this fact is now widely appreciated for correlation (for example, that fact that the number of storks' nests found each year in England is correlated with the number of human births that year does not mean that storks bring babies), it is just as true in the general case for significance. Timely establishment and proof that treatment causes an effect requires an understanding of the underlying mechanism and proof of its validity. At the same time, it is important that we realize that not finding a good correlation or suitable significance associated with a treatment and an effect likewise does not prove that the two are not associated - that a treatment does not cause an effect. At best, it gives us a certain level of confidence that under the conditions of the current test, these items are not associated.

These points will be discussed in greater detail in the "Assumptions" section for each method, along with the other common pitfalls and shortcomings associated with the method.

CHAPTER 2

BASIC PRINCIPLES

Let us first introduce (or review) a few simple terms and concepts which are fundamental to an understanding of statistics.

Each measurement we make - each individual piece of experimental information we gather - is called a datum. It is extremely unusual, however, to either obtain or attempt to analyze a datum. Rather, we gather and analyze multiple pieces at one time, the resulting collection being called data.

Data are collected on the basis of their association with a treatment (intended or otherwise) as an effect (a property) that is measured in the experimental subjects of a study, such as body weights. These identifiers (that is, treatment and effect) are termed variables. Our treatment variables (those that the researcher or nature control, and which can be directly controlled) are termed independent, while our effect variables (such as weight, life span, and number of neoplasms) are termed dependent variables - their outcome is believed to depend on the "treatment" being studied.

All the possible measures of a given set of variables in all the possible subjects that exist is termed the population for those variables. Such a population of variables cannot be truly measured - for example, one would have to obtain, treat and measure the weights of all the Fischer-344 rats that were, are or ever will be. Instead, we deal with a representative group - a sample. If our sample of data is appropriately collected and of sufficient size, it serves to provide good estimates of the characteristics of the parent population from which it was drawn.

Two terms refer to the quality and reproducibility of our measurements of variables. The first, accuracy, is an expression of the closeness of a measured or computed value to its actual or "true" value in nature. The second, precision, reflects the closeness or reproducibility of a series of repeated measurements of the same quantity.

If we arrange all of our measurements of a particular variable in order as a point on an axis marked as to the values of that variable, and if our sample were large enough, the pattern of distribution of the data in the sample would begin to become apparent. This pattern is a representation of the frequency distribution of a given population of data - that is, of the incidence of different measurements, their central tendency, and dispersion.

The most common frequency distribution - and one we will talk about throughout this book - is the normal (or Gaussian) distribution. This distribution is the most common in nature and is such that two-thirds of all values are within one standard deviation (to be defined in chapter two) of the mean (or average value for the entire population) and 95% are within 1.96 standard deviations of the mean. The mathematical equation for the normal curve is

$$y = \frac{1}{\sigma\sqrt{2\pi}} \, e^{-\frac{(x-\mu)^2}{2\sigma^2}}$$

where μ is the mean and σ is the standard deviation.

There are other frequency distributions, such as the binomial, Poisson and chi square.

In all areas of biological research, optimal design and appropriate interpretation of experiments require that the researcher understand both the biological and technological underpinnings of the system being studied and of the data being generated. From the point of view of the statistician, it is vitally important that the experimenter both know and be able to communicate the nature of the data, and understand its limitations. One classification of data types is presented in Table 1.

The nature of the data collected is determined by three considerations. These are the biological source of the data (the system being studied), the instrumentation and techniques being used to make measurements, and the design of the experiment. The researcher has some degree of control over each of these - least over the biological system (he/she normally has a choice of only one of several models to study) and most over the design of the experiment or study. Such choices, in fact, dictate the type of data generated by a study.

Statistical methods are based on specific assumptions. Parametric statistics - those that are most familiar to the majority of scientists -have more stringent underlying assumptions than do nonparametric statistics. Among the underlying assumptions for many parametric statistical methods (such as the analysis of variance) is that the data are continuous. The nature of the data associated with a variable (as described above) imparts a "value" to that data, the value being the power of the statistical tests which can be employed.

Continuous variables are those which can at least theoretically assume any of an infinite number of values between any two fixed

TABLE 1

TYPES OF VARIABLES (DATA) AND EXAMPLES OF EACH TYPE

Classified By		Type	Example[a]
Scale	Continuous	Scalar	Body weight
		Ranked	Severity of a lesion
	Discontinuous	Scalar	Weeks until the first observation of a tumor in a carcinogenicity study
		Ranked	Clinical observations in animals
		Attribute	Eye colors in fruit flies
		Quantal	Dead/alive or present/absent
Frequency Distribution		Normal	Body weights
		Bimodal	Some clinical chemistry parameters
		Others	Measures of time-to-incapacitation

[a]It should be kept in mind that though these examples are most commonly of the data types assigned above, it is not always the case.

points (such as measurements of body weight between 2.0 and 3.0 kilograms). Discontinuous variables, meanwhile, are those which can have only certain fixed values, with no possible intermediate values (such as counts of 5 and 6 dead animals, respectively).

Limitations on our ability to measure constrain the extent to which the real-world situation approaches the theoretical, but many of the variables studied in toxicology are in fact continuous. Examples of these are lengths, weights, concentrations, temperatures, periods of time and percentages. For these continuous variables, we may describe the character of a sample with measures of central tendency and dispersion that we are most familiar with - the mean, denoted by the symbol $\overline{X}$ and also called the arithmetic average, and the standard deviation SD, which is denoted by the symbol σ; and is calculated as being equal to

$$\sqrt{\frac{\Sigma X^2 - \frac{(\Sigma X)^2}{N}}{N - 1}}$$

where X is the individual datum and N is the total number of data in the group.

Contrasted with these continuous data, however, we have discontinuous (or discrete) data, which can only assume certain fixed numerical values. In these cases our choice of statistical tools or tests is, as we will find later, more limited.

Probability

Probability is simply the likelihood that in a sufficiently large sample a particular event will occur or a particular value be found. Hypothesis testing, for example, is generally structured so that the likelihood of a treatment group being the same as a control group (the so called "null hypothesis") can be assessed as being less than a selected low level (very frequently 5%, which implies that we are $1.0 - \alpha$ (that is $1.0 - 0.05$ or 95% sure) that the groups are *not* equivalent).

Functions of Statistics

Statistical methods may serve to do any combination of three possible tasks. The one we are most familiar with is hypothesis testing - that is, determining if two (or more) groups of data differ from each other at a predetermined level of confidence. A second function is the construction and use of models which may be used to predict future outcomes of chemical - biological interactions. This is most commonly seen in linear regression or in the derivation of some form of correlation coefficient. Model fitting allows us to relate one variable (typically a treatment or "independent" variable) to another. The third function, reduction of dimensionality, continues to be less commonly utilized than the first two. This final category includes methods for reducing the number of variables in a system while only minimally reducing the amount of information, therefore making a problem easier to visualize and to understand. Examples of such techniques are factor analysis and cluster analysis. A subset of this last function, discussed later under descriptive statistics, is the reduction of raw data to single expressions of central tendency and variability (such as the mean and standard deviation).

There is also a special subset of statistical techniques which is part of both the second and third functions of statistics. This is data transformation, which includes such things as the conversion of numbers to log or probit values.

As a matter of practicality, the contents of this book are primarily designed to address the first of the three functions of statistical methods that we presented (hypothesis testing). The second function, modeling - especially in the form of risk assessment, is becoming increasingly important as the science continues to evolve from the descriptive phase to a mechanistic phase (i.e. the elucidation of mechanisms of action), and as such is addressed in some detail. Likewise, because the interrelation of multiple factors is becoming a real concern, a discussion of reduction of dimensionality has been included.

Descriptive Statistics

Descriptive statistics are used to convey, in summary, the general nature of the data. As such, the parameters describing any single group of data have two components. One of these describes the location of the data, while the other gives a measure of the dispersion of the data in and about this location. Often overlooked is the fact that the choice of which parameters are used to give these pieces of information implies a particular type of distribution for the data.

Most commonly, location is described by giving the (arithmetic) mean and dispersion by giving the standard deviation (SD) or the standard error of the mean (SEM). The calculation of the first two of these has already been described. If we again denote the total number of data in a group as N, then the SEM would be calculated as

$$SEM = \frac{SD}{\sqrt{N}}$$

The use of the mean with either the SD or SEM implies, however, that we have reason to believe that the data being summarized are from a population which is at least approximately normally distributed. If this is not the case, then we should rather use a set of statistical quantities which do not require a normal distribution. These are the median, for location, and the semiquartile distance, for a measure of dispersion. These somewhat less familiar parameters are characterized as follows.

MEDIAN: When all the numbers in a group are arranged in a ranked order (that is, from smallest to largest), the median is the middle value. If there is an odd number of values in a group then the middle value is obvious (in the case of 13 values, for example, the seventh largest is the median). When the number of values in the sample is even, the median is calculated as the midpoint between the (N/2)th and the ([N/2] + 1)th number. For example, in the series of numbers 7, 12, 13, 19 the median value would be the midpoint between 12 and 13, which is 12.5.

The standard deviation and the standard error of the mean are related to each other but yet are quite different. To compare these two, let us first demonstrate their calculation from the same set of fifteen observations.

$$Sum\,(\Sigma)$$

Data Points (X_i): 1, 2, 3, 4, 4, 5, 5, 5, 6, 6, 6, 7, 7, 8, 9,   78

Squares (X_i^2): 1, 4, 9, 16, 16, 25, 25, 25, 36, 36, 36, 49, 49, 64, 81 472

The standard deviation can then be calculated as:

$$SD = \sqrt{\dfrac{472 - \dfrac{(78)^2}{15}}{15 - 1}} = \sqrt{\dfrac{472 - \dfrac{(6084)}{15}}{14}}$$

$$= \sqrt{\dfrac{472 - 405.6}{14}} = \sqrt{4.7428571} = 2.1778$$

with a mean $(\overline{X})$ of $\dfrac{78}{15}$ = 5.2 for the data group. The SEM for the same set of data, however, is

$$SEM = \dfrac{2.1778}{\sqrt{15}} = \dfrac{2.1778}{3.8730} = 0.562301$$

The SEM is quite a bit smaller than the SD, making it very attractive to use in reporting data. This size difference is because the SEM actually is an estimate of the error (or variability) involved in measuring the means of samples, and not an estimate of the error (or variability) involved in measuring the data from which means are calculated. This is implied by the Central Limit Theorem, which tells us three major things.

- The distribution of sample means will be approximately normal regardless of the distribution of values in the original population from which the samples were drawn.

- The mean value of the collection of all possible sample means will equal the mean of the original population.

- The standard deviation of the collection of all possible means of samples of a given size, called the standard error of the mean, depends on both the standard deviation of the original population and the size of the sample.

The SEM should be used only when the uncertainty of the estimate of the mean is of concern - which is almost never the case in toxicology. Rather, we are concerned with an estimate of the variability of the population - for which the standard deviation is appropriate.

SEMI-QUARTILE DISTANCE: When all the data in a group are ranked, a quartile of the data contains one ordered quarter of the values. Typically, we are most interested in the borders of the middle two quartiles, Q_1 and Q_2, which together represent the semi-quartile distance and which contain the median as their center. Given that there are N values in an ordered group of data, the upper limit of the jth quartile (Q_j) may be computed as being equal to the $[j(N + 1)/4th]$ value. Once we have used this formula to calculate the upper limits of Q_1 and Q_3, we can then compute the semiquartile distance (which is also called the quartile deviation, and as such is abbreviated as the QD) with the formula $QD = (Q_3 - Q_1)/2$.

For example, for the fifteen value data set 1, 2, 3, 4, 4, 5, 5, 5, 6, 6, 6, 7, 7, 8, 9, we can calculate the upper limits of Q_1 and Q_3 as

$$Q_1 = \frac{1(15 + 1)}{4} = \frac{16}{4} = 4$$

$$Q_3 = \frac{3(15 + 1)}{4} = \frac{48}{4} = 12$$

The 4th and 12th values in this data set are 4 and 7, respectively. The semiquartile distance can then be calculated as

$$QD = \frac{12 - 4}{2} = 4$$

One final sample parameter which sees some use in toxicology (primarily in inhalation studies) is the geometric mean, denoted by the term $\overline{X}g$. This is calculated as

$$\overline{X}_g = (X_1 . X_2 ... X_N)^{1/N}$$

and has the attractive feature that it does not give excessive weight to extreme values (or "outliers"), such as the mass of a single very large particle in a dust sample. In effect, it "folds" extreme values in towards the center of the distribution, decreasing the sensitivity of the parameter to the undue influence of the outlier. This is particularly important in the case of aerosol samples where a few very large particles would cause the arithmetic mean of particle diameters to present a misleading picture of the nature of the "average" particle.

There are times when it is desired to describe the relative variability of one or more sets of data. The most common way of doing this to compute the coefficient of variation (CV), which is calculated simply as the ratio of the standard deviation to the mean, or

$$CV = \frac{SD}{\overline{X}}$$

A CV of 0.2 or 20% thus means that the standard deviation is 20% of the mean. In toxicology the CV is frequently between 20 and 50% and may at times exceed 100%.

Outliers and Rounding of Numbers

These two considerations in the handling of numerical data can be, on occasion, of major concern to the toxicologist because of their pivotal nature in borderline cases. Outliers should also be of concern for other reasons, however. On the principle that one should always have a plan to deal with all reasonably likely contingencies in advance of their happening, early decisions should be made to select a policy for handling both outliers and the rounding of numbers.

Outliers are extreme (high or low) values which are widely divergent from the main body of a group of data and from what is our common experience. They may arise from an instrument (such as a balance) being faulty, the apparently natural urge of some animals to frustrate research, or they may be indicative of a "real" value. Outlying values can be detected by visual inspection of the data, use of a scattergram (described later), or (if the data set is small enough, which is usually the case in toxicology) by a large increase in the parameter estimating the dispersion of data, such as the standard deviation.

When we can solidly tie one of the above error-producing processes (such as a balance being faulty) to an outlier, we can safely delete it from consideration. But if we cannot solidly tie such a cause to an outlier (even if we have strong suspicions), we have a much more complicated problem, for then such a value may be one of several other things. It could be the result of a particular cause that is the grounds for the entire study - that is, the very "effect" that we are looking for, or it could be because of the collection of legitimate effects which constitute sample error. As will be discussed later (under exploratory data analysis), and as is now more widely appreciated, outliers can be an indication of a biologically significant effect which is not yet statistically significant. Variance inflation can be the result of such outliers, and can be used to detect them. Outliers, in fact, by increasing the variability within a sample, decrease the sensitivity of our statistical tests and actually preclude our having a statistically significant result (Beckman and Cook (1983)).

Alternatively the outlier may be the result of, for example, an unobserved technician error, and may be such as to change the decisions made from a set of data. In this case we want to reject the data point - to exclude it from consideration with the rest of the data. But how can one identify these legitimate statistical rejection cases?

There are a wide variety of techniques for data rejection. Their proper use depends on one's having an understanding of the nature of the distribution of the data. For normally distributed data with a single extreme value, a simple method such as Chauvenet's Criterion (Meyer, 1975) may legitimately be employed. This states that if the probability of a value deviating from the mean is greater than ½ N, one should consider that there are adequate grounds for its rejection.

In practice, this approach is demonstrated below.

USE OF CHAUVENET'S CRITERION

Having collected twenty values as a data set, we find they include the following values: 1, 6, 7, 8, 8, 9, 9, 9, 10, 10, 10, 10, 10, 11, 11, 11, 12, 12, 13 and 14. Was the lowest value (1) erroneous and should it be rejected as an outlier? Some simple calculations are performed, as

Mean (X) = 9.55
Standard deviation (SD) = 2.80
Chauvenet's Criterion Value = ½ N = $\frac{20}{2}$ = 10

So we would reject the value of "1" if its probability of occurrence were less than 10%. Going to a table of Z scores (such as Table H in Appendix I), we see that 10% of the values in a normal distribution are beyond ± 1.645 standard deviations of the mean. Multiplying this by the standard deviation for the sample, we get (1.645) (2.80) = 4.606. This means we would reject values beyond this range from the mean - that is, less than (9.55 - 4.606) = 4.944 or greater than (9.55 + 4.606) = 14.156. We therefore reject the value of "1".

One should note that as the sample size gets bigger, the rejection zone for Chauvenet's Criterion will also increase. Indeed, an N of 20 is about as large as this method is useful for.

A second relatively straightforward approach, for use when the data are normally distributed but contain several extreme values, is to winsorize the data. Though there are a number of variations to this approach, the simplest (called the G-1 method) calls for replacing the highest and lowest values in a set of data. In a group of data consisting of the values 54, 22, 18, 15, 14, 13, 11 and 4, we would replace 54 with a second 22, and 4 with a replicate 11. This would give us a group consisting of 22, 22, 18, 15, 14, 14, 13, 11 and 11, which we would then treat as our original data. Winsorizing should not be performed, however, if the extreme values constitute more than a small minority of the entire data set.

Another approach is to use Dixon's Test (Dixon and Maney, 1969) to determine if extreme values should be rejected. In Dixon's test, the set of observations is first ordered according to their magnitude (as we did earlier for the data set used to demonstrate Chauvenet's Criterion, though there this step was simply to make the case clearer). The ratio of the difference of an extreme value from one of its nearest neighbor values in the range of values in the sample is then calculated, using a formula which varies with sample size. This ratio is then compared to a table value, and if found to be equal or greater, is considered to be an outlier at the $p \le 0.05$ level. The formula for the ratio varies with sample size and according to whether it is the smallest or largest value that is suspect.

If we have more information as to the nature of the data or the type of analysis to be performed, there are yet better techniques to handle outliers. Extensive discussions of these may be found elsewhere (Barnett and Lewis (1984), Grubbs (1969), Beckman and Cook (1983), Snedecor and Cochran (1980)).

When the number of digits in a number is to be reduced (due to limitations of space or to reflect the extent of significance of a number) we must carry out the process of rounding off a number. Failure to have a rule for performing this operation can lead to both confusion and embarrassment for a facility (during such times as study audits). One common rule follows.

A digit to be rounded is not changed if it is followed by a digit less than 5 - the digits following it are simply dropped off ("truncated"). If the number is followed by a digit greater than 5 or by a 5 followed by other nonzero digits, it is increased to the next highest number. When the digit to be rounded is followed by 5 alone or by 5 followed by zeros, it is unchanged if it is even but increased by one if it is odd. Examples of this rule in effect are (in a case where we must reduce to 3 digits)

1374 becomes 137
1376 becomes 138
13852 becomes 139

1375   becomes 138
and 1385   becomes 138

The rationale behind this procedure is that over a period of time, the results should even out - as many digits will be increased as are decreased.

Sampling

Sampling - the selection of which individual data points will be collected, whether in the form of selecting which animals to collect blood from or to remove a portion of a diet mix from for analysis - is an essential step upon which all other efforts towards a good experiment or study are based.

There are three assumptions about sampling which are common to most of the statistical analysis techniques that are used in toxicology. These are that sample is collected without bias, that each member of a sample is collected independently of the others and that members of a sample are collected with replacements. Precluding bias, both intentional and unintentional, means that at the time of selection of a sample to measure, each portion of the population from which that selection is to be made has an equal chance of being selected. Ways of precluding bias are discussed in detail in the chapter on experimental design.

Independence means that the selection of any portion of the sample is not affected by and does not affect the selection or measurement of any other portion.

Finally, sampling with replacement means that in theory, after each portion is selected and measured, it is returned to the total sample pool and thus has the opportunity to be selected again. This is a corrolary of the assumption of independence. Violation of this assumption (which is almost always the case in toxicology and all the life sciences) does not have serious consequences if the total pool from which samples are sufficiently large (say 20 or greater) that the chance of reselecting that portion is small anyway.

There are four major types of sampling methods - random, stratified, systematic and cluster. Random is by far the most commonly employed method in toxicology. It stresses the fulfillment of the assumption of avoiding bias. When the entire pool of possibilities is mixed or randomized (procedures for randomization are presented in a later chapter), then the members of the group are selected in the order they are drawn from the pool.

Stratified sampling is performed by first dividing the entire pool into subsets or strata, then doing randomized sampling from each strata. This method is employed when the total pool contains subsets which are distinctly different but in which each subset contains similar members. An example is a large batch of a powdered pesticide in which it is desired to determine the nature of the particle size distribution. Larger pieces or particles are on the top, while progressively smaller particles have settled lower in the container and at the very bottom, the material has been packed and compressed into aggregates. To determine a timely representative answer, proportionately sized subsets from each layer or strata should be selected, mixed and randomly sampled. This method is used most commonly in diet studies.

In systematic sampling, a sample is taken at set intervals (such as every fifth container of reagent or taking a sample of water from a fixed sample point in a flowing stream every hour). This is most commonly employed in quality assurance or (in the clinical chemistry lab) in quality control.

In cluster sampling, the pool is already divided into numerous separate groups (such as bottles of tablets), and we select small sets of groups (such as several bottles of tablets) then select a few members from each set. What one gets then is a cluster of measures. Again, this is a method most commonly used in quality control or in environmental studies when the effort and expense of physically collecting a small group of units is significant.

In classical toxicology studies sampling arises in a practical sense in a limited number of situations. The most common of these are as follows:

(1) Selecting a subset of animals or test systems from a study to make some measurement (which either destroys or stresses the measured system, or is expensive) at an interval during a study. This may include such cases as doing interim necropsies in a chronic study or collecting and analyzing blood samples from some animals during a subchronic study.

(2) Analyzing inhalation chamber atmospheres to characterize aerosol distributions with a new generation system.

(3) Analyzing diet in which test material has been incorporated.

(4) Performing quality control on an analytical chemistry operation by having duplicate analyses performed on some materials.

(5) Selecting data to audit for quality assurance purposes.

Generalized Methodology Selection

One approach for the selection of appropriate techniques to employ in a particular situation is to use a decision-tree method. Figure 1 is a decision tree that leads to the choice of one of three other trees to assist in technique selection, with each of the subsequent trees addressing one of the three functions of statistics that was defined earlier in this chapter. Figure 2 is for the selection of hypothesis-testing procedures, Figure 3 for modeling procedures, and Figure 4 for reduction of dimensionality procedures. For the vast majority of situations, these trees will guide the user into the choice of the proper technique. The tests and terms in these trees will be explained subsequently.

REFERENCES

Barnett, V., and Lewis, T. (1984): *Outliers in Statistical Data,* 2nd Ed. John Wiley, New York

Beckman, R.J. and Cook, R.D. (1983): Outliers, *Technometrics* 25:119-163.

Dixon, W.J. and Massey, F.J., Jr. (1969): *Introduction to Statistical Analysis,* 3rd ed., McGraw-Hill, New York

Grubbs, F.E. (1969): Procedure for Detecting Outlying Observations in Samples, *Technometrics* 11:1-21.

Meyer, S.L. (1975): *Data Analysis for Scientists and Engineers,* pp. 17–18. John Wiley, New York.

Snedecor, G.W. and Cochran, W.G. (1980): *Statistical Methods,* Seventh ed. Iowa State University Press, Ames.

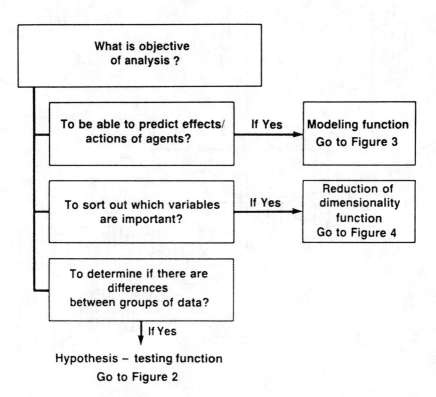

Figure 1   Overall Decision Tree for Selecting Statistical Procedures

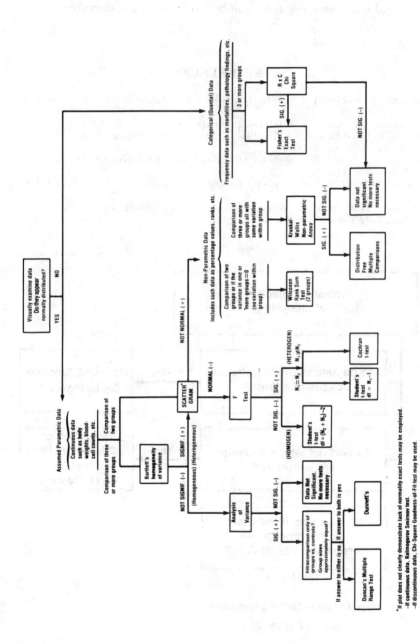

FIG. 2. Decision Tree for Selecting Hypothesis-testing Procedures

*If plot does not clearly demonstrate lack of normality exact tests may be employed.
—If continuous data, Kolmogorov Smirnov test.
—If discontinuous data, Chi-Square Goodness-of-Fit test may be used.

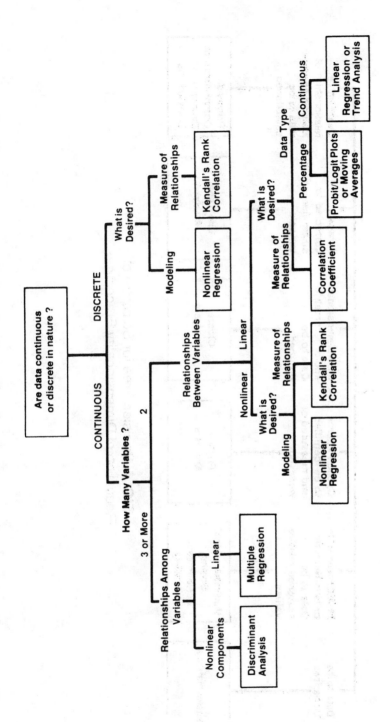

Figure 3 Decision Tree for Selecting Modeling Procedures

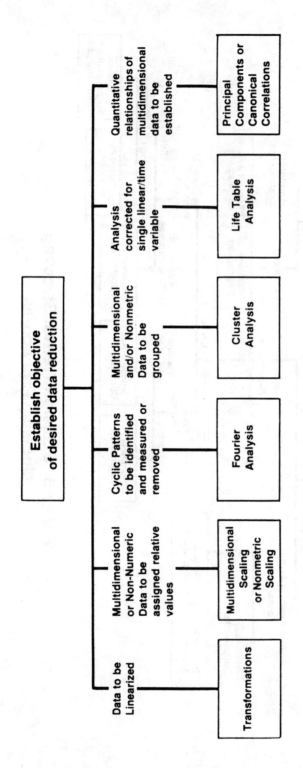

FIG. 4. Decision Tree for Selection of Reduction of Dimensionality Procedures

CHAPTER 3

EXPERIMENTAL DESIGN

Toxicological experiments generally have a twofold purpose. The first question is whether or not an agent results in an effect on a biological system. The second question, never far behind, is how much of an effect is present. Both the cost to perform research to answer such questions and the value that society places upon the results of such efforts have continued to increase rapidly. Additionally, it has become increasingly desirable that the results and conclusions of studies aimed at assessing the effects of environmental agents be as clear and unequivocal as possible. It is essential that every experiment and study yield as much information as possible, and that (more specifically) the results of each study have the greatest possible chance of answering the questions it was conducted to address. The statistical aspects of such efforts, so far as they are aimed at structuring experiments to maximize the possibilities of success, are called experimental design.

We have now become accustomed to developing exhaustively detailed protocols for an experiment or study prior to its conduct. But, typically, such protocols do not include or reflect a detailed plan for the statistical analysis of the data generated by the study and certainly even less frequently, reflect such considerations in their design. A priori selection of statistical methodology (as opposed to the post hoc approach) is as significant a portion of the process of protocol development and experimental design as any other and can measurably enhance the value of the experiment or study. Prior selection of statistical methodologies is essential for proper design of other portions of a protocol such as the number of animals per group or the sampling intervals for body weight. Implied in such a selection is the notion that the toxicologist has both an in-depth knowledge of the area of investigation and an understanding of the general principles of experimental design, for the analysis of any set of data is dictated to a large extent by the manner in which the data are obtained.

The four basic statistical principles of experimental design are replication, randomization, concurrent ("local") control and balance. In abbreviated form, these may be summarized as follows.

Replication: Any treatment must be applied to more than one experimental unit (animal, plate of cells, litter of offspring, etc.). This provides more accuracy in the measurement of a response than can be obtained from a single observation, since underlying experimental errors tend to cancel each other out. It also supplies an estimate of the experimental error derived from the variability among each of the measurements taken (or "replicates"). In practice, this means that an experiment should have enough experimental units in each treatment group (that is, a large enough "N") so that reasonably sensitive statistical analysis of data can be performed. The estimation of sample size is addressed in detail later in this chapter.

Randomization: This is practiced to ensure that every treatment shall have its fair share of extreme high and extreme low values. It also serves to allow the toxicologist to proceed as if the assumption of "independence" is valid. That is, there is no avoidable (known) systematic bias in how one obtains data.

Concurrent Control: Comparisons between treatments should be made to the maximum extent possible between experimental units from the same closely defined population. Therefore, animals used as a "control" group should come from the same source, lot, age, etc. as test group animals. Except for the treatment being evaluated, test and control animals should be maintained and handled in exactly the same manner.

Balance: If the effect of several different factors is being evaluated simultaneously, the experiment should be laid out in such a way that the contributions of the different factors can be separately distinguished and estimated. There are several ways of accomplishing this using one of several different forms of design, as will be discussed below.

There are four basic experimental design types used in toxicology. These are the randomized block, latin square, factorial design, and nested design. Other designs that are used are really combinations of these basic designs, and are very rarely employed in toxicology. Before examining these four basic types, however, we must first examine the basic concept of blocking.

Blocking is, simply put, the arrangement or sorting of the members of a population (such as all of an available group of test animals) into groups based on certain characteristics which may (but are not sure to) alter an experimental outcome. Such characteristics which may cause a treatment to give a differential effect include genetic background, age, sex, overall activity levels and so on. The process of blocking then acts (or attempts to act), so that each experimental group (or block) is assigned its fair share of the members of each of these subgroups.

We should now recall that randomization is aimed at spreading out the effect of undetectable or unsuspected characteristics in a population of animals or some portion of this population. The merging of the two concepts or randomization and blocking leads to the first basic experimental design, the randomized block. This type of design requires that each treatment group have at least one member of each recognized group (such as age), the exact members of each block being assigned in an unbiased (or random) fashion.

The second type of experimental design assumes that we can characterize treatments (whether intended or otherwise) as belonging clearly to separate sets. In the simplest case, these categories are arranged into two sets which may be thought of as rows (for, say, source litter of test animal, with the first litter as row 1, the next as row 2, etc.) and the secondary set of categories as columns (for, say, our ages of test animals, with 6-8 weeks as column 1, 8-10 weeks as column 2 and so on). Experimental units are then assigned so that each major treatment (control, low dose, intermediate dose, etc.) appears once and only once in each row and each column. If we denote our test groups as A (control), B (low), C (intermediate) and D (high), such an assignment would appear as below:

		Age			
Litter	Source	6-8 Weeks	8-10 Weeks	10-12 Weeks	12-14 Weeks
1	:	A	B	C	D
2	:	B	C	D	A
3	:	C	D	A	B
4	:	D	A	B	C

The third type of experimental design is the factorial design, in which there are two or more clearly understood treatments, such as exposure level to test chemical, animal age or temperature. The classical approach to this situation (and to that described under the latin square) is to hold all but one of the treatments constant; and at any one time to vary just that one factor. Instead, in the factorial design all levels of a given factor are combined with all levels of every other factor in the experiment. When a change in one factor produces a different change in the response variable at one level of a factor than at other levels of this factor, there is an interaction between these two factors which can then be analyzed as an interaction effect.

The last of the major varieties of experimental design are the nested designs, where the levels of one factor are nested within (or are subsamples of) another factor. That is, each subfactor is evaluated only within the limits of its single larger factor.

A second concept and its understanding are essential to the design of experiments in toxicology, that of censoring. Censoring is the exclusion of measurements from certain experimental units, or indeed of the experimental units themselves, from consideration in data analysis or inclusion in the experiment at all. Censoring may occur either prior to initiation of an experiment (where, in modern toxicology, this is almost always a planned procedure), during the course of an experiment (when they are almost universally unplanned, resulting from such as the death of animals on test), or after the conclusion of an experiment (when usually data are excluded because of being identified as some form of outlier).

In practice, *a priori* censoring in toxicology studies occurs in the assignment of experimental units (such as animals) to test groups. The most familiar example is in the common practice of assignment of test animals to acute, subacute, subchronic and chronic studies, where the results of otherwise random assignments are evaluated for body weights of the assigned members. If the mean weights are found not to be comparable by some preestablished criterion (such as a 90% probability of difference by analysis of variance) then members are reassigned (censored) to achieve comparability in terms of starting body weights. Such a procedure of animal assignment to groups is known as a *censored randomization*.

The first precise or calculable aspect of experimental design encountered is determining sufficient test and control group sizes to allow one to have an adequate level of confidence in the results of a study. This number (N) can be calculated using the formula

$$N = \frac{(t_1 + t_2)^2}{d^2} \; S$$

where t_1 is the one-tailed t value with N-1 degrees of freedom corresponding to the desired level of confidence, t_2 is the one-tailed t value with N-1 degrees of freedom corresponding to the probability that the sample size will be adequate to achieve the desired precision, S is the sample standard deviation, derived typically from historical data and calculated as

$$S = \sqrt{\frac{1}{N-1} \; \Sigma \, (V_1 - V_2)^2}$$

V being the variable of interest and d the acceptable range of variation in the variable of interest.

A good approximation can be generated by substituting the t

values (from a table such as Table F in Appendix 1) for an infinite number of degrees of freedom. This entire process is demonstrated in Example 1.

Example 1

In a subchronic dermal study in rabbits, the principal point of concern is the extent to which the compound causes oxidative damage to erythrocytes. To quantitate this, the laboratory will be measuring the numbers of reticulocytes in the blood. What then would be an adequate sample size to allow the question at hand to be addressed with reasonable certitude?

To do this, we use the one-tailed t value for an infinite number of degrees of freedom at the 95% confidence level (that is, $p \leq 0.05$). Going to a set of t tables, we find this number to be 1.645. From prior experience, we know that the usual values for reticulocytes in rabbit blood are from 0.5 to 1.9×10^6/ml. The acceptable range of variation, 0, is therefore equal to the span of this range, or 1.4. Likewise, examining the control data from previous rabbit studies, we find our sample standard deviation to be 0.825. When we insert all of these numbers into the equation (presented above) for sample size, we can calculate the required sample size (N) to be

$$= \frac{(1.645 + 1.645)^2}{(1.4)^2} \ 0.825$$

$$= \frac{10.824}{1.96} \ (0.825)$$

$$= 4.556$$

In other words, in this case where there is little natural variability, measuring the reticulocyte counts of groups of only five animals each should be sufficient.

There are a number of aspects of experimental design which are specific to the practice of toxicology. Before we look at a suggestion for step-by-step development of experimental designs, these aspects should first be considered as follows.

1) Frequently, the data gathered from specific measurements of animal characteristics are such that there is wide variability in the data. Often, such wide variability is not present in a control or low dose group, but in an intermediate dosage group variance inflation may occur. That is, there may be a large standard deviation associated with the measurements from this intermediate group. In the face of such a set of data, the conclusion that there is no biological effect based on a finding of no statistically significant effect might well be erroneous.

2) In designing experiments, a toxicologist should keep in mind the potential effect of involuntary censoring on sample size. In other words, though the study described in Example 1 might start with five dogs per group, this provides no margin should any die before the study is ended and blood samples are collected and analyzed. Just enough experimental units per group frequently leaves too few at the end to allow meaningful statistical analysis, and allowances should be made accordingly in establishing group sizes.

3) It is certainly possible to pool the data from several identical toxicological studies. For example, after first having performed an acute inhalation study where only three treatment group animals survived to the point at which a critical measure (such as analysis of blood samples) was performed, we would not have enough data to perform a meaningful statistical analysis. We could then repeat the protocol with new control and treatment group animals from the same source. At the end, after assuring ourselves that the two sets of data are comparable, we could combine (or pool) the data from survivors of the second study with those from the first. The costs of this approach, however, would then be both a greater degree of effort expended (than if we had performed a single study with larger groups) and increased variability in the pooled samples (decreasing the power of our statistical methods).

4) Another frequently overlooked design option in toxicology is the use of an unbalanced design - that is, of different group sizes for different levels of treatment.

There is no requirement that each group in a study (control, low dose, intermediate dose and high dose) have an equal number of experimental units assigned to it. Indeed, there are frequently good reasons to assign more experimental units to one group than to others, and, as we shall see later in this book, all the major statistical methodologies have provisions to adjust for such inequalities, within certain limits. The two most common uses of the unbalanced design have larger groups assigned to either the highest dose, to compensate for losses due to possible deaths during the study, or to the lowest dose to give more sensitivity in detecting effects at levels close to an effect threshold - or more confidence to the assertion that no effect exists.

5) We are frequently confronted with the situation where an undesired variable is influencing our experimental results in a nonrandom fashion. Such a variable is called a confounding variable - its presence, as discussed earlier, makes the clear attribution and analysis of effects at best difficult, and at worst impossible. Sometimes such confounding variables are the result of conscious design or management decisions, such as the use of different instruments, personnel, facilities, or procedures for different test groups within the same study.

Occassionally, however, such confounding variables are the result of unintentional factors or actions, in which case it is called a lurking variable. Examples of such variables are almost always the result of standard operating procedures being violated - water not being connected to a rack of animals over a weekend, a set of racks not being cleaned as frequently as others, or a contaminated batch of feed being used.

6) Finally, some thought must be given to the clear definition of what is meant by experimental unit and concurrent control.

The experimental unit in toxicology encompasses a wide variety of possibilities. It may be cells, plates of microorganisms, individual animals, litters of animals, etc. The importance of clearly defining the experimental unit is that the number of such units per group is the "N" which is used in statistical calculations or analyses , and critically affects such calculations.

The experimental unit is the unit which receives treatments and yields a response which is measured and becomes a datum. What this means in practice is that, for example, in reproduction or teratology studies where we treat the parental generation females and then determine results by counting or evaluating offspring, the experimental unit is still the parent. Therefore, the number of litters, not the number of offspring, is the N (Weil, 1970).

A true concurrent control is one that is identical in every manner with the treatment groups except for the treatment being evaluated. This means that all manipulations, including gavaging with equivalent volumes of vehicle or exposing to equivalent rates of air exchanges in an inhalation chamber, should be duplicated in control groups just as they occur in treatment groups.

The goal of the four principles of experimental design is statistical efficiency and the economizing of resources. It is possible to think of design as a logic flow analysis. Such an analysis is conducted in three steps, and should be performed every time any major study or project is initiated or indeed, at regular periods during the course of conduct of a series of "standard" smaller studies. These steps are detailed below.

I. Define the objective of the study - get a clear statement of what questions are being asked.

– Can the question, in fact, be broken down into a set of subquestions?

– Are we asking one or more of these questions repeatedly? For example, does "X" (an event or effect) develop at 30, 60, 90 + days and/or does it progress/regress or recover?

–What is our model to be in answering this/these questions? Is it appropriate and acceptably sensitive?

II. For each subquestion (i.e. separate major variable to be studied):

– How is the variable of interest to be measured?

– What is the nature of the data generated by the measure? Are we getting an *efficient* set of data? Are we buying too little information, (would another technique improve the quality of the information generated to the point that it becomes a higher "class" of data?), or too much information, i.e., does some underlying aspect of the measure limit the class of data obtainable within the bounds of feasibility of effort?

– Are there possible interactions between measurements? Can they be separated/identified?

– Is our N (sample size) both sufficient and efficient?

– What is the control - formal or informal? Is it appropriate?

– Are we needlessly adding confounding variables (asking inadvertent or unwanted questions)?

– Are there "lurking variables" present? These are undesired and not readily recognized differences which can affect results, such as different technicians observing different groups of animals.

– How large an effect will be considered biologically significant? This is a question which can only be resolved by reference to experience or historical control data.

III. What are the possible outcomes of the study - i.e., what answers are possible to both our subquestions and to our major question?

– How do we use these answers?

– Do the possible answers offer a reasonable expectation of achieving the objectives that caused us to initiate the study?

– What new questions may these answers cause us to ask? Can the study be redesigned, before it is actually started, so that these "revealed" questions may be answered in the original study?

A practical example of the application of this approach can be demonstrated in the process of designing a chronic inhalation study. Although in such a situation the primary question being asked is usually "does the chemical result in cancer by this route?", even at the beginning there are a number of other questions that it is expected the study will answer. Two such are (1) if cancer is caused, what is the relative risk associated with it and (2) are there other expressions of toxicity associated with chronic exposure? Several, if not all, of these three questions are actually to be asked repeatedly during the course of the study. Before the study starts, a plan and arrangements must be formed to make measurements to allow us to answer these questions.

When considering the last portion of our logic analysis, however, we must start by considering each of the things which may go wrong during the study. These include the occurrence of an infectious disease the finding that extreme nasal and respiratory irritation was occurring in test animals, or the uncovering of a hidden variable. Do we continue or stop exposures? How will we now separate those portions of observed effects which are due to the chemical under study and those portions which are due to the disease process? Can we preclude (or minimize) the possibility of a disease outbreak by doing a more extensive health surveillance and quarantine on our test animals prior to the start of the study? Could we select a better test model - one that is not as sensitive to upper respiratory or nasal irritation?

For the reader who would like to further explore experimental design, there are a number of more detailed texts available which include more extensive treatments of the statistical aspects of experimental design. Among those recommended are Cochran and Cox (1975); Diamond (1981); Federer (1955); Hicks (1982); and Myers (1972).

REFERENCES

Cochran, W.G. and Cox, G.M. (1975): *Experimental Designs*, John Wiley, New York.
Diamond W.J. (1981): *Practical Experimental Designs*, Lifetime Learning Publications, Belmont, CA.
Federer, W.T. (1955): *Experimental Design*, Macmillan, New York.
Gad. S.C. (1982): Statistical analysis of behavioral toxicology data and studies, *Arch. Toxicol. Suppl.* 5 256-266.
Hicks, C.R. (1982): *Fundamental Concepts in the Design of Experiments*, Holt, Rinehart and Winston, New York.
Myers, J.L. (1972): *Fundamentals of Experimental Design*, Allyn and Bacon, Boston.
Weil, C.S. (1970): Selection of the valid number of sampling units and a consideration of their combination in toxicological studies involving reproduction, teratogenesis or carcinogenesis, *Food Cosmet. Toxicol.* 8 177-182.

CHAPTER 4

COMPUTATIONAL DEVICES

The range, scope and availability of aids for the calculation of mathematical techniques in general and for statistical techniques in particular have increased at an almost geometric rate since the mid-70's. There is no longer any reason to use paper and pencil to perform such calculations; the capabilities of electronic systems are sufficiently developed at each level (as discussed below) and the costs, compared to labor savings, are minimal.

There are now four tiers of computational support available for statistical analysis, (though it may be argued that the middle two tiers are becoming indistinguishable), and this chapter will attempt an overview of the major systems available within these tiers and the general characteristics and limitations of each. The four tiers range from programmable calculators (which represent Tier I, and include such devices as the Texas Instruments SR-59 and the Hewlett-Packard HP-41 with their magnetic card storage systems) to complete statistical packages available on mainframe computers (the Tier IV systems, which include such packages as SAS and SPSS).

As a general rule, as one goes from the systems in Tier I to those in Tier IV, the cost, power, and capabilities of the systems increase, while both ease of use ("user friendliness") and flexibility decrease.

There are conventions associated with each system or instrument in these tiers, and these conventions should be known because they can affect both results and the ways in which results are reported.

The first two conventions, which apply to all four tiers, have to do with the length of numbers. The first is that there is a preset number of digits that a machine (or software system) will accept as input, handle in calculations, and report as a result (either on a screen or as a printout). The most common such limit is thirteen digits - that is, a number such as 12345.67890123. If, in the course of performing calculations, a longer string of digits is produced (for example, by dividing our example number by four, which should produce the actual number 3086.4197253075, a 14 digit number, a 13 digit system would then handle the last ("extra") digit in one of two ways. It would either truncate it (that is, just drop off the last digit) or it would round it by some rule (rounding was discussed in an earlier chapter). Truncation, particularly on the result of a long series of calculations (as is often the case in statistics) is more likely to produce erroneous results. Rounding is much less likely to produce errors, but knowledge of the rounding method utilized can be helpful.

The second convention which applies to all systems is that there is also a limit to how long a series of digits any system will report out, and there are different ways in which systems report out, and there are different ways in which systems report longer digit series. The first, less common, is truncation. The second is rounding combined with presentation of the results as an exponential. Exponentials are a series of digits followed by an expression of the appropriate powers of ten. Examples of such exponential expressions are:

$$a)\ 1.234567 \times 10^{16}$$
$$b)\ 1.234567 \times 10^{-16}$$
$$c)\ 1.234567\ E\ 16$$
$$d)\ 1.234567\ E\text{-}16$$

a) and c) are the same number represented two different ways, as are b) and d).

Tier I Systems (Programmable Calculators)

The two major Tier I systems (described more fully below) can readily perform all of the univariate (that is, two variable) procedures described in this book. Libraries of programs, stored on magnetic cards, are available and well documented. Data sets may also be stored on magnetic cards, and by clever coding programs and data sets of extreme length may be processed. But longer programs or larger data sets run extremely slowly. Accordingly, use of these instruments is limited, in practice, to univariate procedures and small data sets.

The two Tier I systems are the Texas Instruments SR-59 and the Hewlett-Packard HP-41. These differ mainly in that the HP programs and data entry systems are in reverse Polish notation (RPN) form, while the TI has a straightforward entry form. There are printers available for both units to provide hard copy. Both have unique but simple programming languages.

Tier II (Microcomputers and Software)

At levels above Tier I there are additional conventions as to the way systems operate and handle data. Additionally, there are a larger number and options for both machines and software systems because only a few common programming languages are involved.

The first common convention which must be understood and considered is that the systems actually perform a statistical operation in one of two modes, batch or interactive. In batch mode, the entire desired sequence of analysis is specified, then the entire set of data is processed in accordance with this specified sequence. The drawback to this approach is that if a result early in the sequence indicates that an alternative latter set of procedures should be performed, there is no opportunity to change to these alternative (as opposed to the originally specified) procedures. In the interactive mode, procedures are specified (and results calculated) one step at a time, usually by the use of a series of menus.

The second convention concerns the structure of commonly-used software systems. They are almost always divided into three separate parts or modules. The first module is a data base manager, which allows the person using the system to store data in (and recall it from) a desired format, to perform a transformation(s) or arithmetic manipulation(s), and to pass the data along to either one of the other two modules or to another software system.

The second module performs the actual analysis of the data. Such modules also allow one to tailor reports to one's specifications.

The last module (which is not always present) is a graphics module, which presents (on a display screen) and prints out in any of a wide range of graphs and charts. The range may be limited to line, bar and pie charts, or may extend to contour, cluster and more exotic plots.

There are a wide variety of microcomputers available which support extensive statistical packages. These include the Apple II series, Kaypro, Commodore, TRS-80, IBM PC, Atari 800, Northstar, PET, and numerous systems that use the CPM operating system. Each of these has at least 64K memory, and printers and plotters are available. Each of these machines also has its own peculiarities.

Before reviewing software packages, several considerations should be presented. First, systems perform in one of two modes - either as libraries of programs, each of which can be selected to perform an individual procedure or as an integrated system, where a single loading of the file allows access to each and every procedure. In the first mode, each step in an analysis (such as Bartlett's test, analysis of variance and Duncan's) requires loading a separate file and then executing the procedure. Secondly, the machine must have adequate memory available to use the software. Generally, this requirement is for only 48 or 64K, which is not usually a problem.

Third, the available range of transformations should be carefully considered. At least a small number (log, reciprocal, probit, addition, subtraction, multiplication, division and absolute value) are essential.

If unusual data sets are to be handled or exploratory data analysis (discussed later) performed regularly, a more extensive set is required. Some of the packages (such as STATPRO) offer literally hundreds of transformations.

Fourth, all the packages listed in Table 2 have at least a basic set of capabilities. They can each perform, besides data base management and basic transformation and graphic functions, the following simple tests (all discussed in later chapters).

−Analysis of Variance (ANOVA)
−2 x 2 Chi Square
−Linear Regression
−Student's t - Test

Table 2 presents an overview of 37 commercially available statistical packages for microcomputers which the authors are familiar with. There are at least 120 additional packages available. Woodward *et al.* (1985) presents an overview of many of these. For each package, the following information is presented.

TITLE	–	The name of the package.
MACHINE	–	Which systems the package will operate on.
NPAR	–	Will the package perform nonparametric analysis?
ANCOVA	–	Will the package perform analysis of covariance?
EDA	–	Does the system perform exploratory data analysis?
MULTIVAR	–	Does the system perform multivariate analysis?
GRAPHICS	–	What graphic functions does the package perform?
MODE	–	Is the package integrated or a library?
NOTES	–	Any special characteristics.

Tier III (Minicomputers and Software Packages)

The distinction between the microcomputer and the minicomputer is fading rapidly. As hard discs are generally available for many of the "personal computers" and these machines advance to being 16 bit machines, the division may now refer only to a cost difference. The mini in general, however, can still handle larger data sets and more complicated analyses and perform more rapidly than the micro. Two examples of such systems are the HP series (HP 9816, 9826 and 9836) and the STAT CAT. Hewlett-Packard also sells a Statistical Library package (to run on its three machines) which performs the full range of methods presented in this book except for life table analysis. The STAT CAT is a made-to-order minicomputer which has SPSS (a main frame statistical package discussed below) built into it. It will perform all the procedures described in this book.

TABLE 2
MICROCOMPUTER STATISTICAL PACKAGES

TITLE	MACHINE	NPAR	ANCOVA	EDA	MULTIVAR	GRAPHICS	MODE	NOTES
ABSTAT	CPM					Histogram Plots	I	Menu Driven
AIDA	APPLE	X			X	Histogram Plots	I	Menu Driven
A-STAT	CPM APPLE PET		X				I	Menu Driven
ASYST	IBM					Full	I	Command Driven
APP-STAT	APPLE	X	X			Histogram Plots	I	Menu Driven
COMPSTAT	NORTHSTAR CPM	X		X	X		L	Command Driven
DAISY	APPLE	X				Histogram Plots	L	Command Driven
DYNACOMP SERIES	APPLE ATARI TRS-80 PET	X	X		X	Plots	L	Menu Driven

	Machine				Graphics		Interface
EXPLORATORY DATA ANALYSIS	APPLE		X			—	Command Driven
ELF	APPLE, CPM, IBM			(Some)	Histogram Plots	—	Menu Driven
EPISTAT	APPLE, IBM	X			Histogram Plots	—	Menu Driven
HSD STATISTICS SERIES	APPLE	X			Histogram Plots	—	Menu Driven
INTER-STAT	APPLE				Plots	L	Command Driven
LISREL	APPLE, IBM	X		X		—	
MASS	CPM	X	Discrim		Time Series Plots	—	Menu Driven
MICROSTAT	CPM, IBM	X			Histogram Plots	—	Menu Driven
MICRO TSP	CPM, APPLE, IBM			X	Histogram Plots	—	Menu Driven

TABLE 2 (Continued)

MICROCOMPUTER STATISTICAL PACKAGES

TITLE	MACHINE	NPAR	ANCOVA	EDA	MULTIVAR	GRAPHICS	MODE	NOTES
MSU STAT	IBM CPM	X	X		X	Histogram Plots	I	Menu Driven
NWA STATISTICS PACKAGE	CPM					Histogram	L	Command Driven
NUMBER CRUNCHER	IBM COMMODORE MACHIN-TOSH	X	X		X	Histogram Plots	I	Transformations Menu Driven Time Series
SCA SYSTEM	IBM			X		Plots	I	Menu Driven
SAM	IBM				Discrim Cluster	Plots	I	Menu Driven
SIGSTAT	IBM HP-150		X	X	X		I	Menu Life table micro version of BMD

Program	System					Interface
SPEEDSTAT	APPLE CPM	X			L	Command Driven
SPSS/PC	IBM	X	X	Full	I	Micro version of SPSS command driven
STAN	IBM CPM		X	Full	I	Menu Driven
STATMAT	CPM KAYPRO RAINBOW				I	Menu Driven
STAT-GRAPHICS	IBM	X		X	Full	I	Time series Menu Driven
STATA	IBM		X		I	Menu Driven
STATPRO	IBM APPLE	X		X	Full	I	Menu Driven
STATIS-TICIAN	TRS-80 CPM IBM	X		X		I	Menu Driven
STATISTICAL ANALYSIS	CPM			Histogram Plots	I	Menu Driven

TABLE 2 (Continued)

MICROCOMPUTER STATISTICAL PACKAGES

TITLE	MACHINE	NPAR	ANCOVA	EDA	MULTIVAR	GRAPHICS	MODE	NOTES
STATISTICAL MICRO PROGRAMS	APPLE						I	Menu Driven
STATISTICS PACKAGE	CPM					Histogram	L	Command Driven
STATVIEW	MACINTOSH	X				Full	I	Mouse Driven
SYSTAT	CPM	X	X		X	Full	L	Command Driven
TWG/ARIMA	APPLE CPM			X			I	Menu Driven
X-STAT	IBM			X		Full	I	Menu Driven

Tier IV (Main frame Programs)

The tier four system programs are all large commercial software packages which run on large computer systems on a time sharing basis. By definition, this means that these programs operate in a batch mode and use a unique (for each package) code language. Five of these libraries are briefly described below.

PACKAGE	REFERENCE	DESCRIPTION
SPSS	Nie *et. al..*, 1975	With manipulation, SPSS will perform all the procedures described in this book and the full range of graphics.
BMD	Dixon, 1974	Has generally wider capabilities than SPSS (which are constantly being added to) and easily manipulated.
SAS	SAS Institute, 1979	Widely available. Easier to format and very strong on data summarization. Has its own higher level programming language.
MINITAB	Ryan *et. al.*, 1982	Easiest to use and least expensive of these six, but does not have the full range of capabilities.
STAT/ PROTRAN		Newest of the packages, offering a full range of capabilities

The difficulty with the recently-achieved, wide availability of automated analysis systems is that it has become increasingly easy to perform the wrong tests on the wrong data and from there to proceed to the wrong conclusions. This serves to make at least a basic understanding of the procedures and discipline of statistics a vital necessity for the research toxicologist.

REFERENCES

Dixon, W.J. (1974): *BMD-Biomedical Computer Programs*, University of California Press, Berkeley.

Nie, N.H., Hall, C.H., Jenkins, J.G., Steinbrenner, K., and Bent, D.H. (1975): *Statistical Package for the Social Sciences*, McGraw-Hill, New York.

Ryan, T.A.; Joiner, B.L. and Ryan, B.F. (1982): *Minitab Reference Manual*, Duxbury Press, Boston.

SAS Institute (1979): *SAS User's Guide 1979 Edition*, SAS Institute, Raleigh.

Woodward, W.A.; Elliott, A.C. And Gray, H.L. (1985) *Directory of Statistical Microcomputer Software*, Marcel Dekker, Inc., New York.

CHAPTER 5

METHODS FOR DATA PREPARATION
AND EXPLORATION

The data from toxicology studies should always be examined before any formal analysis is performed. Such examinations should be directed to determining if the data are suitable for analysis, and if so what form the analysis should take (see Figure 2.) If the data as collected are not suitable for analysis, or if they are only suitable for low-powered analytical techniques, one may wish to use one of many forms of data transformation to change the data characteristics so that they are more amenable to analysis.

The above two objectives, data examination and preparation, are the primary focus of this chapter. For data examination, two major techniques are presented—the scattergram and Bartlett's test. Likewise, for data preparation (with the issues of rounding and outliers having been addressed in a previous chapter) two techniques are presented—randomization (including a test for randomness in a sample of data) and transformation.

Finally, at the end of this chapter the concept of exploratory data analysis (EDA) is presented and briefly reviewed. This is a relatively new collection of techniques and approaches to "probe" data - that is, to both examine and to perform some initial, flexible analysis of the data.

Scattergram

Two of the major points to be made throughout this volume are (a) the use of the appropriate statistical tests, and (b) the effects of small sample sizes (as is often the case in toxicology) on our selection of statistical techniques. Frequently, simple examination of the nature and distribution of data collected from a study can also suggest patterns and results which were unanticipated and for which the use of additional or alternative statistical methodology is warranted. It was these three points which caused the authors to consider a section on scatter-grams and their use essential for toxicologists.

We will show that Bartlett's test may be used to determine if the values in groups of data are homogeneous. If they are, this (along with the knowledge that they are from a continuous distribution) demonstrates that parametric methods are applicable.

But, if the values in the (continuous data) groups fail Bartlett's test (i.e., are heterogeneous), we cannot be secure in our belief that parametric methods are appropriate until we gain some confidence that the values are normally distributed. With large groups of data, we can compute parameters of the population (kurtosis and skewness, in particular) and from these parameters determine if the population is normal (with a certain level of confidence). If our concern is espe-cially marked, we can use a chi-square goodness-of-fit test for normal-ity. But when each group of data consists of 25 or fewer values, these measures or tests (kurtosis, skewness, and chi-square goodness-of-fit) are not accurate indicators of normality. Instead, in these cases we should prepare a scattergram of the data, then evaluate the scattergram to estimate if the data are normally distributed. This procedure consists of developing a histogram of the data, then examining the histogram to get a visual appreciation of the location and distribution of the data.

The abscissa (or horizontal scale) should be in the same scale as the values, and should be divided so that the entire range of observed values is covered by the scale of the abscissa. Across such a scale we then simply enter symbols for each of our values. Example 2 shows such a plot.

Example 2 is a traditional and rather limited form of scatterplot but such plots can reveal significant information about the amount and types of association between the two variables, the existence and nature of outliers, the clustering of data, and a number of other two-dimensional factors (Anscombe, 1973; Chambers et al., 1983).

Current technology now allows us to add significantly more graphi-cal information to scatterplots by means of graphic symbols (letters, faces, different shapes - such as squares, colors, etc.) for the plotted data points. One relatively simple example of this approach is shown in Figure 5, where the simple case of dose (in a dermal study), dermal irritation, and white blood cell count is presented. This graph quite clearly suggest that as dose (variable x) is increased, dermal irritation (variable y) also increases; and as irritation becomes more severe, white blood cell count (variable z) an indicator of immune system involve-ment, suggesting infection or persistent inflammation, also increases. There is no direct association of variables x and z, however.

Recently, Cleveland and McGill (1984) presented an excellent, detailed overview of the expanded capabilities of the scatterplot, and the interested reader should refer to that article.

FIGURE 5

Correlative Plots

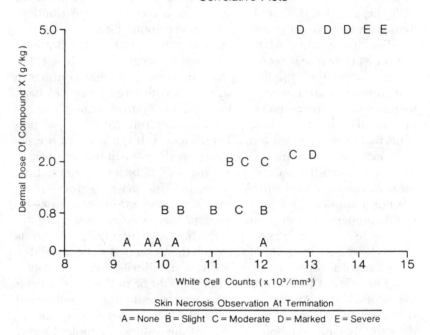

White Cell Counts (x 10³/mm³)

Skin Necrosis Observation At Termination

A = None B = Slight C = Moderate D = Marked E = Severe

EXAMPLE 2

Suppose we have the two data sets below:

Group 1: 4.5, 5.4, 5.9, 6.0, 6.4, 6.5, 6.9, 7.0, 7.1, 7.0, 7.4, 7.5, 7.5, 7.5, 7.6, 8.0, 8.1, 8.4, 8.5, 8.6, 9.0, 9.4, 9.5 and 10.4.

Group 2: 4.0, 4.5, 5.0, 5.1, 5.4, 5.5., 5.6, 6.5, 6.5, 7.0, 7.4, 7.5, 7.5, 8.0, 8.1, 8.5, 8.5, 9.0, 9.1, 9.5, 9.5, 10.1, 10.0 and 10.4.

Both of these groups contain 24 values and cover the same range. From them we can prepare the following scattergrams.

Group 1:

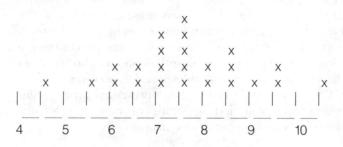

Group 2:

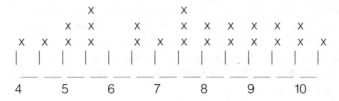

```
            X                   X
       X    X        X          X    X    X    X    X    X
  X    X    X    X        X    X    X    X    X    X    X    X    X
  |    |    |    |    |    |    |    |    |    |    |    |    |    |
```
```
  4         5         6         7         8         9         10
```

Group 1 can be seen to approximate a normal distribution (bell-shaped curve); we can proceed to perform the appropriate parametric tests with such data. But group 2 clearly does not appear to be normally distributed. In this case, the appropriate nonparametric technique must be used.

Bartlett's Test for Homogeneity of Variance

Bartlett's test (see Sokal and Rohlf (1981), pp. 403–407) is used to compare the variances (values reflecting the degree of variability in data sets) among three or more groups of data, where the data in the groups are continuous sets (such as body weights, organ weights, red blood cell counts, or diet consumption measurements). It is expected that such data will be suitable for parametric methods, and Bartlett's is frequently used as a test for the assumption of equivalent variances.

Bartlett's is based on the calculation of the corrected X^2 (chi square) value by the formula:

$$X^2_{corr} = 2.3026 \frac{\Sigma df \left(\log_{10}\left[\frac{\Sigma[df(S^2)]}{\Sigma df} \right] \right) - \Sigma[df(\log_{10}S^2)]}{1 + \frac{1}{3(K-1)}\left[\Sigma \frac{1}{df} - \frac{1}{\Sigma df} \right]}$$

where S^2 = variance = $\dfrac{N\Sigma X)^2 - (\Sigma X)^2}{N}$
$\dfrac{}{N-1}$

X = individual datum within each group.
N = number of data within each group.
K = number of groups being compared.
df = degrees of freedom for each group = $(N - 1)$.

The corrected X^2 value yielded by the above calculations is compared to the values listed in the chi square table according to the numbers of degrees of freedom [such as found in Snedecor and Cochran, pp. 470–471].

If the calculated value is smaller than the table value at the selected p level (traditionally 0.05) the groups are accepted to be homogeneous and the use of ANOVA is assumed proper. If the calculated X^2 is greater than the table value, the groups are heterogeneous and other tests (as indicated in Fig. 2, the decision tree) are necessary. This is demonstrated in Example 3.

EXAMPLE 3

If monocytes in rat blood taken in the course of an inhalation study were counted, the results might appear as follows:

400 ppm		200 ppm		0 ppm	
(X_1)	$(X_1)^2$	(X_2)	(X_2)	(X_3)	$(X_2)^2$
9	81	5	25	7	49
5	25	5	25	6	36
5	25	4	16	5	25
4	16	6	36	7	49
		7	49	$\Sigma X_3 = 25$	$\Sigma X_3^2 = 159$
$\Sigma X_1 = 23$	$\Sigma X_1^2 = 147$	$\Sigma X_2 = 27$	$\Sigma X_3^2 = 151$		

$$S_1^2 = \frac{\dfrac{4(147) - (23)^2}{4}}{4-1} = 4.9167 \quad S_2^2 = \frac{\dfrac{5(151) - (27)^2}{5}}{5-1} = 1.3000$$

$$S_3^2 = \frac{\dfrac{4(159) - (25)^2}{4}}{4-1} = 0.9167$$

In continuing the calculations, it is helpful to set up a table such as follows:

Concentration	N	df = (N–1)	S^2	$(df)(S^2)$	log S^2
400 ppm	4	3	4.9167	14.7501	0.6917
200 ppm	5	4	1.3000	5.2000	0.1139
0 ppm	4	3	0.9167	2.7501	–0.0378
Sums (Σ)	13	10		22.7002	

EXAMPLE 3 (continued)

Concentration	$(df)(\log S^2)$	$\dfrac{1}{df}$
400 ppm	2.0751	0.3333
200 ppm	0.4556	0.2500
0 ppm	−0.1134	0.3333
Sums (Σ)	2.4173	0.9166

Now we substitute into our original formula for corrected X^2

$$X^2 = 2.3026 \frac{10[\log_{10}\left(\dfrac{22.7002}{10}\right) - 2.4173]}{\dfrac{1}{3(3-1)}\left(0.9166 - \dfrac{1}{10}\right)}$$

$$= 2.3026 \frac{10(0.3560) - 2.4173}{1 + 0.1667\,(0.8166)}$$

$$= 2.32$$

The table value for two degrees of freedom at the 0.05 level is 5.99. As our calculated value is less than this, the corrected X^2 is not significant and the variances are accepted as homogeneous. We may thus use parametric methods (such as ANOVA) for further comparisons.

ASSUMPTIONS AND LIMITATIONS

1. Bartlett's test does not test for normality, but rather homogeneity of variance (also called equality of variances or homoscedasticity).
2. Homoscedasticity is an important assumption for Student's t-test, analysis of variance, and analysis of covariance.
3. The F-test (covered in the next chapter) is actually a test for the two sample (that is, control and one test group) case of homoscedasticity. Bartlett's is designed for three or more samples.
4. Bartlett's is very sensitive to departures from normality. As a result, a finding of a significant chi square value in Bartlett's may indicate non-normality rather than heteroscedasticity. Such a finding can be brought about by outliers, and the sensitivity to such erroneous findings is extreme with small sample sizes.

Randomization

Randomization is the act of assigning a number of items (plates of bacteria or test animals, for example) to groups in such a manner that there is an equal chance for any one item to end up in any one group. This is a control against any possible bias in assignment of subjects to test groups. A variation on this is censored randomization, which insures that the groups are equivalent in some aspect after the assignment process is complete. The most common example of a censored randomization is one in which it is insured that the body weights of test animals in each group are not significantly different from those in the other groups. This is done by analyzing group weights both for homogeneity of variance and by analysis of variance after animal assignment, then rerandomizing if there is a significant difference at some nominal level, such as $p \leq 0.10$. The process is repeated until there is no difference.

There are several methods for actually performing the randomization process. The three most commonly used are card assignment, use of a random number table, and use of a computerized algorithm.

For the card-based method, individual identification numbers for items (plates or animals, for example) are placed on separate index cards. These cards are then shuffled, placed one at a time in succession into piles corresponding to the required test groups. The results are a random group assignment.

The random number table method requires only that one have unique numbers assigned to test subjects and access to a random number table. One simply sets up a table with a column for each group to which subjects are to be assigned. We start from the head of any one column of numbers in the random table (each time the table is used, a new starting point should be utilized). If our test subjects number less than 100, we utilize only the last two digits in each random number in the table. If they n umber more than 99 but less than 1000, we use only the last three digits. To generate group assignments, we read down a column, one number at a time. As we come across digits which correspond to a subject number, we assign that subject to a group (enter its identifying number in a column) proceeding to assign subjects to groups from left to right filling one row at a time. After a number is assigned to an animal, any duplication of its unique number is ignored. We use as many successive columns of random numbers as we may need to complete the process.

The third (and now most common) method is to use a random number generator that is built into a calculator or computer program. Procedures for generating these are generally documented in user manuals.

One is also occasionally required to evaluate whether a series of numbers (such as an assignment of animals to test groups) is random.

This requires the use of a randomization test, of which there are a large variety. The chi-square test, described later, can be used to evaluate the goodness-of-fit to a random assignment. If the result is not critical, a simple sign test will work. For the sign test, we first determine the middle value in the numbers being checked for randomness. We then go through a list of the numbers assigned to each group, scoring each as a " + " (greater than our middle number) or " − " (less than our middle number). The number of pluses and minuses in each group should be approximately equal. This is demonstrated in Example 4.

EXAMPLE 4

In auditing a study performed at another lab, we wish to ensure that their assignment of animals to test groups was random. Thirty-three animals numbered 1 to 33 were assigned to groups of eleven animals each. Using the middle value in this series (17) as our check point, we assign signs as below.

Control Animal Number	Sign	Test Group A Animal Number	Sign	Test Group B Animal Number	Sign
17	0	18	+	11	−
14	−	1	−	2	−
7	−	12	−	22	+
26	+	9	−	28	+
21	+	5	−	19	+
15	−	20	+	3	−
16	−	33	+	29	+
6	−	27	+	10	−
25	+	8	−	23	+
32	+	24	+	30	+
4	−	31	+	13	−
Sums of signs	− 2		+ 1		+ 1

Note that 17 is scored as a zero, insuring (as a check on results) that the sum of the sums of the three columns would be zero. The results in this case clearly demonstrate that there is no systematic bias in animal number assignments.

Transformations

If our initial inspection of a data set reveals it to have an unusual or undesired set of characteristics (or to lack a desired set of characteristics), we have a choice of three courses of action. We may proceed to select a method or test appropriate to this new set of conditions, or abandon the entire exercise, or transform the variable(s) under consideration in such a manner that the resulting transformed variates (X' and Y', for example, as opposed to the original variates X and Y) meet the assumptions or have the characteristics that are desired.

The key to all this is that the scale of measurement of most (if not all) variables is arbitrary. That is, although we are most familiar with a linear scale of measurement, there is nothing which makes this the "correct" scale on its own, as opposed to a logarithmic scale (familiar logarithmic measurements are that of pH values, or earthquake intensity (Richter scale)). Transforming a set of data (converting X to X') is really as simple as changing the scale of measurement.

There are at least four good reasons to transform data. (1) To normalize the data, making them suitable for analysis by our most common parametric techniques such as analysis of variance ANOVA. A simple test of whether a selected transformation will yield a distribution of data which satisfies the underlying assumptions for ANOVA is to plot the cumulative distribution of samples on probability paper (that is a commercially - available paper which has the probability function scale as one axis). One can then alter the scale of the second axis (that is, the axis other than the one which is on a probability scale) from linear to any other (logarithmic, reciprocal, square root, etc.) and see if a previously curved line indicating a skewed distribution becomes linear to indicate normality. The slope of the transformed line gives us an estimate of the standard deviation. And if the slopes of the lines of several samples or groups of data are similar, we accordingly know that the variances of the different groups are homogeneous.

(2) To linearize the relationship between a paired set of data, such as dose and response. This is the most common use in toxicology for transformations and is demonstrated in the section under probit/logit plots.

(3) To adjust data for the influence of another variable. This is an alternative in some situations to the more complicated process of analysis of covariance. A ready example of this usage is the calculation of organ weight to body weight ratios in *in vivo* toxicity studies, with the resulting ratios serving as the raw data for an analysis of variance performed to identify possible target organs. This use is discussed in detail later in this chapter.

(4) Finally, to make the relationships between variables clearer by removing or adjusting for interactions with third, fourth, etc. uncontrolled variables which influence the pair of variables of interest. This case is discussed in detail under time series analysis.

Common transformations are presented in Table 3 below.

Table 3: Common Data Transformations

Transformation	How Calculated[1]	Example of Use
Arithmetic	$x^1 = \dfrac{x}{y}$ or $x^1 = x + c$	Organ weight/ Body weight
Reciprocals	$x^1 = \dfrac{1}{x}$	Linearizing data, particularly rate phenomena
Arcsine (also called Angular)	$x^1 = \text{arcsine } \sqrt{x}$	Normalizing dominant lethal and mutation rate data
Logarithmic	$x^1 = \log x$	pH values
Probability (Probit)	$x^1 = \text{probability } X$	Percentage responding
Square Roots	$x^1 = \sqrt{x}$	Surface area of animal from body weights
Box Cox	$x^1 = (x^v - 1) v:$ for $v \neq 0$ $x' = 1n\, x$: for $v = 0$	A family of transforms For use when one has no prior knowledge of the appropriate transformation to use

[1] x and y are original variables, x' and y' transformed values. "c" stands for a constant.
[2] Plotting a double reciprocal (that is, $\frac{1}{x}$ vs. $\frac{1}{y}$) will linearize almost any data set. So will plotting the log transforms of a set of variables.

Exploratory Data Analysis

Over the past ten years, an entirely new approach has been developed to get the most information out of the increasingly larger and more complex data sets that scientists are faced with. This approach involves the use of a very diverse set of fairly simple techniques which comprise exploratory data analysis (EDA). As expounded by Tukey (Tukey, 1977), there are four major ingredients to EDA:

Displays: These visually reveal the behavior of the data and suggest a framework for analysis. The scatterplot (presented earlier) is an example of this approach.

Residuals: These are what remain of a set of data after a fitted model (such as a linear regression) or some similar level of analysis has been removed.

Reexpressions: These involve questions of what scale would serve to best simplify and improve the analysis of the data. Simple transformations, such as those presented earlier in this chapter, are used to simplify data behavior (for example, linearizing or normalizing) and clarify analysis.

Resistance: This is a matter of decreasing the sensitivity of analysis and summary of data to misbehavior, so that the occurrence of a few outliers, for example, will not complicate or invalidate the methods used to analyze the data. For example, in summarizing the location of a set of data, the median (but not the arithmetic mean) is highly resistant.

These four ingredients are utilized in a process falling into two broad phases: an exploratory phase and a confirmatory phase. The exploratory phase isolates patterns in and features of, the data and reveals them, allowing an inspection of the data before there is any firm choice of actual hypothesis testing or modeling methods has been made.

Confirmatory analysis allows evaluation of the reproducibility of the patterns or effects. Its role is close to that of classical hypothesis testing, but also often includes steps such as (a) incorporating information from an analysis of another, closely related set of data and (b) validating a result by assembling and analyzing additional data. These techniques are in general beyond the scope of this text. However, Velleman and Hoaglin (1981) and Hoaglin *et al.* (1983) present a clear overview of the more important methods, along with codes for their execution on a microcomputer (they have also now been incorporated into Minitab). A short examination of a single case of the use of these methods, however, is in order.

Toxicology has long recognized that no population - animal or human - is completely uniform in its response to any particular toxicant. Rather, a population is composed of a (presumably normal) distribution of individuals - some resistant to intoxication (hyporesponders), the bulk that respond close to a central value (such as an LD_{50}), and some that are very sensitive to intoxication (hyperresponders). This population distribution can, in fact, result in additional statistical techniques. The sensitivity of techniques such as ANOVA is reduced markedly by the occurrence of outliers (extreme high or low values - including hyper and hypo responders) which, in fact, serve to markedly inflate the variance (standard deviation) associated with a sample. Such variance inflation is particularly common in small groups that are exposed or dosed at just over or under a threshold level, causing a small number of individuals in the sample (who are more sensitive than the other members) to respond markedly. Such a situation is displayed in Figure 6 which plots the mean and standard deviations of methemoglobin levels in a series of groups of animals exposed to successively higher levels of a hemolytic agent.

Though the mean level of methemoglobin in group C is more than double that of the control group (A), no hypothesis test will show this difference to be significant because it has such a large standard deviation associated with it. Yet this "inflated" variance exists because a single individual has such a marked response. The occurrence of the inflation is certainly an indicator that the data need to be examined closely. Indeed, all tabular data in toxicology should be visually inspected for both trend and variance inflation.

A concept related (but not identical) to resistance and exploratory data analysis is that of robustness. Robustness generally implies insensitivity to departures from assumptiuons surrounding an underlying model, such as normality.

In summarizing the location of data the median, though highly resistant, is not extremely robust. But the mean is both nonresistant and nonrobust.

Figure 6. Variance Inflation

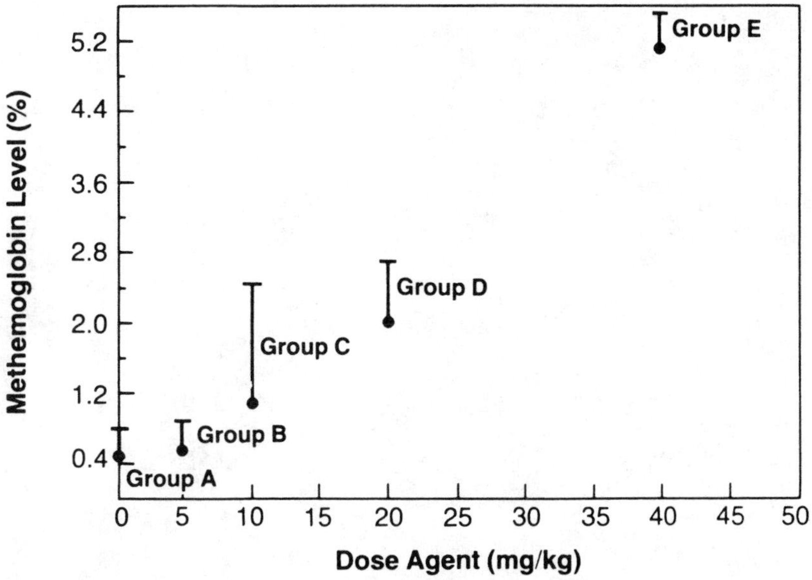

(Points Are Means – Error Bars Are + One Standard Deviation)

REFERENCES

Anscombe, F.J. (1973): Graphs in Statistical Analysis, *The American Statistician* 27: 17–21.

Chambers, J.M., Cleveland, W.S., Kleiner, B., and Tukey, P.A. (1983): *Graphical Methods for Data Analysis*, Wadsworth, Belmont.

Cleveland, W.S. and McGill, R. (1984): Graphical Perception: Theory, Experimentation, and Application to the Development of Graphical Methods, *Journal of the American Statistical Association*, 79: 531–554.

Hoaglin, D.C.; Mosteller, F. and Tukey, J.W. (1983): *Understanding Robust and Explanatory Data Analysis*, John Wiley, New York.

Snedecor, G.W. and Cochran, W.G. (1980): *Statistical Methods*, Seventh edition, Iowa State University Press, Ames.

Sokal, R.R., and Rohlf, F.J. (1981): *Biometry*. W.H. Freeman, San Francisco.

Tukey, J.W., (1977): *Exploratory Data Analysis*. Addison-Wesley Publishing Co., Reading.

Velleman, P.F. and Hoaglin, D.C. (1981): *Applications, Basics and Computing of Exploratory Data Analysis*, Duxbury Press, Boston.

CHAPTER 6

HYPOTHESIS TESTING OF CATEGORICAL AND RANKED DATA

The test methods presented in this chapter are designed to maximize the analysis of low information-value data while also maintaining acceptable levels of resistance. In general, the assumptions necessary for the use of these methods are less rigorous than those underlying the methods to be discussed in Chapter VII.

Categorical (or contingency table) presentations of data can contain any single type of data, but generally the contents are collected and arranged so that they can be classified as belonging to treatment and control groups, with the members of each of these groups then classified as belonging to one of two or more response categories (such as tumor/no tumor or normal/hyperplastic/neoplastic). For these cases, two forms of analysis are presented - Fisher's Exact Test (for the 2 x 2 contingency table) and the RXC chi square test (for large tables). It should be noted, however, that there are versions of both of these tests which permit the analysis of any size of contingency table.

The analysis of rank data - what is generally called nonparametric statistical analysis - is an exact parallel of the more traditional (and familiar) parametric methods. There are methods for the single comparison case (just as Student's t-test is used) and for the multiple comparison case (just as analysis of variance is used) with appropriate *post hoc* tests for exact identification of the significance with a set of groups. Four tests are presented for evaluating statistical significance in rank data - the Wilcoxon Rank Sum Test, distribution-free multiple comparisons, Mann-Witney U Test, and the Kruskall-Wallis nonparametric analysis of variance. For each of these tests, as for those in the next chapter, tables of distribution values for the evaluation of results are presented in Appendix I.

It should be clearly understood that for data which do not fulfill the necessary assumptions for parametric analysis, these nonparametric methods are either as powerful or in fact, more powerful than the equivalent parametric test.

Fisher's Exact Test

Fisher's exact test should be used to compare two sets of discontinuous, quantal (all or none) data. Small sets of such data can be checked by contingency data tables, such as those of Finney *et al.* (1963). Larger sets, however, require computation. These include frequency data such as incidences of mortality or certain histopathological findings, etc. Thus, the data can be expressed as ratios. These data do not fit on a continuous scale of measurement but usually involve numbers of responses classified as either negative or positive — that is, a contingency table situation [Sokal and Rohlf (1981), pp. 738–743].

The analysis is started by setting up a 2x2 contingency table to summarize the numbers of "positive" and "negative" responses as well as the totals of these, as follows:

	"Positive"	"Negative"	Total
Group I	A	B	A + B
Group II	C	D	C + D
Totals	A + C	B + D	$A + B + C + D = N_{total}$

Using the above set of symbols, the formula for P appears as follows:

$$P = \frac{(A+B)! \, (C+D)! \, (A+C)! \, (B+D)!}{N!A!B!C!D!}$$

The exact test produces a probability (P) which is the sum of the above calculation repeated for each possible arrangement of the numbers in the above cells (that is, A, B, C and D) showing an association equal to or stronger than that between the two variables.

The P resulting from these computations will be the exact one-or two-tailed probability depending on which of these two approaches is being employed. This value tells us if the groups differ significantly (with a probability less than 0.05, say) and the degree of significance. This is demonstrated in Example 5.

EXAMPLE 5

The pathology reports from 22 control and 48 treated animals show that 1 control and 3 treated animals have tumors of the spleen. Setting this up as a contingency table we see:

	Tumor-bearing	No tumors	Total
Control	1	21	22
Treated	3	45	48
Total	4	66	70

A! is A factorial. For 4! - as an example this would be (4) (3) (2) (1) = 24

The probability for the worst case on this calculates as:

$$P = \frac{(1+21)! \, (3+45)! \, (1+3)! \, (21+45)!}{70! \, 1! \, 2! \text{... } 45!}$$

$$P = \frac{22! \, 48! \, 4! \, 66!}{70! \, 1! \, 21! \, 3! \, 45!}$$

$$= 0.415002$$

All other possible stronger combinations must in turn be computed (in this case, 0, 22, 4, 44 is the only other such combination and it computes as P = 0.212216970). The probabilities must be summed to give the total P = 0.627 (single-tailed probability, to be discussed later).

ASSUMPTIONS AND LIMITATIONS

1. Tables are available which provide individual exact probabilities for small sample size contingency tables. See Zar, pp. 518–542 (1974).
2. Fisher's exact must be used in preference to the chi-square test when there are small cell sizes.
3. The probability resulting from a two-tailed test is exactly double that of a one-tailed for the same data.
4. Ghent has developed and proposed a good (though, if performed by hand, laborious) method extending the calculation of exact probabilities to 2 x 3, 3 x 3, and RXC contingency tables (Ghent, 1972).

2 x 2 Chi Square

Though Fisher's Exact Test is preferable for analysis of most 2 x 2 contingency tables in toxicology, the chi square test is still widely used and is preferable in a few unusual situations (particularly if cell sizes are large yet only limited computational support is available).

The formula is simply:

$$X^2 = \frac{(O_1 - E_1)^2}{E_1} + \frac{(O_2 - E_2)^2}{E_2}$$

$$= \sum \frac{(O_i - E_i)^2}{E_i}$$

where 0 are observed numbers (or counts) and E are expected numbers. The common practice in toxicology is for the observed figures to be test or treatment group counts. The expected figure is calculated as

$$E = \frac{\text{(column total) (row total)}}{\text{grand total}}$$

for each box or cell in a contingency table.

EXAMPLE 6

In an subacute toxicity study, there were 25 animals in the control group and 25 animals in the treatment group. Seven days after dosing, control and 13 treatment animals were observed to be exhibiting fine muscle tremors. All other animals had no tremors. Do significantly more treatment animals have tremors?

	Tremors		No tremors		Σ
	Observed	(Expected)	Observed	(Expected)	
Control	5	(8.5)	20	(16.5)	25
Treated	12	(8.5)	13	(16.5)	25
Σ	17		22		40

$$X^2 = \frac{(5\text{-}8.5)^2}{8.5} + \frac{(12\text{-}8.5)^2}{8.5} + \frac{(20\text{-}16.5)^2}{16.5} + \frac{(13\text{-}16.5)^2}{16.5}$$

$$= \frac{12.25}{8.5} + \frac{12.25}{8.5} + \frac{3.5}{16.5} + \frac{3.5}{16.5}$$

$$= 1.441 + 1.441 + 0.742 + 0.742$$

$$= 4.366$$

Our degrees of freedom are $(R\text{-}1)(C\text{-}1) = (2\text{-}1)(2\text{-}1) = 1$. Looking at a chi square table (such as in Table C of Appendix I) for one degree of freedom we see that this is greater than the test statistic at 0.05 (3.84) but less than that at 0.01 (6.63) so that $0.05 > p > 0.01$.

ASSUMPTIONS AND LIMITATIONS

ASSUMPTIONS: (1) Data are univariate and categorical
(2) Data are from a multinomial population
(3) Data are collected by random, independent sampling
(4) Groups being compared are of approximately the same size.

WHEN TO USE:	(1)	When the data are of a categorical (or frequency) nature
	(2)	When the data fit the assumptions above
	(3)	To test goodness-of-fit to a known distribution
	(4)	When cell sizes are large and computational support is limited.
WHEN NOT TO USE:	(1)	When the data are continuous rather than categorical
	(2)	When the sample sizes are very unequal
	(3)	When sample sizes are too small (for example, when total N is less than 50 or if any expected value is less than 5)
	(4)	For any 2 x 2 comparison when another method is available

R X C Chi Square

The RxC chi-square test can be used to analyze discontinuous (frequency) data as in the Fisher's exact or 2 X 2 chi-square tests. However, in the RxC test (R = row, C = column) we wish to compare three or more sets of data. An example would be comparison of the incidence of tumors among mice on three or more oral dosage levels. We can consider the data as "positive" (tumors) or "negative" (no tumors). The expected frequency for any box is equal to: (row total) (column total)/(N_{total}).

As in the Fisher's exact test, the initial step is setting up a table (this time a RxC contingency table). This table would appear as follows:

	"Positive"	"Negative"	Total
Group I	A_1	B_1	$A_1 + B_1 = N$
Group II	A_2	B_2	$A_2 + B_2 = N$
	1	1	
Group R	A_R	B_R	$A_R + B_R = N_A$
Totals	N_A	N_B	N_{total}

Using these symbols, the formula for chi-square (X^2) is:

$$X^2 = \frac{N_{tot}^2}{N_A N_B N_K} \left(\frac{A_1^2}{N_1} + \frac{A_2^2}{N_2} + \dots \frac{A_K^2}{N_K} - \frac{N_A^2}{N_{tot}} \right)$$

This resulting X^2 value is compared to table values [as in Snedecor and Cochran, pp. 470–471 or Table C) according to the number of degrees of freedom, which is equal to (R-1) (C-1). If X^2 is smaller than the table value at the 0.05 probability level, the groups are not significantly different. If the calculated X^2 is larger, there is some difference among the groups and 2 x R chi square or Fisher's exact tests will have to be completed to determine which group(s) differ from which other group(s). Example 7 demonstrates this.

EXAMPLE 7

The RxC chi-square can be used to analyze tumor incidence data gathered during a mouse feeding study as follows:

Dosage (mg/kg)	No. of mice with tumors	No. of mice without tumors	Total no. of mice
2.00	19	16	35
1.00	13	24	37
0.50	17	20	37
0.25	22	12	34
0.00	20	23	43
Totals	91	95	186

$$X^2 = \frac{(186)^2}{91(95)} \left[\frac{19^2}{35} + \frac{13^2}{37} + \frac{17^2}{37} + \frac{22^2}{34} + \frac{20^2}{43} - \frac{91^2}{186} \right]$$
$$= (4.00)(1.71)$$
$$= 6.84$$

The smallest expected frequency would be (91) (34)/186 + 16.6; well above 5.0. The number of degrees of freedom is (5 - 1) (2 - 1) = 4. The chi-square table value for four degrees of freedom is 9.49 at the 0.05 probability level. Therefore, there is no significant association between tumor incidence and dose or concentration.

ASSUMPTIONS AND LIMITATIONS

(1) Based on data being organized in a table (such as below) so that there are *cells* (in below, A, B, C and D are "cells").

	Columns (C)		
	Control	Treated	Total
No Effect	A	B	A + B
Rows (R)			
Effect	C	D	C + D
Total	A + C	B + D	A + B + C + D

(2) None of the "expected" frequency values should be less than 5.0.

(3) Chi square test is always one tailed.

(4) Without the use of some form of correction, the test becomes less accurate as the differences between group sizes increases.

(5) The results from each additional column (group) are approximately additive. Due to this characteristic, chi square can be readily used for evaluating any R x C combination.

(6) The results of the chi square calculation must be a positive number.

(7) Test is weak with either small sample sizes or when the expected frequency in any cell is less than 5 (this latter limitation can be overcome by "pooling" - combining cells).

(8) Test results are independent of order of cells, unlike Kolmogorov-Smirnov.

(9) Can be used to test the probability of validity of any distribution.

RELATED TESTS:

Fisher's Exact
G of likelihood ratio
Kolmogorov-Smirnov

Wilcoxon Rank-Sum Test

The Wilcoxon rank-sum test is commonly used for the comparison of two groups of nonparametric (interval or not normally distributed) data, such as those which are not measured exactly but rather as falling within certain limits (for example, how many animals died during each hour of an acute study). The test is also used when there is no variability (variance = 0) within one or more of the groups we wish to compare [Sokal and Rohlf, pp. 432–437].

The data in both groups being compared are initially arranged and listed in order of increasing value. Then each number in the two groups must receive a rank value. Beginning with the smallest number in either group (which is given a rank of 1.0), each number is assigned a rank. If there are duplicate numbers (called "ties"), then each value of equal size will receive the median rank for the entire identically-sized group. Thus if the lowest number appears twice, both figures receive the rank of 1.5. This, in turn, means that the ranks of 1.0 and 2.0 have been used and that the next highest number has a rank of 3.0. If the lowest number appears three times, then each is ranked as 2.0 and the next number has a rank of 4.0. Thus, each tied number gets a "median" rank. This process continues until all the numbers are ranked. Each of the two columns of ranks (one for each group) is totalled giving the "sum of ranks" for each group being compared. As a check, we can calculate the value:

$$\frac{(N)\,(N\,+\,1)}{2}$$

where N is the total number of data in both groups. The result should be equal to the sum of the sum of ranks for both groups.

The sum of rank values are compared to table values [such as Beyer, pp. 409–413 or Table J) to determine the degree of significant differences, if any. These tables include two limits (an upper and a lower) that are dependent upon the probability level. If the number of data is the same in both groups ($N_1 = N_2$), both of the calculated sums of ranks must fall within the two limit values. If this is the case, the two groups are not statistically different. If one or both of the sums of ranks is equal to or falls outside the table limits, the groups are different at that probability level. If the numbers of data in the two groups are not equal ($N_1 \neq N_2$), then the lesser sum of ranks (smaller N) is compared to the table limits to find the degree of significance. Normally the comparison of the two groups ends here and the degree of significant difference can be reported. This is demonstrated in Example 8.

EXAMPLE 8

If we recorded the approximate times to death (in hours) of rats dosed with 5.0 g/kg (Group A) or 2.5 g/kg (Group B) of a given material, we might obtain the following results:

Hours to death (Group A)	Hours to death (Group B)	Group A ranks	Group B ranks
1	1	2.5	2.5
1	2	2.5	6.0
1	4	2.5	9.5
2	4	6.0	9.5
2	5	6.0	11.5
3	7	8.0	14.5
5	7	11.5	14.5
6	8	13.0	16.0
Sums		52.0	84.0

Sum of sums $= 52.0 + 84.0 = 136$

$$\text{Check} = \frac{16(17)}{2} = 136$$

From the probability table (Table J), for $N_1 = 8$ we read the limit values (at 0.05) of 49 and 87. Since the calculated sums fall between these numbers, the two groups are not considered significantly different at $p = 0.05$.

ASSUMPTIONS AND LIMITATIONS

1. The model assumes no set distribution or form of data, but is in fact most appropriate for discontinuous or rank type data.
2. The occurrence of too many ties (that is, of ties in 10% or more of the cases in the sample) causes this test to overestimate alpha (that is, to have an inflated false negative rate). The test should not be used in such cases.

Distribution-Free Multiple Comparison

The distribution-free multiple comparison test should be used to compare three or more groups of nonparametric data. These groups are then analyzed two at a time for any significant differences [Hollander and Wolfe (1973), pp 124–129]. The test can be used for data similar to those compared by the rank-sum test. We often employ this test for reproduction and mutagenicity studies (such as comparing survival rates of offspring of rats fed various amounts of test materials in the diet).

As shown in Example 9, two values must be calculated for each pair of groups; the difference in mean ranks, and the probability level value against which the difference will be compared. To determine the difference in mean ranks we must first arrange the data within each of the groups in order of increasing values. Then we must assign rank values, beginning with the smallest overall figure. Note that this ranking is similar to that in the Wilcoxon test except that it applies to more than two groups.

The ranks are then added for each of the groups. As a check, the sum of these should equal

$$\frac{N_{tot}(N_{tot} + 1)}{2}$$

where N_{tot} is the total number of figures from all groups. Next we can find the mean rank (R) for each group by dividing the sum of ranks by the number of data (N) in the group. These mean ranks are then taken in those pairs which we want to compare (usually each test group versus the control) and the differences are found ($| R_1 - R_2 |$). This value is expressed as an absolute figure; that is, it is always a positive number.

The second value for each pair of groups (the probability value) is calculated from the expression:

$$^z[(a/K(K-1)]\sqrt{\frac{N_{tot}(N_{tot}+1)}{12}}\sqrt{\frac{1}{N_1}\frac{1}{N_2}}$$

where a is the level of significance for the comparison (usually 0.05, 0.01, 0.001, etc.), K is the total number of groups, and Z is a figure obtained from a normal probability table. This last figure is found by reading the result of $\propto (K/K - 1)$ within the table and determining the corresponding "Z-score" from Table H.

The result of the probability value calculation for each pair of groups is compared to the corresponding mean difference $| R_1 - R_2 |$. If $| R_1 - R_2 |$ is smaller, there is no significant difference between the groups. If it is larger, the groups are different and $| R_1 - R_2|$ must be compared to the calculated probability values for a = 0.01 and a = 0.001 to find the degree of significance.

EXAMPLE 9

Consider the following set of data (ranked in increasing order), which could represent the proportion of rats surviving given periods of time during diet inclusion of a test chemical at four dosage levels (survival index).

	I 5.0 mg/kg		II 2.5 mg/kg		III 1.25 mg/kg		IV 0.0 mg/kg	
	% value	rank	% value	rank	% value	rank	% value	rank
	40	2.0	40	2.0	50	5.5	60	9.0
	40	2.0	50	5.5	50	5.5	60	9.0
	50	5.5	80	12.0	60	9.0	80	12.0
	100	17.5	80	12.0	100	17.5	90	14.0
			100	17.5	100	17.5	100	17.5
							100	17.5
Sum of ranks		27.0		49.0		55.0		79.0
	$N_1 = 4$		$N_n = 5$		$N_m = 5$		$N_{iv} = 6$	
							$N_{tot} = 20$	

Check sum of sums = 210, $\dfrac{20(21)}{2} = 210$

Mean ranks (R): $R_1 = \dfrac{27.0}{4} = 6.75$ $R_2 = \dfrac{49.0}{5} = 9.80$

$R_3 = \dfrac{55.0}{5} = 11.00$ $R_4 = \dfrac{79.0}{6} = 13.17$

EXAMPLE 9 (continued)

Comparison groups	$R_1 - R_2$	Probability test values
5.0 vs 0.0	6.42	$(0.05/4(3)) = Z_{0.00417} = 2.637 \sqrt{\dfrac{(20)(21)}{12}} \sqrt{\dfrac{1}{4} + \dfrac{1}{6}} = 10.07$
2.5 vs 0.0	3.37	$(0.05/4(3)) = Z_{0.00417} = 2.637 \sqrt{\dfrac{(20)(21)}{12}} \sqrt{\dfrac{1}{5} + \dfrac{1}{6}} = 9.45$
1.25 vs 0.0	2.17	$(0.05/4(3)) = Z_{0.00417} = 2.637 \sqrt{\dfrac{(20)(21)}{12}} \sqrt{\dfrac{1}{5} + \dfrac{1}{6}} = 9.45$

Since each of the $|R_1 - R_2|$ values is smaller than the corresponding probability calculation, the pairs of groups compared are not different at the 0.05 level of significance.

ASSUMPTIONS AND LIMITATIONS

1. As with the Wilcoxon Rank-Sum, too many tied ranks inflate the false positive
2. Generally, this test should be used as a *post hoc* comparison after Kruskall-Wallis.

Mann-Whitney U Test

This is a non-parametric test in which the data in each group are first ordered from lowest to highest values, then the entire set (both control and treated values) is ranked, with the average rank being assigned to tied values. The ranks are then summed for each group and U is determined according to

$$U_t = n_e n_t + \frac{n_t(n_t + 1)}{2} - R_t$$

and

$$U_c = n_c n_t + \frac{n_c(n_c + 1)}{2} - R_c$$

where n_c, n_t = sample size for control and treated groups; and R_c, R_t = sum of ranks for the control and treated groups.

For the level of significance for a comparison of the two groups, the larger value of U_c or U_t is used. This is compared to critical values as found in tables (such as in Siegel, 1956 or in Table E).

With the above discussion and methods in mind, we may now examine the actual variables that we encounter in teratology studies. These variables can be readily divided into two groups—measures of lethality and measures of teratogenic effect (Gaylor, 1978). Measures of lethality include: (a) corpora lutea per pregnant female, (b) implants per pregnant female, (c) live fetuses per pregnant female, (d) percentage of preimplantation loss per pregnant female, (e) percentage of resorptions per pregnant female, and (f) percentage of dead fetuses per pregnant female. Measures of teratogenic effect include: (a) percentage of abnormal fetuses per litter, (b) percentage of litter with abnormal fetuses, and (c) fetal weight gain. As demonstrated in Example 10, the Mann-Whitney U test is employed for the count data, but which test should be employed for the percentage variables should be decided on the same grounds as described later under reproduction studies in the applications chapter.

EXAMPLE 10

In a two week study, the levels of serum cholesterol in treatment and control animals are successfully measured and assigned ranks as below:

	Treatment		Control	
	Value	Rank	Value	Rank
	10	1	19	4
	18	3	28	13
	26	10.5	29	14.5
	31	16	26	10.5
	15	2	35	19
	24	8	23	7
	22	6	29	14.5
	33	17	34	18
	21	5	38	20
	25	9	27	12
SUM OF RANKS		77.5		132.5

The critical value for a one tailed $p \leq 0.05$ is $U \geq 73$. We then calculate

$$U_t = (10)(10) + \frac{10(10+1)}{2} - 77.5$$

$$= 100 + \frac{110}{2} - 77.5 = 77.5$$

$$U_c = (10)(10) + \frac{10(10+1)}{2} - 132.5 = 22.5$$

As 77.5 is greater than 73, these groups are significantly different at the 0.05 level.

ASSUMPTIONS AND LIMITATIONS

1. It does not matter whether the observations are ranked from smallest to largest or vice versa.
2. This test should not be used for paired observations.
3. The test statistics from a Mann-Whitney are linearly related to those of the Wilcoxon. The two tests will always yield the same result. The Mann-Whitney is presented here for historical completeness, as it has been much favored in reproductive and developmental toxicology studies. However, it should be noted that the authors do not include it in the decision tree for method selection (Figure 2).

Kruskal-Wallis Nonparametric ANOVA

The Kruskal-Wallis nonparametric one-way analysis of variance should be the initial analysis performed when we have three or more groups of data which are by nature nonparametric (either not a normally distributed population, or of a discontinuous nature, or all the groups being analyzed are not from the same population) but not of a categorical (or quantal) nature. Commonly these will be either rank type evaluation data (such as behavioral toxicity observation scores) or reproduction study data. The analysis is initiated [Pollard, 1977, pp. 170–173] by ranking all the observations from the combined groups to be analyzed. Ties are given the average rank of the tied values (that is, if two values which would tie for 12th rank—and therefore would be ranked 12th and 13th—both would be assigned the average rank of 12.5).

The sum of ranks of each group (r_1, r_2,....r_k) is computed by adding all the rank values for each group. The test value H is then computed as

$$H = \frac{12}{n(n+1)} \Sigma r_1^2/n_1 + \Sigma r_2^2/n_2$$
$$+ ... + \Sigma r_k^2/n_k)\text{-}3(n+1)$$

where n_1, n_2, . . . n_k are the number of observations in each group. The test statistic is then compared with a table of H values (such as in Table D). If the calculated value of H is greater than the table value for the appropriate number of observations in each group, there is a significant difference between the groups, but further testing (using the distribution-free multiple comparisons method) is necessary to determine where the difference lies (as demonstrated in example 11).

EXAMPLE 11

As part of a neurobehavioral toxicology study, righting reflex values whole numbers ranging from 0 to 10) were determined for each of five rats in each of three groups. The values observed, and their ranks, are as follows:

Control group		5 mg/kg group		10 mg/kg group	
Reflex Score	Rank	Reflex score	Rank	Reflex score	Rank
0	2	1	5	4	11
0	2	2	7.5	4	11
0	2	2	7.5	5	13
1	5	3	9	8	14.5
1	5	4	11	8	14.5
Sums of of ranks (r)	16		40		64

From these the H value is calculated as

$$H = \frac{12}{15(15+1)} \left[\frac{16^2 +}{5} \quad \frac{40^2 +}{5} \quad \frac{64^2}{5} \right] - 3(15+1)$$

$$= \frac{12}{240} \quad \frac{(256 + 1600 + 4096)}{5} \quad -48$$

$$= \frac{1}{20} (1190.4) - 48$$

$$= 59.52 - 48$$

$$= 11.52$$

Consulting a table of values for H, we find that for the case where we have three groups of five observations each, the test values are 4.56 (for p = 0.10), 5.78 (for p = 0.05), and 7.98 (for p = 0.01). As our calculated H is greater than the p = 0.01 test value, we have determined that there is a significant difference between these groups at the level of $p < 0.01$, and would now have to continue to a multiple comparisons test to determine where the difference is.

ASSUMPTIONS AND LIMITATIONS

1. The test statistic H is used for both small and large samples.
2. When we find a significant difference, we do not know which groups are different. It is not correct to then perform a Mann-Whitney U test on all possible combinations - rather, a multiple comparison method must be used, such as the distribution-free multiple comparisons.
3. Data must be independent for the test to be valid.
4. Too many tied ranks will decrease the power of this test and also lead to increased false positive levels.

REFERENCES

Finney, D.J., Latscha, R., Bennet, B.M., and Hsu, P. (1963): *Tables for Testing Significance in a 2 x 2 Contingency Table*. Cambridge University Press, Cambridge.

Gaylor, D.W. (1978): Methods and concepts of biometrics applied to teratology. In: *Handbook of Teratology*, Vol. 4, edited by J.G. Wilson and F.C. Fraser, pp. 429-444. Plenum Press, New York.

Ghent, A.W. (1972): A Method for Exact Testing of 2 x 2, 2 x 3, 3 x 3 and Other Contingency Tables, Employing Binomiate Coefficients. *American Midland Naturalist.* 88:15–27.

Hollander, M., and Wolfe, D.A. (1973): *Nonparametric Statistical Methods*, pp. 124–129. John Wiley, New York

Pollard, J.H. (1977): *Numerical and Statistical Techniques*. Cambridge University Press, New York.

Siegel, S. (1956): *Nonparametric Statistics for the Behavioral Sciences*. McGraw-Hill, New York.

Snedecor, G.W. and Cochran, W.G. (1980): *Statistical Methods*, Seventh edition, Iowa State University Press, Ames.

Sokal, R.R., and Rohlf, F.J. (1981): *Biometry*. W.H. Freeman, San Francisco.

Zar, J.H. (1974): *Biostatistical Analysis*, p. 50. Prentice-Hall, Englewood.

CHAPTER 7

HYPOTHESIS TESTING: UNIVARIATE PARAMETRIC TESTS

In this chapter we consider test methods for univariate case[1] data from normally distributed populations. Such data generally have a higher information value associated with them but the traditional hypothesis testing techniques (which include all the methods described in this chapter) are generally neither resistant nor robust. All the data analyzed by these methods are also, effectively, continuous - that is, at least for practical purposes, the data may be represented by any number and each such data number has a measurable relationship to other data numbers.

Student's t-Test (Unpaired t-Test)

Pairs of groups of continuous, randomly distributed data are compared via this test. We can use this test to compare three or more groups of data, but they must be intercompared by examination of two groups taken at a time and are preferentially compared by analysis of variance (ANOVA). Usually this means comparison of a test group versus a control group, although two test groups may be compared as well. To determine which of the three types of t-tests described in this chapter should be empoloyed, the F-test is usually performed first. This will tell us if the variances of the data are approximately equal, which is a requirement for the use of a parametric method. If the F test indicates homogeneous variances and the numbers of data within the groups (N) are equal, then the Student's t-test is the appropriate procedure [Sokal and Rohlf, 1981, pp. 226-231]. If the F is significant (the data are heterogeneous) and the two groups have equal numbers of data, the modified Student's t-test is applicable (Diem and Lentner, 1975).

The value of t for Student's t-test is calculated using the formula:

[1]That is, where each datum is defined by one treatment and one effect variable.

$$t = \frac{\bar{X}_1 - \bar{X}_2}{\sqrt{\Sigma D_1^2 + \Sigma D_3^2}} \qquad \sqrt{\frac{N_1 N_2}{N_1 + N_2}(N_1 + N_2 - 2)}$$

where the value of $\Sigma D^2 = \dfrac{N\Sigma X^2 - (\Sigma X)^2}{N}$

The value of t obtained from the above calculations is compared to the values in a t-distribution table (such as in Table F) according to the appropriate number of degrees of freedom (df). If the F value is not significant (i.e., variances are homogeneous), the df = $N_1 + N_2 - 2$. If the F. was significant and $N_1 = N_2$, then the df = $N - 1$. Although this case indicates a nonrandom distribution, the modified t-test is still valid. If the calculated value is larger than the table value at p = 0.05, it may then be compared to the appropriate other table values in order of decreasing probability to determine the degree of significance between the two groups. Example 12 demonstrates this methodology.

EXAMPLE 12

Suppose we wish to compare two groups (a test and control group) of dog weights following inhalation of a vapor. First, we would test for homogeneity of variance using the F test. Assuming that this test gave negative (homogeneous) results, we would perform the t-test as follows:

Dog #	Test weight (X_1 in kg)	X_1^2	Control weight (X_2 in kg)	X_2^2
1	8.3	68.89	8.4	70.56
2	8.8	77.44	10.2	104.04
3	9.3	86.49	9.6	92.16
4	9.3	86.49	9.4	88.36
Sums	$\Sigma X_1 = 35.7$	$\Sigma X_1^2 = 319.31$	$\Sigma X_2 = 37.6$	$\Sigma X_2^2 = 355.12$
Means	8.92		9.40	

The difference in means = 9.40 − 8.92 = 0.48

$$\Sigma D_1^2 = \frac{4(319.31) - (35.7)^2}{4} = \frac{2.75}{4} = 0.6875$$

$$\Sigma D_2^2 = \frac{4(355.12) - (37.6)^2}{4} = \frac{6.72}{4} = 1.6800$$

$$t = \frac{0.48}{\sqrt{0.6875 + 1.6800}} \sqrt{\frac{4(4)}{4+4}(4 + 4 - 2)} = 1.08$$

The table value for t at the 0.05 probability level for (4 + 4 − 2), or six degrees of freedom, is 2.447. Therefore, the dog weights are not significantly different at p = 0.05.

ASSUMPTIONS AND LIMITATIONS

1. The test assumes that the data are univariate, continuous and normally distributed.
2. Data are collected by randomly sampling.
3. The test should be used when the assumptions in 1 and 2 are met and there are only two groups to be compared.
4. Do not use when the data are ranked, when the data are not approximately normally distributed, or when there are more than two groups to be compared. Do not use for paired observations.
5. This is the most commonly misused test method, except in those few cases where one is truly only comparing two groups of data and the group sizes are roughly equivalent. Not valid for multiple comparisons (because of resulting additive errors) or where group sizes are very unequal.
6. Test is robust for moderate departures from normality and, when N_1 and N_2 are approximately equal, robust for moderate departures from homogeneity of variances.

Cochran t-test

The Cochran test should be used to compare two groups of continuous data when the variances (as indicated by the F test) are heterogeneous and the numbers of data within the groups are not equal ($N_1 \neq N_2$). This is the situation, for example, when the data, though expected to be randomly distributed, were found not to be [Cochran and Cox, 1975, pp. 100–102].

Two t values are calculated for this test, the "observed" t (t_{obs}) and the "expected" t (t'). The observed t is obtained by:

$$t_{obs} = \frac{\overline{X}_1 - \overline{X}_2}{\sqrt{W_1 + W_2}}$$

where W = SEM^2 (standard error of the mean squared)

$$= S^2/N$$

where S (variance) can be calculated from:

$$S = \frac{\dfrac{N\Sigma X^2 - (\Sigma X)^2}{N}}{N-1}$$

The value for t' is obtained from:

$$t' = \frac{t_1' W_1 + t_2' W_2}{W_1 + W_2}$$

where t'_1 and t'_2 are values for the two groups taken from the t-distribution table corresponding to N - 1 degrees of freedom (for each group) at the 0.05 probability level (or such level as one may select).

The calculated t_{obs} is compared to the calculated t' value (or values, if t' values were prepared for more than one probability level). If t_{obs} is smaller than a t', the groups are not considered to be significantly different at that probability level. This procedure is shown in Example 13.

EXAMPLE 13

Using the red blood cell count comparison from the F test (with $N_1 = 5$, $N_2 = 4$), the following results were determined:

$$X_1 = \frac{37.60}{5} = 7.52 \qquad W_1 = \frac{0.804}{5} = 0.1608$$

$$X_2 = \frac{29.62}{4} = 7.40 \qquad W_2 = \frac{0.025}{4} = 0.0062$$

(Note that S^2 values of 0.804 and 0.025 are calculated in example 14)

$$t_{obs} = \frac{7.52 - 7.40}{\sqrt{0.1608 + 0.0062}} = 0.29$$

From the t-distribution table we use $t_1 = 2.776$ (df = 4) and $t_2 = 3.182$ (df = 3) for the 0.05 level of probability.

$$t_{04}' = \frac{2.776\,(0.1608) + 3.182\,(0.0062)}{0.1608 + 0.0062}$$
$$= 2.79$$

Because t_{obs} is smaller than t' at the 0.05 level of significance, there is no statistical difference at p = 0.05 between the two groups.

ASSUMPTIONS AND LIMITATIONS

1. The test assumes that the data are univariate, continuous, normally distributed and that group sizes are unequal.
2. The test is robust for moderate departures from normality, and very robust for departures from equality of variances.

F Test

This is a test of the homogeneity of variances between two groups of data [Sokal and Rohlf, 1981, pp. 187–188]. It is used in two separate cases. The first is when Bartlett's indicates heterogeneity of variances among three or more groups (i.e., it is used to determine which pairs of groups are heterogeneous). Second, the F test is the initial step in comparing two groups of continuous data which we would expect to be parametric (two groups not usually being compared using ANOVA), the results indicating whether the data are from the same population and whether subsequent parametric comparisons would be valid.

The F is calculated by dividing the larger variance (S_1^2) by the smaller one (S_2^2). S^2 is calculated as

$$S^2 = \frac{N\Sigma X^2 - (\Sigma X)^2}{N - 1}$$

where N is the number of data in the group and X represents the individual values within the group. Frequently, S^2 values may be obtained from ANOVA calculations. Use of this is demonstrated in Example 14.

The calculated F value is compared to the appropriate number in an F value table (such as Table G) for the appropriate degrees of freedom (N - 1) in the numerator (along the top of the table) and in the denominator (along the side of the table). If the calculated value is smaller, it is not significant and the variances are considered homogeneous (and the Student's t-test would be appropriate for further comparison). If the calculated F value is greater, F is significant and the variances are heterogeneous (and the next test would be modified Student's t-test if $N_1 = N_2$ or the Cochran t-test if $N_1 \neq N_2$; see Figure 2 to review decision tree).

EXAMPLE 14

If we wished to compare the red blood cell counts (RBC) of rats receiving a test material in their diet with the RBCs of control rats we might obtain the following results:

Test RBC (X_1)	X_1^2	Control RBC (X_2)	X_2^2
8.23	67.73	7.22	52.13
8.59	73.79	7.55	57.00
7.51	56.40	7.53	56.70
6.60	43.56	7.32	53.58
6.67	44.49		
$\Sigma X_1 = 37.60$	$\Sigma X_1^2 = 285.97$	$\Sigma X_2 = 29.62$	$\Sigma X_2^2 = 219.41$

$$\text{Variance for } X_1 = S_1^2 = \frac{5(285.97) - (37.60)^2}{5 - 1}$$

$$= 0.804$$

$$\text{Variance for } X_2 = S_3^2 = \frac{4(219.41) - (29.62)^2}{4 - 1}$$

$$= 0.025$$

$$F = \frac{0.804}{0.025} = 32.16$$

From the table for F values, for 4 (numerator) versus 3 (denominator) df, we read the limit of 15.1 at the 0.05 level. As our calculated value is larger (and, therefore, significant), the variances are heterogeneous and the Cochran t-test would be appropriate for comparison of the two groups of data.

ASSUMPTIONS AND LIMITATIONS

1. This test could be considered as a two group equivalent of the Bartlett's test.
2. If the test statistic is close to 1.0, the results are (of course) not significant.
3. The test assumes normality and independence of data.

Analysis of Variance (ANOVA)

ANOVA is used for the comparison of three or more groups of continuous data when the variances are homogeneous and the data are independent and normally distributed.

A series of calculations are required for ANOVA, starting with the values within each group being added (ΣX) and then these sums being added ($\Sigma\Sigma X$). Each figure within the groups is squared, and these squares are then summed (ΣX^2) and these sums added ($\Sigma\Sigma X^2$).

Next the "correction factor" (CF) can be calculated from the following formula.

$$CF = \frac{\left(\sum\limits_{1}^{K} \sum\limits_{1}^{N} X \right)^{2}}{N_1 + N_2 + ...N_k}$$

where N is the number of values in each group and K is the number of groups. The total sum of squares (SS) is then determined as follows:

$$SS_{total} = \sum\limits_{1}^{K} \sum\limits_{1}^{N} X^2 - CF$$

In turn, the sum of squares between groups (bg) is found from:

$$SS_{bg} = \frac{(\Sigma X_1)^2}{N_1} + \frac{(\Sigma X_2)^2}{N_2} + ... \frac{(\Sigma X_k)^2}{N_k} - CF$$

The sum of squares within group (wg) is then the difference between the last two figures, or:

$$SS_{wg} = SS_{total} - SS_{bg}$$

Now, there are three types of degrees of freedom to determine. The first, total df, is the total number of data within all groups under analysis minus one ($N_1 + N_2 + ... N_K - 1$). The second figure (the df between groups) is the number of groups minus one ($K - 1$). The last figure (the df within groups or "error df") is the difference between the first two figures ($df_{total} - df_{bg}$).

The next set of calculations requires determination of the two mean squares (MS_{bg} and MS_{wg}). These are the respective sum of square values divided by the corresponding df figures ($MS = SS/df$). The final calculation is that of the F ratio. For this, the MS between groups is divided by the MS within groups ($F = MS_{bg}/MS_{wg}$).

A table of the results of these calculations (using data from Example 15 at the end of this section) would appear as follows:

	df	SS	MS	F
Bg	3	0.04075	0.01358	4.94
Wg	12	0.03305	0.00275	
Total	15	0.07380		

For interpretation, the F ratio value obtained in the ANOVA is compared to a table of F values (Table G). If $F \leq 1.0$, the results are not significant and comparison with the table values is not necessary. The degrees of freedom (df) for the greater mean square (MS_{bg}) are indicated along the top of the table. Then read down the side of the table to the line corresponding to the df for the lesser mean square

(MS_{wg}). The figure shown at the desired significance level (traditionally 0.05) is compared to the calculated F value. If the calculated number is smaller, there are no significant differences among the groups being compared. If the calculated value is larger, there is some difference but further (*post hoc*) testing will be required before we know which groups differ significantly.

EXAMPLE 15

Suppose we want to compare four groups of dog kidney weights, expressed as percentage of body weights, following an inhalation study. Assuming homogeneity of variance (from Bartlett's test), we could complete the following calculations:

	400 ppm	200 ppm	100 ppm	0 ppm
	0.43	0.49	0.34	0.34
	0.52	0.48	0.40	0.32
	0.43	0.40	0.42	0.33
	0.55	0.34	0.40	0.39
ΣX	1.93	1.71	1.56	1.38

$$\Sigma\Sigma X = 1.93 + 1.71 + 1.56 + 1.38 = 6.58$$

Next, the preceeding figures are squared:

	400 ppm	200 ppm	100 ppm	0 ppm
	0.1849	0.2401	0.1156	0.1156
	0.2704	0.2304	0.1600	0.1024
	0.1849	0.1600	0.1764	0.1089
	0.3025	0.1156	0.1600	0.1521
ΣX^2	0.9427	0.7461	0.6120	0.4790

$$\Sigma\Sigma X^2 = 0.9427 + 0.7461 + 0.6120 + 0.4790 = 2.7798$$

$$CF = \frac{(6.58)^2}{4 + 4 + 4 + 4} = 2.7060$$

$$SS_{total} = 2.7798 - 2.7060 = 0.0738$$

$$SS_{bg} = \frac{(1.93)^2}{4} + \frac{(1.71)^2}{4} + \frac{(1.56)^2}{4} + \frac{(1.38)^2}{4} - 2.7060$$

$$= 0.04075$$

$$SS_{wg} = 0.07380 - 0.04075 = 0.03305$$

The total degrees of freedom $(df) = 4 + 4 + 4 + 4 - 1 = 15$

$$df_{bg} = 4 - 1 = 3 \quad df_{wg} = 15 - 3 = 12$$

$$MS_{bg} = \frac{0.4075}{3} = 0.01358$$

$$MS_{wg} = \frac{0.03305}{12} = 0.00275$$

$$F = \frac{0.01358}{0.00275} = 4.94$$

Going to an F value table we find that for 3 df_{bg} (greater mean square) and 12 df_{wg} (lesser mean square), the 0.05 value of F is 3.49. As our calculated value is greater, there is a difference among groups at the 0.05 probability level. To determine where the difference is, further comparisons by a *post hoc* test will be necessary.

ASSUMPTIONS AND LIMITATIONS

1. What is presented here is the workhorse of toxicology - the one way analysis of variance. Many other forms exist for more complicated experimental designs.
2. The test is robust for moderate departures from normality if the sample sizes are large enough. Unfortunately, this is rarely the case in toxicology.
3. ANOVA is robust for moderate departures from equality of variances (as determined by Bartlett's test) if the sample sizes are apprroximately equal.
4. It is not appropriate to use a t-test (or a 2 groups at a time version of ANOVA) to identify where significant differences are within the design. A multiple - comparison *post hoc* method must be used.

Post Hoc Tests

There is a wide variety of *post hoc* tests available to analyze data after finding a significant result in an ANOVA. Each of these tests has advantages and disadvantages, proponents and critics. Four of the tests are commonly used in toxicology and will be presented or reviewed here. These are Dunnett's t-test and Williams' t-test. Two other tests which are available in many of the mainframe statistical packages are Turkey's method and the Student-Newman-Keuls method (Zar, 1974, 151–161).

If ANOVA reveals no significance it is not appropriate to proceed to perform a *post hoc* test in hope of finding differences. To do so would only be another form of multiple comparisons, increasing the type I error rate beyond the desired level.

Duncan's Multiple Range Test

Duncan's (Duncan, 1955) is used to compare groups of continuous and randomly distributed data (such as body weights, organ weights, etc.). The test normally involves three or more groups taken one pair at a time. It should only follow observation of a significant F value in the ANOVA, and can serve to determine which group (or groups) differs significantly from which other group (or groups).

There are two alternative methods of calculation. The selection of the proper one is based on whether the number of data (N) are equal or unequal in the groups.

Groups with Equal Number of Data ($N_1 = N_2$)

Two sets of calculations must be carried out; first, the determination of the difference between the means of pairs of groups; second, the preparation of a probability table against which each difference in means is compared (as shown in the first of the two examples in this section).

The means (averages) are determined (or taken from the ANOVA calculation) and ranked in either decreasing or increasing order. If two means are the same, they take up two equal positions (thus, for four means we could have ranks of 1, 2, 2, and 4 rather than 1, 2, 3, and 4). The groups are then taken in pairs and the differences between the means ($\overline{X}_1 - \overline{X}_2$), expressed as positive numbers, are calculated. Usually, each pair consists of a test group and the control group, through multiple test groups may be intracompared if so desired. The relative rank of the two groups being compared must be considered. If a test group is ranked "2" and the control group is ranked "1", then we say that there are two places between them, while if the test group were ranked "3", then there would be three places between it and the control.

To establish the probability table, the standard error of the mean (SEM) must be calculated. This can be done as presented in Chapter 2 or shown as

$$\sqrt{\frac{\text{error mean square}}{N}}$$

$$= \sqrt{\frac{\text{mean square within group}}{N}}$$

where N is the number of animals or replications per dose level. The mean square within groups (MS_{wg}) can be calculated from the information given in the ANOVA procedure (refer to the earlier section on ANOVA). The SEM is then multiplied by a series of table values [as in Harter, 1960 or Beyer 1976, pp. 369–378] to set up a probability table. The table values used for the calculations are chosen according to the probability levels (note that the tables have sections for 0.05, 0.01, and 0.001 levels) and the number of means apart for the groups being compared and the number of "error" degrees of freedom (df). The "error" df is the number of df within the groups. This last figure is determined from the ANOVA calculation and can be taken from ANOVA output. For some values of df, the table values are not given and should thus be interpolated. Example 16 demonstrates this case.

EXAMPLE 16

Using the data given in example 15 (4 groups of dogs, with 4 dogs in each group), we can make the following calculations:

Ranks	1	2	3	4
Concentration	0 ppm	100 ppm	200 ppm	400 ppm
Mean kidney weight ($\bar{X}$)	0.345	0.390	0.428	0.483

Groups compared	$\bar{X}_1 - \bar{X}_2$	No of means apart
2 vs. 1 (100 vs. 0 ppm)	0.045	2
3 vs. 1 (200 vs 0 ppm)	0.083	3
4 vs. 1 (400 vs 0 ppm)	0.138	4
4 vs. 2 (400 vs. 100 ppm)	0.093	3

The mean square within groups from the ANOVA example was 0.00275. Therefore, the SEM = $\sqrt{0.00275/4}$ = 0.02622. The "error" df (df_{wg}) was 12 so the following table values are used.

No. of means apart	Probability levels		
	0.05	0.01	0.001
2	3.082	4.320	6.106
3	3.225	4.504	6.340
4	3.313	4.622	6.494

When these are multiplied by the SEM we get the following probability table:

No. of means apart	Probability levels		
	0.05	0.01	0.001
2	0.0808	0.1133	0.1601
3	0.0846	0.1181	0.1662
4	0.0869	0.1212	0.1703

Groups with Unequal Numbers of Data ($N_1 \neq N_2$)

This procedure is very similar to that discussed above. As before, the means are ranked and the differences between the means are determined ($\overline{X}_1 - \overline{X}_2$). Next, weighting values ("a_{ij}" values) are calculated for the pairs of groups being compared in accordance with

$$\alpha_v = \sqrt{\frac{2N_i N_j}{(N_i + N_j)}} = \sqrt{\frac{2N_1 N_2}{(N_1 + N_2)}}$$

This weighting value for each pair of groups is multiplied by $\overline{X}_1 - \overline{X}_2$ for each value to arrive at a "t" value. It is this "t" that will later be compared to a probability table.

The probability table is set up as above except that instead of multiplying the appropriate table values by SEM, SEM^2 is used. This is equal to $\sqrt{MS_{wg}}$.

For the desired comparison of two groups at a time, either the $\overline{X}_1 - \overline{X}_2$ value (if $N_1 = N_2$) or the "t" value (if $N_1 = N_2$) is compared to the appropriate probability table. Each comparison must be made according to the number of places between the means. If the table value is larger at the 0.05 level, the two groups are not considered to be statistically different. If the table value is smaller, the groups are different and the comparison is repeated at lower levels of significance. Thus, the degree of significance may be determined. We might have significant differences at 0.05 but not at 0.01, in which case the probability would be represented as $0.05 > p > 0.01$. Example 17 demonstrates this case.

EXAMPLE 17

Suppose that the 400 ppm level from the above example had only 3 dogs, but that the mean for the group and the mean square within groups were the same. To continue Duncan's we would calculate the weighing factors as follows:

100 ppm vs. 0 ppm

200 ppm vs. 0 ppm $\quad N_1 = 4; N_2 = 4 \; \alpha v = \sqrt{\dfrac{2(4)(4)}{4+4}} = 2.00$

400 ppm vs. 0 ppm $\quad N_2 = 3; N_4 = 4 \; \alpha v = \sqrt{\dfrac{2(3)(4)}{3+4}} = 1.852$

400 ppm vs 100 ppm

Using the $\overline{X}_1 - \overline{X}_2$ from the above example we can set up the following tables:

[2]Where K = the number of groups and N = the total number of data.

Concentrations ppm	No. of means apart	$\bar{X}_1 - \bar{X}_2$	α_v	$(\bar{X}_1 - \bar{X}_2)\alpha_v$
100 vs 0	2	0.045	2.000	2.000 (.045) = .090
200 vs. 0	3	0.083	2.000	2.000 (.083) = .166
400 vs. 0	4	0.138	1.852	1.852 (.138) = .256
400 vs. 100	3	0.093	1.852	1.852 (.093) = .172

Next we calculate SEM^2 as being 0.00275 = 0.05244. This is multiplied by the appropriate table values chosen for 11 df (df_{wg} for this example). This gives the following probability table:

No. of means apart	Probability levels		
	0.05	0.01	0.001
2	0.1632	0.2303	0.3291
3	0.1707	0.2401	0.3417
4	0.1753	0.2463	0.3501

Comparing the "t" values with the probability table values we get the following:

Comparison	Probability
100 ppm vs. 0 ppm	$p > 0.05$
200 ppm vs. 0 ppm	$p > 0.05$
400 ppm vs. 0 ppm	$0.01 > p > 0.001$
400 ppm vs. 100 ppm	$0.05 > p > 0.01$

ASSUMPTION AND LIMITATIONS

1. Duncan's assures a set alpha level or type I error rate for all tests when means are separated by no more than ordered step increases. Preserving this alpha level means that the test is less sensitive than some others, such as the Student-Newman-Keuls. The test is inherently conservative and not resistant or robust.

Scheffe's Multiple Comparisons

Scheffe's is another *post hoc* comparison method for groups of continuous and randomly distributed data. It also normally involves three or more groups [Scheffe, 1959 and Harris, 1975]. It is widely considered a more powerful significance test than Duncan's.

Each *post hoc* comparison is tested by comparing an obtained test value (F_{contr}) with the appropriate critical F value at the selected level of significance (the table F value multiplied by K - 1 for an F with K - 1 and N - K degrees of freedom[2]). F_{contr} is computed as follows:

(a) Compute the mean for each sample (group);

(b) Denote the residual mean square by MS_{wg};

(c) Compute the test statistic as

$$F_{contr} = \frac{(C_1 \bar{X}_1 + C_2 \bar{X}_2 + \cdots + C_K \bar{X}_K)^2}{(K-1) MS_{wg} (C_1^2/n_1 + \cdots + C_K^2/n_k)}$$

where C_k is the comparison number such that the sum of C_1, C_2 ... $C_k = 0$. (See Example 18).

EXAMPLE 18

At the end of a short-term feeding study the following body weight changes were recorded:

	Group 1	Group 2	Group 3
	10.2	12.2	9.2
	8.2	10.6	10.5
	8.9	9.9	9.2
	8.0	13.0	8.7
	8.3	8.1	9.0
	8.0	10.8	
		11.5	
Totals	51.6	76.1	46.6
Means	8.60	10.87	9.32

$MS_{wg} = 1.395$

To avoid logical inconsistencies with pair-wise comparisons, we compare the group having the largest sample mean (group 2) with that having the smallest sample mean (group 1), then with the group having the next smallest sample mean, and so on. As soon as we find a nonsignificant comparison in this process (or no group with a smaller sample mean remains), we replace the group having the largest sample mean with that having the second largest sample mean and repeat the comparison process.

Accordingly, our first comparison is between groups 2 and 1. We set $C_1 = -1$, $C_2 = 1$, and $C_3 = 0$ and calculate our test statistic

$$F_{contr} = \frac{(10.87 - 8.60)^2}{(3-1) \, 1.395 \, (1/6 + 1/7)}$$
$$= 5.97$$

The critical region for F at $p \leqslant 0.05$ for two and eleven degrees of freedom is 3.98. Therefore, these groups are significantly different at this level. We next compare groups 2 and 3, using $C_1 = 0$, $C_2 = 1$, and $C_3 = -1$

$$F_{\text{contr}} = \frac{(10.87 - 9.32)^2}{(3 - 1)\,1.395\,(1/7 + 1/5)} = 2.51$$

This is less than the critical region value, so these groups are not significantly different.

ASSUMPTIONS AND LIMITATIONS

1. The Scheffe procedure is robust to moderate violations of the normality and homogeneity of variance assumptions.
2. It is not formulated on the basis of groups with equal numbers (as one of the Duncan procedures is), and if $N_1 = N_2$ there is no separate weighing procedure.
3. It tests all linear contrasts among the population means (the other three methods confine themselves to pairwise comparison, except when they use a Bonferroni type correlation procedure).
4. The Scheffe procedure is powerful because of its robustness, yet is still conservative. Type I error (the false positive rate) is held constant at the selected test level for each comparison.

Dunnett's t-Test

Dunnett's t-test (Dunnett, 1955 and Dunnett, 1964) has as its starting point the assumption that what is desired is a comparison of each of several means with one other mean and only one other mean; in other words, that one wishes to compare each and every treatment group with the control group, but not compare treatment groups with each other. The problem here is that, in toxicology, one is frequently interested in comparing treatment groups with other treatment groups. However, if one does want only to compare treatment groups versus a control group, Dunnett's is a useful approach. In a study with K groups (one of them being the control) we will wish to make K-1 comparisons. In such a situation, we want to have a P level for the entire set of K-1 decisions (not for each individual decision). The Dunnett's t distribution is predicated on this assumption. The parameters for utilizing a Dunnett's t table, such as found in his original article, are K (as above) and the number of degrees of freedom for mean square within groups (MS_{wg}). The test value is calculated as

$$t = \frac{|T_j - T_i|}{2\,MS_{wg/n}}$$

where n is the number of observations in each of the groups. The mean square within group (MS_{wg}) is as we have defined it previously; T_j is the control group mean and T_i is the mean of, in order, each successive test group observation. Note that one uses the absolute value of the number resulting from subtracting T_i from T_j. This is to ensure a positive number for our final t.

Example 19 demonstrates this test, again with the data from Example 15.

EXAMPLE 19

The means, N's and sums for the groups previously presented in Example 15 are:

	Control	100 ppm	200 ppm	400 ppm
Sum (ΣX)	1.38	1.56	1.71	1.93
N	4	4	4	4
Mean	0.345	0.39	0.4275	0.4825

The MS_{wg} was 0.00275, and our test t for 4 groups and 12 df is 2.41. Substituting in the equation, we calculate our t for the control versus the 400 ppm to be

$$= \frac{|\ 0.345 - 0.4825\ |}{\sqrt{2(0.00275)/4}}$$

$$= \frac{0.1375}{\sqrt{0.001375}}$$

$$= \frac{0.1375}{\sqrt{0.03781}} = 3.637$$

which exceeds our test value of 2.41, showing that these two groups are significantly different at $p \leq 0.05$. The values for the comparisons of the control versus the 200 and 100 ppm groups are then found to be, respectively, 2.182 and 1.190. Both of these are less than our test value, and therefore the groups are not significantly different.

ASSUMPTIONS AND LIMITATIONS

1. Dunnett's seeks to ensure that the type I error rate will be fixed at the desired level by incorporating correction factors into the design of the test value table.
2. Group sizes must be equal.

Williams' t-Test

Williams' t-test (Williams, 1971 and Williams, 1972) has also become popular, although the following discussion will show that its use is quite limited in toxicology. It is designed to detect the highest level (in a set of dose/exposure levels) at which there is no significant effect. It assumes that the response of interest (such as change in body weights) occurs at higher levels, but not at lower levels, and that the responses are monotonically ordered so that $X_o \leqslant X_1 \ldots \leqslant X_k$. This is, however, frequently not the case. The Williams' technique handles the occurrence of such discontinuities in a response series by replacing the offending value and the value immediately preceding it with weighted average values. The test also is adversely affected by any mortality at high dose levels. Such mortalities "impose a severe penalty, reducing the power of detecting an effect not only at level K but also at all lower doses" (Williams, 1972, p. 529). Accordingly, it is not generally applicable in toxicological studies.

Analysis of Covariance

Analysis of covariance (ANCOVA) is a method for comparing sets of data which consist of two variables (treatment and effect, with our effect variable being called the "variate"), when a third variable (called the "covariate") exists which can be measured but not controlled and which has a definite effect on the variable of interest. In other words, it provides an indirect type of statistical control, allowing us to increase the precision of a study and to remove a potential source of bias. One common example of this is in the analysis of organ weights in toxicity studies. Our true interest here is the effect of our dose or exposure level on the specific organ weights, but most organ weights also increase (in the young, growing animals most commonly used in such studies) in proportion to increases in animal body weight. As we are not here interested in the effect of this covariate (body weight), we measure it to allow adjustment of the measurement of the variate in which we are interested (the organ weights). Analysis of covariance allows us to make this adjustment. We must be careful before using ANCOVA, however, to ensure that the underlying nature of the correspondence between the variate and covariate is such that we can rely on it as a tool for adjustments (Anderson *et al.*, 1980 and Kotz and Johnson, 1982).

Calculation is performed in two steps. The first is a type of linear regression between the variate Y and the covariate X.

This regression, performed as described under the linear regression section, gives us the model

$$Y = \alpha_1 + \beta X + e$$

which in turn allows us to define adjusted means ($\bar{Y}$ and $\bar{X}$) such that $\bar{Y}_{1a} = \bar{Y}_1 - (\bar{X}_1 - X^*)$.

If we consider the case where K treatments are being compared such that $K = 1, 2, \ldots K$, and we let X_{ik} and Y_{ik} represent the predictor and predicted values for each individual i in group k, we can let X_k and Y_k be the means. Then, we define the between-group (or treatment) sum of squares and cross products as

$$T_{xx} = \sum_{k-1}^{K} n_k \ (\bar{X}^k - \bar{X})^2$$

$$T_{yy} = \sum_{k-1}^{K} n_k \ (\bar{Y} - \bar{Y})^2$$

$$T_{xy} = \sum_{k-1}^{K} n_k \ (\bar{X}_k - \bar{X})(\bar{Y}_k - \bar{Y}_k - \bar{Y})$$

In a like manner, within-group sums of squares and cross products are calculated as

$$\Sigma xx = \sum_{k=1}^{k} \ \sum_{i} \ (X_{ik} - X_k)^2$$

$$\Sigma yy = \sum_{k=1}^{k} \ \sum_{i} \ (Y_{ik} - Y_k)^2$$

$$\Sigma xy = \sum_{k=1}^{k} \ \sum_{i} \ (X_{ik} - X_k)(Y_{ik} - Y_k)$$

Where i indicates the sum from all the individuals within each group. f = total number of subjects minus number of groups

$$S_{xx} = T_{xx} + \Sigma_{yy}$$
$$S_{yy} = T_{yy} + \Sigma_{yy}$$
$$S_{xy} = T_{xy} + \Sigma_{xy}$$

With these in hand, we can then calculate the residual mean squares of treatments (St^2) and error (Se^2)

$$St^2 = \frac{(Tyy - \dfrac{S^2xy}{Sxx} + \dfrac{\Sigma^2xy}{\Sigma xx})}{K - 1}$$

$$Se^2 = \frac{(\Sigma yy - \dfrac{\Sigma^2xy}{\Sigma xx})}{F - 1}$$

These can be used to calculate an F statistic to test the null hypothesis that all treatment effects are equal.

$$F = \frac{S^2 t}{S^2 e}$$

The estimated regression coefficient of Y or X is

$$B = \frac{\Sigma xy}{\Sigma xx}$$

The estimated standard error for the adjusted difference between two groups is given by

$$Sd = Se \; \frac{1}{n_0} + \frac{1}{n_1} + \frac{(X_1 - X_0)^2}{\Sigma xx}$$

where n_0 and n_1 are the sample sizes of the two groups. A test of the null hypothesis that the adjusted differences between the groups is zero is provided by

$$t = \frac{Y_1 - Y_0 - B(X_1 - X_0)}{Sd}$$

The test value for the t is then looked up in the t-table with f-1 degrees of freedom.

Computation is markedly simplified if all the groups are of equal size, as demonstrated in Example 20.

EXAMPLE 20

As part of a program to characterize the mechanisms of action and biological effects of an ionophore, the transport across an artificial membrane system was measured for four different cations in the presence of different concentrations of the ionophore. Our interest is the differential ability of the ionophore to facilitate transport of the cations, cation transport is our variate, while the concentration of ionophore (which we cannot directly control) is our covariate.

Our data look like this:

CATION	Ionophores									
	I		II		III		IV		V	
	X	Y	X	Y	X	Y	X	Y	X	Y
Sodium	0.47	1.40	0.57	1.75	0.42	1.34	0.63	1.85	0.55	1.61
Potassium	0.65	5.15	0.43	3.52	0.44	3.55	0.48	3.79	0.59	4.72
Calcium	0.54	10.77	0.64	12.36	0.41	8.31	0.59	11.18	0.53	10.37
Magnesium	0.59	0.27	0.68	0.36	0.53	0.28	0.48	0.22	0.43	0.19

X = Concentration of ionophore
Y = Measured transport factor of ion across membrane

	I		II		III		IV		V	
	X	Y	X	Y	X	Y	X	Y	X	Y
Sums										
(X or Y)	2.25	17.59	2.32	17.99	1.80	13.68	2.18	17.04	2.10	16.89
(X^2 or Y^2)	1.28	144.5	1.38	168.35	0.82	83.53	1.21	142.81	1.12	132.44
XY	9.981		10.666		5.680		9.687		9.248	
n	4		4		4		4		4	
Means	0.562	4.398	0.58	4.498	0.45	3.42	0.545	4.26	0.525	4.222

		X	Y
GRAND TOTAL (X or Y)		10.65	83.19
1. Sum of squares (X^2 or Y^2)		5.81	671.68
2. Sum of squared group totals, divided by sample size	$\dfrac{[^n(X \text{ or } Y)]^2}{n}$	5.7118	348.95608
3. Correction term	$\dfrac{[^{a\,n}(Y \text{ or } X)]^2}{a\,n_i}$	5.6711	346.02881
4. SS total = 1-3		0.1389	325.65119
5. SS groups = 2-3		0.0407	2.92727
6. SS within = 4-5		0.0982	322.72392

ANOVA of the dependent variable:

Sources of variation	df	SS	MS	F
Groups	4	2.92727	0.7318175	0.0340
Within	15	322.72392	21.514928	
Total	19	325.65119		

This preliminary ANOVA is not significant

Analysis of Covariance

For each of the five groups we then compute SS_y, SP_{xy} SS_x, $b_{y.x}$, SS_y, $SS_{y.x}$ and $MS_{y.x}$. This procedure is illustrated below for group I.

$$\sum^n y^2 = \sum^n Y_I^2 - \frac{(\sum^n Y_I)^2}{n_I} = 144.55 - \frac{(17.59)^2}{4} = 67.197975$$

$$\sum^n xy = \sum^n X_I Y_I - \frac{(\sum^n X_I)(\sum^n Y_I)}{n} = 9.981 - \frac{(17.59)(2.25)}{4} = 0.086625$$

$$\sum^n x^2 = \sum^n X_I^2 - \frac{(\sum^n X_I)^2}{n} = 1.28 - \frac{(2.25)^2}{4} = 0.014375$$

$$b_I = \frac{\sum^n xy}{\sum^n x^2} = \frac{0.086625}{0.014375} = 6.026087$$

$$\sum_{y}^{n} n_2 = \frac{(\sum^n xy)^2}{\sum^n x_2} = \frac{(.086625)^2}{0.014375} = 0.5220098$$

$$\sum d^2_{y.x} = \sum^n y^2 - \sum^n \hat{y}^2 = 67.197975 - 0.5220098 = 66.675965$$

$$S^2_{y.x} = \frac{\sum^n d^2 y.x}{(n_1 - 2)} = \frac{66.675965}{2} = 33.337982$$

$$F = \frac{\sum^n \hat{y}^2}{S^2 y.x} = \frac{0.522098}{33.337982} = 0.0156608$$

Such an F ratio is not significant. The F ratios for the other groups are in like manner found to be

$$
\begin{aligned}
\text{Group II} &= 0.0363761 \\
\text{Group III} &= 3.2168555 \\
\text{Group IV} &= 0.2325121 \\
\text{Group V} &= 0.3135638
\end{aligned}
$$

Only the F for group III is significant.

$$\sum y^2 \text{ within} = \sum \sum^n y^2 = 67.197975 + 87.439975 + 36.7444 + 70.2196 + 61.121975 = 322.72393$$

$$\sum xy \text{ within} = \sum \sum^n xy = .086625 + .2318 + .476 + .4002 + .38075 = 1.57375$$

$$Sx^2 \text{ within} = .014375 + .0344 + .01 + .0219 + .0175 = 1.57375$$

$$b \text{ within} = \frac{1.57375}{.098175} = 16.030048$$

$$\sum y^2 \text{ within} = \frac{(1.57375)^2}{.098175} = 25.227289$$

$$\sum d^2 y.x \text{ within} = 322.72393 - 25.227289 = 297.49664$$

$$S^2 y.x \text{ within} = \frac{\sum d^2 y.x \text{ within}}{\sum n - a - 1} = \frac{297.49664}{14} = 21.24976$$

$$F_s = \frac{\sum y^2 \text{ within}}{S^2 y.x \text{ within}} = \frac{25.227289}{21.24976} = 1.1871799$$

This pooled regression is not significant.

$$\sum \sum^n d^2 y.x = 0.5220098 + 85.87802 + 14.0868 + 62.906356 + 52.837943 = 216.23113$$

$\Sigma n - 2a = 20 - 10 = 10$

$$S^2 y.x = \frac{\Sigma \overset{n}{d^2} y.x}{\Sigma n - 2a} = \frac{216.23113}{10} = 21.623113$$

$$\text{SS among bs} = \Sigma^{d^2} y.x \text{ within} - \Sigma \overset{n}{\Sigma} d^2 y.x$$

$$= 297.49664 - 21.623113 = 275.87353$$

$$\text{Ms among bs} = \frac{\text{SS among b's}}{a-1} = \frac{275.87353}{4} = 68.968383$$

$$F = \frac{\text{MS among b's}}{S^2 y.x} = \frac{68.968383}{21.623113} = 3.1895677$$

This is significant at the $p \leq 0.05$ level.

ASSUMPTIONS AND LIMITATIONS

1. The underlying assumptions for ANCOVA are fairly rigid and restrictive.
   The assumptions include:
   a. That the slopes of the regression lines of a Y and X are equal from group to group. This can be examined visually or formally (i.e. by a test). If this condition is not met, ANCOVA cannot be used.
   b. That the relationship between X and Y is linear.
   c. That the covariate X is measured without error. Power of the test declines as error increases.
   d. That there are no unmeasured confounding variables.
   e. That the errors inherent in each variable are independent of each other. Lack of independence effectively (but to an immeasurable degree) reduces sample size.
   f. That the variances of the errors in groups are equivalent between groups.
   g. That the measured data which form the groups are normally distributed. ANCOVA is generally robust to departures from normality.

2. Of the seven assumptions above, the most serious are the first four.

3. ANCOVA is currently not widely used in toxicology because it is computationally cumbersome except with computer programs (and, as shown earlier, ANCOVA is not a common feature in available microcomputer packages).

REFERENCES

Anderson, S., Auquier, A., Hauck, W.W., Oakes, D., Vandaele, W. and Weisberg, H.I. (1980): *Statistical Methods for Comparative Studies*. John Wiley & Sons, New York.

Beyer, W.H. (1976): *Handbook of Tables for Probability and Statistics*, pp. 269–378, 409–413. Chemical Rubber co., Boca Raton.

Cochran, W.G., and Cox, G.M. (1975): *Experimental Designs*, pp. 100–102. John Wiley, New York.

Diem, K., and Lentner, C. (1975): *Documenta Geigy Scientific Tables*, pp. 158–159. Geigy, New York.

Duncan, D.B. (1955): Multiple range and multiple F tests. *Biome.*, 11:1–42.

Dunnett, C.W. (1955): A multiple comparison procedure for comparing several treatments with a control. *J. Am. Stat. Assoc.*, 50:1096–1121.

Dunnett, C.W. (1964): New tables for multiple comparison with a control. *Biomet.*, 20:482–492.

Harris, R.J. (1975): *A Primer of Multivariate Statistics*, pp. 96–101. Academic Press, New York.

Harter, A.L. (1960): Critical values for Duncan's new multiple range test. *Biomet.*, 16:671–685.

Kotz, S. And Johnson, N.L., (1982): *Encyclopedia of Statistical Sciences, Vol I.* p. 61–69 John Wiley & Sons, Inc., New York.

Scheffe, H. (1959): *The Analysis of Variance*. Wiley, New York.

Snedecor, G.W. and Cochran, W.G. (1980): *Statistical Methods*, Seventh edition, Iowa State University Press, Ames.

Sokal, R.R., and Rohlf, F.J. (1981): *Biometry*. W.H. Freeman, San Francisco.

Williams, D.A. (1971): A test for differences between treatment means when several dose levels are compared with a zero dose control. *Biomet.*, 27:103–117.

Williams, D.A. (1972): The comparison of several dose levels with a zero dose control. *Biomet.*, 28:519–531.

Zar, J.H. (1974): *Biostatistical Analysis*, p. 50. Prentice-Hall, Englewood.

CHAPTER 8

MODELING

The mathematical modeling of biological systems, restricted even to the field of toxicology, is an extremely large and vigorously growing area. Broadly speaking, modeling is the principal conceptual tool by which toxicology seeks to develop as a mechanistic science. In an iterative process, models are developed or proposed, tested by experiment, reformulated and so on in a continuous cycle. Such a cycle could also be described as two related types of modeling - explanatory (where the concept is formed) and correlative (where data are organized and relationships derived). The outcomes of the cycle are predictions (with cautious extrapolation beyond the range of existing data) and inferences (about analogous situations which are difficult or impossible to measure directly, such as risk of carcingogenesis at extremely low levels of exposure to a material). It is the special area of these last two (prediction and inference) that will be addressed here. An excellent introduction to the broader field of modeling of biological systems can be found in Gold (Gold, 1977).

In toxicology, modeling is of prime interest in seeking to relate a treatment variable with an effect variable and, from the resulting model, predict effects at exact points where no experiment has been done (but in the range where we have performed experiments, such as "determining" LD_{50}'s), to estimate how good our prediction is, and occasionally, simply to determine if a pattern of effect is related to a pattern of treatment. Methods are presented for all three of these objectives under each of several conditions.

For use in prediction, the techniques of linear regression, probit/logit analysis (a special case of linear regression), moving averages (an efficient approximation method), and nonlinear regression (for doses where data cannot be made to fit a linear pattern) are presented. For evaluating the predictive value of these models, both the correlation coefficient (for parametric data) and Kendall's rank correlation (for nonparametric data) are given. And finally, the concept of trend analysis is introduced and a method presented.

Not included here are methods for modeling when there are three or more variables. Rather, two of these methods (discriminant analysis and multiple regression) and a related method (canonical correlation analysis) are discussed in the later chapter on multivariate methods.

When we are trying to establish a pattern between several data points (whether this pattern is in the form of a line or a curve), what we are doing is interpolating. It is possible for any given set of points to produce an infinite set of lines or curves which pass near (for lines) or through (for curves) the data points. In most cases, we cannot actually know the "real" pattern. So we apply a basic principle of science - Occam's razor. We use the simplest explanation (or, in this case, model) which fits the facts (or data). A line is, of course, the simplest pattern to deal with and describe, so fitting the best line (linear regression) is the most common form of modeling in toxicology.

Linear Regression

Foremost among the methods for interpolating within a known data relationship is regression—the fitting of a line or curve to a set of known data points on a graph, and the interpolation ("estimation") of this line or curve in areas where we have no data points. The simplest of these regression models is that of linear regression (valid when increasing the value of one variable changes the value of the related variable in a linear fashion, either postively or negatively). This is the case we will explore here, using the method of least squares.

Given that we have two sets of variables, x (say mg/kg of test material administered) and y (say percentage of animals so dosed that die), what is required is solving for a and b in the equation $Y_i = a + bx_i$ [where the uppercase Y_i is the fitted value of y_i at x_i, and we wish to minimize $(y_i - Y_i)^2$]. So we solve the equations

$$b = \frac{\Sigma x_1 y_1 - n \overline{x}\,\overline{y}}{\Sigma x_1^2 - n \overline{x}^2}$$

$$\text{and } a = \overline{y} - b\overline{x}$$

Where a is the x intercept, b is the slope of the time and n is the number of data points. Use of this is demonstrated in Example 21.

Note that in actuality, dose-response relationships are often not linear and instead we must use either a transform (to linearize the data) or a nonlinear regression method (a good discussion of which may be found in Gallant, 1975 and later in this chapter).

Note also that we can use the correlation test statistic (to be described in the correlation coefficient section) to determine if the regression is significant (and, therefore, valid at a defined level of certainty. A more specific test for significance would be the linear regression analysis of variance (Pollard, 1977). To do so we start by developing the appropriate ANOVA table, as demonstrated in Example 21.

EXAMPLE 21

From a short-term toxicity study we have the following results

Dose administered (mg/kg) x_1	x_1^2	% Animals dead y^1	x_1y_1
1	1	10	10
3	9	20	60
4	16	18	72
5	25	20	100
Sums $x_1 = 13$	$x_1^2 = 51$	$y_1 = 68$	$x_1y_1 = 242$

$\bar{x} = 3.25 \qquad \bar{y} = 17$

$$b = \frac{242 - (4)(3.25)(17)}{51 - (4)(10.5625)} = \frac{21}{8.75} 2.40$$

$a = 17 - (2.4)(3.25) = 9.20$

We therefore see that our fitted line is $Y = 9.2 + 2.4x$.

These ANOVA table data are then used as shown in Example 22.

TABLE 4. Linear regression analysis of variance.

Source of variation (1)	Sum of squares (2)	Degrees of freedom (3)	Mean square (4) $\left(\text{equal to } \frac{(2)}{(3)}\right)$
Regression	$b_1^2(\Sigma x_1^2 - n\bar{x}^2)$	1	By division
Residual	By difference	$n - 2$	By division
Total	$\Sigma y_1^2 - n\bar{y}^2$	$n - 1$	

We then calculate $F_{1,n-2} = \dfrac{\text{regression mean square}}{\text{residual mean square}}$

EXAMPLE 22

We desire to test the significance of the regression line in Example 21.

$\Sigma y_1^2 = 10^2 + 20^2 + 18^2 + 20^2 = 1224$

regression $SS = (2.4)^2 [51 - 4(3.25)^2] = 50.4$

$$\text{total } SS = 1224 - 4(17^2) = 68.0$$
$$\text{residual } SS = 68.0 - 50.4 = 17.6$$
$$\text{and } F_{1,2} = 50.4/8.8 = 5.73$$

This value is not significant at the 0.05 level; therefore, the regression is not significant. A significant F value (as found in an F distribution table for the appropriate degrees of freedom) indicates that the regression line is an accurate prediction of observed values at that confidence level. Note that the portion of the total sum of squares explained by the regression is called the coefficient of determination, denoted by R^2 (the square of the coefficient of correlation, which in the above example is equal to 0.86^2 or 0.74). Calculation of the correlation coefficient is described later in this chapter.

Finally, we might wish to determine the confidence intervals for our regression line—that is, given a regression line with calculated values for Y_i given x_i, within what limits may we be certain (with say a 95% probability) what the real value of Y_i is?

If we denote the residual mean square in the ANOVA by s^2, the 95% confidence limits for a (denoted by A, the notation for the true—as opposed to estimated—value for this parameter) are calculated as [3]:

$$t_n\text{-}2 = \frac{a-A}{\sqrt{\dfrac{s^2(\Sigma x^2)}{n\Sigma x_1^2 - n^2 \bar{x}^2}}}$$

$$\frac{9.2-A}{\sqrt{\dfrac{8.8(51)}{4(51)-(16)(10.562)}}} = \frac{9.2-A}{\sqrt{\dfrac{448.8}{35.006}}}$$

$$= \frac{9.2-A}{3.58} = \pm 4.303$$

$$9.2 - A = \pm 15.405$$
$$A = 9.2 \pm 15.405$$

ASSUMPTIONS AND LIMITATIONS

1. All the regression methods are for interpolation, not extrapolation. That is, they are valid only in the range that we have data - not beyond.
2. The method assumes that the data are normally distributed, and is sensitive to outliers. The x-axis (or horizontal) compo-

nent plays an extremely important part in developing the least square fit. All points have equal weight in determining the height of a regression line, but extreme x-axis values unduly influence the slope of the line.

3. A good fit between a line and a set of data (that is, a strong correlation between treatment and response variables) does not imply any casual relationship.

4. It is assumed that the treatment variable can be measured without error, that each data point is independent, that variances are equivalent, and that a linear relationship does exist between the variables.

5. There are many excellent texts on regression, which is a powerful technique. These include Draper and Smith (1981) and Montgomery and Peck (1982), which are not overly rigorous mathematically.

Probit/Log Transforms and Regression

As we noted in the preceding section, dose-response problems (among the most common interpolation problems encountered in toxicology) rarely are straightforward enough to make a valid linear regression directly from the raw data. The most common valid interpolation methods are based upon probability ("probit") and logarithmic ("log") value scales, with percentage responses (death, tumor incidence, etc.) being expressed on the probit scale while doses (Y_i) are expressed on the log scale. There are two strategies for such an approach. The first is based on transforming the data to these scales, then doing a weighted linear regression on the transformed data (if one does not have access to a computer or a high-powered programmable calculator, the only practical strategy is not to assign weights). The second requires the use of algorithms (approximate calculation techniques) for the probit value and regression process, and is extremely burdensome to perform manually.

Our approach to the first strategy requires that we construct a table with the pairs of values of x_i and y_i listed in order of increasing values of Y_i (percentage response). Beside each of these columns a set of blank columns should be left so that the transformed values may be listed. We then simply add the columns described in the linear regression procedure. Log and probit values may be taken from any of a number of sets of tables (such as provided in Appendix 1) and the rest of the table is then developed from these transformed x'_i and

[3]With t_{n-2} being taken from a table of the upper and lower $2\frac{1}{2}\%$ points of the t distribution

y'i values (denoted as x'_i and y'_i). A standard linear regression is then performed (see example 23).

The second strategy we discussed has been broached by a number of authors (Bliss, 1935; Finney, 1977; Litchfield and Wilcoxon, 1949; Prentice, 1976). All of these methods however, are computationally cumbersome. It is possible to approximate the necessary iterative process using the algorithms developed by Abramowitz and Stegun (1964) but even this merely reduces the complexity to a point where the procedure may be readily programmed on a small computer or programmable calculator.

EXAMPLE 23

Percentage of animals killed x_1	Probit of $x_1 =$	Done of chemical (mg/kg) y_1	Log of $y_1 =$		
	x'_1		y'_1	$(x'_1$F	$x'_1 y'_1$
2	2.9463	3	0.4771	8.6806	1.40567
10	3.7184	5	0.6990	13.8264	2.59916
42	4.7981	10	1.0000	23.0217	4.79810
90	6.2816	20	1.3010	39.45724	8.17223
98	7.0537	30	1.4771	49.75468	10.4190
	$\Sigma x_1 = 24.7981$		$\Sigma y'_1 = 4.9542$	$\Sigma x'_1{}^3 = 134.7461$	$\Sigma x'_1 y'_1 = 27.39416$

Our interpolated log of the LD_{50} (calculated by using $Y = -0.200591 - 0.240226\ x$ where x equals 5.000 — the probit of 50% — in the regression equation) is 1.000539. When we convert this log value to its linear equivalent, we get an LD_{50} of 10.0 mg/kg.

Finally, our calculated correlation coefficient is $r = 0.997$. A goodness-of-fit of the data using chi square may also be calculated.

ASSUMPTIONS AND LIMITATIONS

1. The probit distribution is derived from a common error function, with the mid point (50% point) moved to a score of 5.00.
2. The underlying frequency distribution becomes asymptotic as it approaches the extremes of the range. That is, in the range of 16 to 84%, the corresponding probit values change gradually - the curve is relatively linear. But beyond this range, they change ever more rapidly as they approach either 0% or 100%. In fact, there are no values for either of these numbers.
3. A normally distributed population is assumed, and the results are sensitive to outliers.

Moving Averages

An obvious drawback to the interpolation procedures we have examined to date is that they do take a significant amount of time (though they are simple enough to be done manually), especially if the only result we desire is an LD_{50} or LC_{50}, or LT_{50}.

The method of moving averages (Thompson and Weil, 1952; Weil, 1952) gives a rapid and reasonably accurate estimate of this "median-effective dose" (m) and the estimated standard deviation of its logarithm.

Such methodology requires that the same number of animals be used per dosage level and that the spacing between successive dosage exposure levels be geometrically constant (i.e., levels of 1,2,4, and 8 mg/kg or 1,3,9, and 27 ppm). Given this and access to a table for the computation of moving averages (such as found in Appendix 1) one can readily calculate the median effective dose with the formula (illustrated for dose):

$$\log m = \log D + d(K - 1)/2 + \sigma f$$

where m = median effective dose or exposure
   D = the lowest dose tested
   d = the log of the ratio of successive doses/exposures
   and f = a table value taken from Weil for the proper K (the total number of levels tested minus 1).

Included in Appendix 1 are a complete set of tables covering the full range of possibilities at Ns up to 10 (where N is the number of animals per dosage level). Also included are simplified formulas and calculated values useful if the factor between dosage levels is 2.0 (the logarithm of which is 0.30103 = d in this case).

Example 24 demonstrates the use of this method and the new tables.

EXAMPLE 24

As part of an inhalation study we exposed groups of 5 rats each to levels of 20, 40, 80 and 160 ppm of a chemical vapor. These exposures killed 0, 1, 3, and 5 animals, respectively. From the N = 5, K = 3 tables on the r value 0,1,3,5 line we get an f of 0.7 and an σf[4] of 0.31623. We can then calculate the LC_{50} to be:

$\log LC_{50} = 1.30130 + 0.30103(2)/2 + 0.30103(0.7)$
   $= 1.30103 + 0.51175$
   $= 1.81278$
$\therefore LC_{50} = 65.0$ ppm with 95% confidence intervals
   of $\pm 2.179\, d\sigma f$ or $\pm 2.179\,(0.30103)\,(0.31623)$
   $= \pm 0.20743$

Therefore, the log confidence limits are 1.81278
±0.20743 = 1.60535 to 2.02021; on the linear scale
= 40.3 to 104.8 ppm.

ASSUMPTIONS AND LIMITATIONS

> 1. A common misconception is that the moving average method cannot be used to determine the slope of the reponse curve. This is not true - Weil has published a straightforward method for determining slope in conjunction with a moving average determination of the LD_{50} (Weil, 1983).
> 2. The method also provides confidence intervals.

Nonlinear Regression

More often than not in toxicology (and, in fact, in the biological sciences in general) we find that our data demonstrate a relationship between two variables (such as age and body weight) which is not linear. That is, a change in one variable (say age) does not produce a directly proportional change in the other (e.g. body weight). But some form of relationship between the variables is apparent. If understanding such a relationship and being able to predict unknown points from a limited set of measured data points is of value, we have a pair of options available to us. The first, which was discussed and reviewed earlier, is to use one or more transformations to linearize our data and then to make use of linear regression. This approach, though most commonly used, has a number of drawbacks. Not all data can be suitably transformed; sometimes the transformations necessary to linearize the data require a cumbersome series of calculations; and the resulting linear regression is not always sufficient to account for the differences among sample values—there are significant deviations around the linear regression line (that is, a line may still not give us a good fit to the data or do an adequate job of representing the relationships between the data). In such cases, we have available a second option - the fitting of data to some nonlinear function such as some form of curve. This is, in the general form, nonlinear regression and may involve fitting data to an infinite number of possible functions. But most often we are interested in fitting curves to a polynomial function of the general form.

$$Y = a + bx + cx^2 + dx^3 + \ldots$$

where x is the independent variable. As the number of powers of x increases, the curve becomes increasingly complex and will be able to fit a given set of data increasingly well.

Generally in toxicology, however, if we plot the log of a response (such as body weight) versus a linear scale of our dose or stimulus, we get one of four types of nonlinear curves. These are (Snedecor and Cochran, 1980):

(1) Exponential growth, where
$\log Y = A(B^x)$, such as the growth curve for the log phase of a bacterial culture.
(2) Exponential decay, where
$\log Y = A(B^{-x})$, such as a radioactive decay curve
(3) Asymptotic regression, where
$\log Y = A - B(p^x)$, such as a first order reaction curve
(4) Logistic growth curve, where
$\log Y = A/(1 + Bp^x)$, such as a population growth curve.

In all these cases, A and B are constants while p is a log transform. These curves are illustrated in Figure 7.

FIGURE 7
COMMON CURVILINEAR CURVES

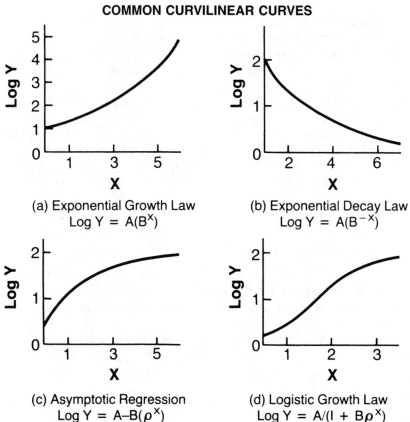

(a) Exponential Growth Law
$\log Y = A(B^x)$

(b) Exponential Decay Law
$\log Y = A(B^{-x})$

(c) Asymptotic Regression
$\log Y = A - B(\rho^x)$

(d) Logistic Growth Law
$\log Y = A/(1 + B\rho^x)$

All four types of curves are fit by iterative processes—that is, best guess numbers are initially chosen for each of the constants and, after a fit is attempted, the constants are modified to improve the fit. This process is repeated until an acceptable fit has been generated. Analysis of variance or covariance can be used to objectively evaluate the acceptability of the fit. Needless to say, the use of a computer generally accelerates such a curve-fitting process.

ASSUMPTIONS AND LIMITATIONS

1. The principle of using least squares may still be applicable in fitting the best curve, if the assumptions of normality, independence, and reasonably error-free measurement of response are valid.
2. Growth curves are best modeled using a nonlinear method.

Correlation Coefficient

The correlation coefficient procedure is used to determine the degree of linear correlation (direct relationship) between two groups of continuous (and normally distributed) variables; it will indicate whether there is any statistical relationship between the variables in the two groups. For example, we may wish to determine if the liver weights of dogs on a feeding study are correlated with their body weights. Thus, we will record the body and liver weights at the time of sacrifice and then calculate the correlation coefficient between these pairs of values to determine if there is some relationship.

A formula for calculating the linear correlation coefficient (r_{xy}) is as follows:

$$ r_{xy} = \frac{N\Sigma XY - (\Sigma X)(\Sigma Y)}{\sqrt{N\Sigma X^2 - (\Sigma X)^2} \ \sqrt{N\Sigma Y^2 - (\Sigma Y)^2}} $$

where X is each value for one variable (such as the dog body weights in the above example), Y is the matching value for the second variable (the liver weights), and N is the number of pairs of X and Y. Once we have obtained r_{xy} it is possible to calculate t_r, which can be used for more precise examination of the degree of significant linear relationship between the two groups. This value is calculated as follows:

$$ t_r = \frac{r_{zy}\sqrt{N-2}}{\sqrt{1 - r_{zy}^2}} $$

This calculation is also equivalent to r = sample covariance/ (S_x S_y), as was seen earlier under ANCOVA.

The value obtained for r_{xy} can be compared to table values [such as Snedecor and Cochran, 1980, p. 477] for the number of pairs of data involved minus two. If the r_{xy} is smaller (at the selected test probability level, such as 0.05), the correlation is not significantly different from zero (no correlation). If r_{xy} is larger than the table value, there is a positive statistical relationship between the groups. Comparisons are then made at lower levels of probability to determine the degree of relationship (note that if r_{xy} = either 1.0 or -1.0, there is complete correlation between the groups). If r_{xy} is a negative number and the absolute value is greater than the table value, there is an inverse relationship between the groups; that is, a change in one group is associated with a change in the opposite direction in the second group of variables. Both computations are demonstrated in Example 25.

Since the comparison of r_{xy} with the table values may be considered a somewhat weak test, it is perhaps more meaningful to compare the t_r value with values in a t-distribution table for N-2 degrees of freedom (df), as is done for the Student's t-test. This will give a more exact determination of the degree of statistical correlation between the two groups.

It should be noted that this method examines only possible linear relationships between sets of continuous, normally distributed data. Other mathematical relationships (log, log/linear, exponential, etc.) between data sets exist which require either the use of another correlation testing method or that one or more of the data sets be transformed so that they are of linear nature. This second approach requires, of course, that one know the nature of the data so that an appropriate transform may be used. Some few transforms were discussed earlier in the sections on linear regression and probit/log analysis.

EXAMPLE 25

If we computed the dog body weight versus dog liver weight for a study we could have the following results:

Dog #	Body weight (kgj) X	X^2	Liver weight (g) Y	Y^2	XY
1	8.4	70.56	243	59049	2041.2
2	8.5	72.25	225	50625	1912.5
3	9.3	86.49	241	58081	2241.3
4	9.5	90.25	263	69169	2498.5
5	10.5	110.25	256	65536	2688.0
6	8.6	73.96	266	70756	2287.6
Sums	$\Sigma X = 54.8$	$\Sigma X^2 = 503.76$	$\Sigma Y = 1494$	$\Sigma Y^2 = 373216$	$\Sigma XY = 13669.1$

$$r_{xy} = \frac{6(13669.1)}{\sqrt{6(503.76)-(54.8)^2}} \quad - \quad \frac{(54.8)(1494)}{\sqrt{6(373216)-(1494)^2}}$$

$$= 0.381$$

The table value for six pairs of data (read beside the N - 2 value, or 6 - 2 = 4) is 0.811 at a 0.05 probability level. Thus, there is a lack of statistical correlation (at $p = 0.05$) between the body weights and liver weights for this group of dogs.

The t_r value for these data would be calculated as follows:

$$t_r = \frac{0.381 \sqrt{6-2}}{\sqrt{1-(0.381)^2}} = 0.824$$

The value for the t-distribution table for four df at the 0.05 level is 2.776; therefore, this again suggests a lack of significant correlation at $p = 0.05$.

ASSUMPTION AND LIMITATIONS

1. A strong correlation does not imply that a treatment causes an effect.
2. The distances of data points from the regression line are the portions of the data not "explained" by the model. These are called residuals. Poor correlation coefficents imply high residuals, which may be due to many small contributions (variations of data from the regression line) or a few large ones. Extreme values (outliers) greatly reduce correlation.
3. X and Y are assumed to be independent.
4. Feinstein (1979) has provided a fine discussion of the difference between correlation (or association of variables) and causation.

Kendall's Coefficient of Rank Correlation

Kendall's rank correlation, represented by t (tau), should be used to evaluate the degree of association between two sets of data when the nature of the data is such that the relationship may not be linear. Most commonly, this is when the data are not continuous and/or normally distributed. An example of such a case is when we are trying to determine if there is a relationship between length of hydra and their survival time in a test medium in hours, as is presented in Example 26. Both of our variables here are discontinuous, yet we suspect a relationship exists. Another common use is in comparing the subjective scoring done by two different observers.

Tau is calculated as $t = N/n(n - 1)$ where n is the sample size and

N is the count of ranks, calculated as $N = 4 \, (^n C_i)-n(n-1)$, with the computing of $^n C_i$ being demonstrated in the example.

If a second variable Y_2 is exactly correlated with the first variable Y_1, then the variates Y_2 should be in the same order as the Y_1-variates. However, if the correlation is less than exact, the order of the variates Y_2 will not correspond entirely to that of Y. The quantity N measures how well the second variable corresponds to the order of the first. It has a maximum value of $n(n-1)$ and a minimum value of $-n(n-1)$.

A table of data is set up with each of the two variables being ranked separately. Tied ranks are assigned as demonstrated earlier under the Kruskall Wallis test. From this point, disregard the original variates and deal only with the ranks. Place the ranks of one of the two variables in rank order (from lowest to highest), paired with the rank values assigned for the other variable. If one (but not the other) variable has tied ranks, order the pairs by the variable without ties (Sokal and Rohlf, 1981, p. 601–607).

The most common way to compute a sum of the counts is also demonstrated in Example 26.

The resulting value of tau will range from -1 to +1, as does the familiar parametric correlation coefficient, r.

EXAMPLE 26

During the validation of an *in vitro* method, it was noticed that larger hydra seem to survive longer in test media than do small individuals. To evaluate this, 15 hydra of random size were measured (mm), then placed in test media. How many hours each individual survives was recorded over a 24 hr. period. These data are presented below, along with ranks for each variable.

Length	Rank(R_1)	Survival	Rank(R_2)
3	6.5	19	9
4	10	17	7
6	15	11	1
1	1.5	25	15
3	6.5	18	8
3	6.5	22	6
1	1.5	24	14
4	10	16	12
4	10	15	5
2	3.5	21	11
5	13	13	3
5	13	14	4
3	6.5	20	10
2	3.5	23	13
5	13	12	2

We then arrange this based on the order of the rank of survival time, (there are no ties here). We then calculate our count of ranks. The conventional method is to obtain a sum of the counts C_i, as follows; examine the first value in the column of ranks paired with the ordered column. In the case below, this is rank 15. Count all ranks subsequent to it that are higher than the rank being considered. Thus, in this case, count all ranks greater than 15. There are 14 ranks following the 2 and all of them are less than 15. Therefore, we count a score of $C_1 = 0$. We repeat this process for each subsequent rank of R_1, giving us a final score of 1 (By this point it is obvious that our original hypothesis - that larger hydrae live longer in test media than do small individuals - was in error).

R_2	R_1	Following (R_2) ranks greater than (R_1)	Counts (C_i)
1	15	------	$C_1 = 0$
2	13	------	$C_2 = 0$
3	13	------	$C_3 = 0$
4	13	------	$C_4 = 0$
5	10	------	$C_5 = 0$
6	6.5	10	$C_6 = 1$
7	10	------	$C_7 = 0$
8	6.5	------	$C_8 = 0$
9	6.5	------	$C_9 = 0$
10	6.5	------	$C_{10} = 0$
11	3.5	10	$C_{11} = 1$
12	6.5	------	$C_{12} = 0$
13	3.5	------	$C_{13} = 0$
14	1.5	------	$C_{14} = 0$
15	1.5	------	$C_{15} = 0$
			$\overset{M}{C_i} = 2$

Our count of ranks, N, is then calculated as

$$N = 4(2) - 15(15 - 1)$$
$$= 8 - 15(14)$$
$$= -202$$

We can then calculate tau as

$$= \frac{-202}{15(15 - 1)}$$
$$= \frac{-202}{210}$$

$$= -0.9619$$

In other words, there is a strong negative correlation between our variables.

ASSUMPTIONS AND LIMITATIONS

---

1. A very robust estimator which does not assume normality, linearity, or minimal error of measurement.

Trend Analysis

A variation on the theme of regression testing which has gained popularity in toxicology over the last ten years is trend analysis. In the broadest sense, this is used to determine whether a sequence of observations taken over a period of time (say the cumulative proportions of groups of animals which have tumors of a particular sort) exhibits some sort of pattern of change—either an increase (an upward trend) or a decrease (a downward trend) associated with dosage. There are a number of tests which can be used to evaluate data to determine if a trend exists. The most popular in toxicology is currently that presented by Tarone in 1975 because it is that used by the National Cancer Institute in the analysis of carcinogenicity data. A simple, but efficient alternative is the Cox and Stuart test (Cox and Stuart, 1955) which is a modification of the sign test. For each point at which we have a measure (such as the incidence of animals observed with tumors) we form a pair of observations - one from each of the groups we wish to compare. In a traditional NCI bioassay this would mean pairing control with low dose and low dose with high dose (to explore a dose-related trend) or each time period observation in a dose group (except the first) with its predecessor (to evaluate time-related trend). When the second observation in a pair exceeds the earlier observation, we record a plus sign for that pair. When the first observation is greater than the second, we record a minus sign for that pair. A preponderance of plus signs suggests a downward trend while an excess of minus signs suggests an upward trend. A formal test at a preselected confidence level can then be performed.

More formally put, after having defined what trend we want to test for, we first match pairs as $(X_1 + X_{1+c})$, (X_2, X_{2+c}), ... $(X_{n' - c}, X_{n'})$ where $c = n'/2$ when n' is even and $c = (n' + 1)/2$ when n' is odd (where n' is the number of observations in a set). The hypothesis is then tested by comparing the resulting number of excess positive or negative signs against a sign test table such as are found in Beyer.

We can, of course, combine a number of observations to allow ourselves to actively test for a set of trends, such as the existence of a trend of increasing difference between two groups of animals over a period of time. This is demonstrated in Example 27.

EXAMPLE 27

In a chronic feeding study in rats, we tested the hypothesis that, in the second year of the study, there was a dose responsive increase in tumor incidence associated with the test compound. We utilize, below, a Cox-Stuart test for trend to address this question. All groups start the second year with an equal number of animals.

Month of Study	Control		Low Doses			High Doses		
	Total X Animals with Tumors	Change $[X_{A-B}]$	Total Y Animals with Tumors	Change $[Y_{A-B}]$	Compared to Control $(Y-X)$	Total Z Animals with Tumors	Change $[Z_{A-B}]$	Compared to Control $(Z-X)$
12 (A)	1	NA	0	NA	NA	5	NA	NA
13 (B)	1	0	0	0	0	7	2	(+)2
14 (C)	3	2	1	1	(-)1	11	4	(+)2
15 (D)	3	0	1	0	0	11	0	0
16 (E)	4	1	1	0	(-)1	13	2	(+)1
17 (F)	5	1	3	2	(+)1	14	1	0
18 (G)	5	0	3	0	0	15	1	(+)1
19 (H)	5	0	5	2	(+)2	18	3	(+)3
20 (I)	6	1	6	1	0	19	1	0
21 (J)	8	2	7	1	(-)1	22	3	(+)1
22 (K)	12	4	9	2	(-)2	26	4	0
23 (L)	14	2	12	3	(+)1	28	2	0
24 (M)	18	4	17	5	(+)1	31	3	(-)1
			Sum of signs $Y-X$		4+ 4- =0 (No trend)	Sum of signs $Z-X$		6+ 1- =5

Reference to a sign table is not necessary for the low dose comparison (where there is no trend) but clearly shows the high dose to be significant at the $p \leq 0.05$ level.

ASSUMPTIONS AND LIMITATIONS

1. Trend tests seek to evaluate whether there is a monotonic tendency in response to a change in treatment. That is, the dose response direction is absolute - as dose goes up; the incidence of tumors increases. Thus the test loses power rapidly in response to the occurrences of "reversals" - for example, a low dose group with a decreased tumor incidence. There are methods (such as those of Dykstra and Robertson, 1983) which "smooth the bumps" of reversals in long data series. In toxicology, however, most data series are short (that is, there are only a few dose levels).

REFERENCES

Abramowitz, M., and Stegun, I.A. (1964): *Handbook of Mathematical Functions,* pp. 925–964. National Bureau of Standards, Washington.

Beyer, W.H. (1976): *Handbook of Tables for Probability and Statistics,* Chemical Rubber Co., Boca Raton.

Bliss, C.I. (1935): The calculation of the dosage-mortality curve. *Ann. Appl. Biol.,* 22:134–167.

Cox, D.R. and Stuart, A. (1955): Some Quick Tests for Trend in Location and Dispersion. *Biomet.,* 42:80–95.

Draper, N.R. and Smith, H. (1981): *Applied Regression Analysis,* John Wiley, New York.

Dykstra, R.L. and Robertson, T. (1983): On Testing Monotone Tendencies, *J. Amer. Stat. Assoc.,* 78: 342–350.

Feinstein, A.R. (1979): Scientific standards vs. statistical associations and biological logic in the analysis of causation, *Clin Pharmacol Therapeu.,* 25: 481–492.

Finney, D.K. (1977): *Probit Analysis,* third ed. Cambridge University Press, Cambridge.

Gallant, A.R. (1975): Nonlinear regression. *Am. Stat.,* 29:73–81.

Gold, H.J. (1977): *Mathematical Modeling of Biological Systems - An Introductory Guidebook,* John Wiley, New York.

Litchfield, J.T. and Wilcoxon, F. (1949): A simplified method of evaluating dose effect experiments. *J. Pharmacol. Exp. Ther.,* 96:99–113.

Montgomery, D.C. and Smith, E.A. (1983): *Introduction to Linear Regression Analysis.* John Wiley, New York.

Pollard, J.H. (1977): *Numerical and Statistical Techniques.* Cambridge University Press, New York.

Prentice, R.L. (1976): A generalization of the probit and logit methods for dose response curves. *Biomet.,* 32:761–768.

Snedecor, G.W. and Cochran, W.G. (1980): *Statistical Methods,* Seventh ed. Iowa State University Press, Ames.

Sokal, R.R., and Rohlf, F.J. (1981): *Biometry.* W.H. Freeman, San Francisco.

Tarone, R.E. (1975): Tests for trend in life table analysis. *Biometrika,* 62: 679–682.

Thompson, W.R., and Weil, C.S. (1952): On the construction of tables for moving average interpolation. *Biomet.,* 8:51–54.

Weil, C.S. (1952): Tables for convenient calculation of median-effective dose (LD_{50} or ED_{50}) and instructions in their use. *Biomet.*, 8: 249–263.

Weil, C.S. (1983): Economical LD_{50} and Slope Determinations. *Drug Chem. Toxicol.*, 6:595–603.

CHAPTER 9

METHODS FOR THE REDUCTION OF DIMENSIONALITY

Techniques for the reduction of dimensionality are those that simplify the understanding of data, either visually or numerically, while causing only minimal reductions in the amount of information present. These techniques operate primarily by pooling or combining groups of variables into single variables, but may also entail the identification and elimination of low-information-content (or irrelevant) variables.

In an early chapter we presented the descriptive statistics (calculations of means, standard deviations, etc.) which are the simplest and most familiar form of reduction of dimensionality. The first topic we will address in this chapter is classification, which provides the general conceptual tools for identifying and quantifying similarities and differences between groups of things which have more than a single linear scale of measurement in common (for example, which have both been determined to have or lack a number of enzyme activities).

Two common methodology sets will then be presented and reviewed. Both, table preparation and statistical graphics, are familiar activities for most toxicologists, but are much misused. Guidelines for the proper preparation of tables and graphs are presented, along with some of the more recent improvements in presentation techniques that are available. Both tables and graphs can address two objectives, presentation (communication of information) and analysis.

We will then move on to two collections of methodologies which combine graphic and computational methods, multidimensional/nonmetric scaling and cluster analysis. Multidimensional scaling (MDS) is a set of techniques for quantitatively analyzing similarities, dissimilarities and distances between data in a display-like manner. Nonmetric scaling is an analogous set of methods for displaying and relating data when measurements are non-quantative (the data are described by attributes or ranks). Cluster analysis is a collection of graphic and numerical methodologies for classifying things based on the relationships between the values of the variables that they share.

The final pair of methods for reduction of dimensionality which will be tackled in this chapter are Fourier analysis and life table analysis. Fourier analysis seeks to identify cyclic patterns in data and then either analyze the patterns or the residuals after the patterns are taken out. Life table analysis techniques are directed to identifying and quantitating the time course of risks (such as death, or the occurrence of tumors).

Three purely multivariate techniques for the reduction of dimensionality (principal components analysis, factor analysis and canonical correlation analysis) are discussed in a later chapter on multivariate analysis.

Classification

Classification is both a basic concept and a collection of techniques which are necessary prerequisites for further analysis of data when the members of a set of data are (or can be) each described by several variables. At least some degree of classification (which is broadly defined as the dividing of the members of a group into smaller groups in accordance with a set of decision rules) is necessary prior to any data collection. Whether formally or informally, an investigator has to decide which things are similar enough to be counted as the same and develop rules governing collection procedures. Such rules can be as simple as "measure and record body weights only of live animals on study", or as complex as that demonstrated by the expanded weighting classification presented in example 28. Such a classification also demonstrates that the selection of which variables to measure will determine the final classification of data.

EXAMPLE 28

I.	Is animal of desired species?	Yes/No
II.	Is animal member of study group?	Yes/No
III.	Is animal alive?	Yes/No
IV.	Which group does animal belong to?	
	A. Control	
	B. Low Dose	
	C. Intermediate Dose	
	D. High Dose	
V.	What sex is animal?	Male/Female
VI.	Is the measured weight in acceptable range?	Yes/No

Classifications of data have two purposes (Hartigan, 1983; Gordon, 1981); data simplification (also called a descriptive function) and prediction. Simplification is necessary because there is a limit to both the volume and complexity of data that the human mind can comprehend and deal with conceptually. Classification allows us to attach a label (or name) to each group of data, to summarize the data (that is, assign individual elements of data to groups and to characterize the population of the group), and to define the relationships between groups (that is, develop a taxonomy).

Prediction, meanwhile, is the use of summaries of data and knowledge of the relationships between groups to develop hypotheses as to what will happen when further data are collected (as when more animals or people are exposed to an agent under defined conditions) and as to the mechanisms which cause such relationships to develop. Indeed, classification is the prime device for the discovery of mechanisms in all of science. A classic example of this was Darwin's realization that there were reasons (the mechanisms of evolution) behind the differences and similarities in species which had caused Linnaeus to earlier develop his initial modern classification scheme (or taxonomy) for animals.

To develop a classification, one first sets bounds wide enough to encompass the entire range of data to be considered but not unnecessarily wide. This is typically done by selecting some global variables (variables every piece of data have in common) and limiting the range of each so that it just encompasses all the cases on hand. Then one selects a set of local variables (characteristics which only some of the cases have, say the occurrence of certain tumor types, enzyme activity levels or dietary preferences) and which thus serve to differentiate between groups. Data are then collected, and a system for measuring differences and similarities is developed. Such measurements are based on some form of measurement of distance between two cases (x and y) in terms of each single variable scale. If the variable is a continuous one, then the simplest measure of distance between two pieces of data is the Euclidean distance, (d [x, y]) defined as:

$$d(x, y) = \sqrt{(x_i - y_i)^2}$$

For categorical or discontinuous data, the simplest distance measure is the matching distance, defined as:

$$d(x, y) = \text{number of times } x_i \neq y_i.$$

After we have developed a table of such distance measurements for each of the local variables, some weighting factor is assigned to each variable. A weighting factor seeks to give greater importance to those variables which are believed to have more relevance or predictive value. The weighted variables are then used to assign each piece of data to a group. The actual act of developing numerically based classifications and assigning data members to them is the realm of cluster analysis, and will be discussed later in this chapter. Classification of biological data based on qualitative factors has been well discussed by Glass (1975), and Gordon (1981) does an excellent job of introducing the entire field and mathematical concepts.

Relevant examples of the use of classification techniques range from the simple to the complex. Schaper *et al.* (1985) developed and used a very simple classification of response methodology to identify those airborne chemicals which alter the normal respiratory response induced by CO_2. At the other end of the spectrum, Kowalski and Bender (1972) developed a more mathematically based system to classify chemical data (a methodology they termed pattern recognition).

Table Preparation

Tables are the most common means of presenting data (in both raw and summarized forms) in toxicology. There are some general principles which should be adhered to in the construction and use of tables. However, these are not commonly followed, or even understood. Some of these principles also apply to graphs and their use, which is a major reason for placing this discussion of tables in this section of the book.

1. Tables should be used when some form of repetitive data must be presented. They should be explained in the accompanying text, but their contents should not be repeated in the text.

2. If only a few (two or three) pieces of data are to be presented, give them in the text (not as a table).

3. Tables should be self-contained but should not try to repeat the materials and methods portion of a report in the tables contents.

4. Column headings in tables should always specify the units of measure. The contents should be arranged so that like elements read down in a table, not across. And the contents should be arranged so that there is an order to the elements (such as ascending dose or increase in time of exposure). This helps in mentally summarizing and understanding the table contents.

5. Standard conditions which apply to all the data elements presented in a table or the columns or rows of tables should be presented in footnotes, and not in the columns of a table. The footnotes should be denoted by superscript symbols which are clear and consistent.

6. Symbols (such as ascending numbers, letters or sets of asterisks) should be assigned in the order they will be encoun-

tered in reading the table. For example, the first footnote encountered should be denoted by 1, the second by 2, etc.

7. There are common conventions which set aside certain groups of footnote symbols for particular uses. In toxicology, statistical significance is very commonly denoted by the use of superscript a's, b's, c's, denoting $p \leq 0.05$, $p \leq 0.01$ and $p \leq 0.001$, respectively. The use of these same symbols for other footnotes should be avoided as it may lead to confusion.

8. Any table which presents a large number of identical entries as results should be reconsidered. For example, presenting a table of the effects of 15 different dose levels on body weight where 6 of the doses had no effect (a 0% change), 8 cut weight gain in half (a 50% response) and one dose did something in between is wasteful; this result could be presented very clearly by a single sentence of text.

9. The table legend (title) should clearly label (summarize) the contents or intent of the table.

10. Do not use more significant figures than are necessary or appropriate for the precision of the data-to do so misleads the reader. And the number of significant figures presented in a column (also called the level of decimalization) should be constant for the column and all equivalent data sets presented in a column. If three columns all present mean rabbit weights, for example, than all should report weights to the gram (or tenths of grams, tens of grams, etc.). If some of the members of a column were actually measured to a different level of precision (such as happens when different scales are used to weigh different groups of animals), those with more precision should be rounded for inclusion in the table.

11. Do not present descriptive statistics (such as means and standard deviation) that are labeled in a misleading manner. Examples of this are presenting the arithmetic average of two numbers as a mean and calculating and presenting a standard deviation for these two numbers. Similarly, presenting SEM's (standard error of measurements) without also presenting the size of the groups that they are calculated for is incorrect and makes evaluation of the presented data difficult.

Statistical Graphics

The use of graphics of one form or another in statistics is the single most effective and robust statistical tool and at the same time, one of the most poorly understood and improperly-used.

Graphs are used in statistics (and in toxicology) for one of four major purposes. Each of the four is a variation on the central theme of making complex data easier to understand and use. These four major functions are exploration, analysis, communication and display of data, and graphical aids. Exploration (which may be simply summarizing data or trying to expose the relationships between variables) is determining the characteristics of data sets and deciding on one or more appropriate forms of further analysis, such as the scatter plot. Analysis is the use of graphs to formally evaluate some aspect of the data, such as whether there are outliers present or if an underlying assumption of a population distribution is fulfilled. As long ago as 1960 (Anderson, 1960), some 18 graphical methods for analyzing multivariate data relationships were developed and proposed.

Communication and display of data is the most commonly-used function of statistical graphics in toxicology, whether used for internal reports, presentations at meetings, or formal publications in the professional literature. In communicating data, graphs should not be used to duplicate data that are presented in tables, but rather to show important trends and/or relationships in the data. Though such communication is most commonly of a quantitative compilation of actual data, it can also be used to summarize and present the results of statistical analysis. The fourth and final function of graphics is one that is largely becoming outdated as microcomputers become more widely available. Graphical aids to calculation include nomograms (the classic example in toxicology of a nomogram is that presented by Litchfield and Wilcoxon for determining median effective doses) and extrapolating and interpolating data graphically based on plotted data.

There are many forms of statistical graphics (a partial list, classified by function, is presented in Table 4), and a number of these (such as scatter plots and histograms) can be used for each of a number of possible functions. Most of these plots are based on a Cartesian system (that is, they use a set of rectangular coordinates), and our review of construction and use will focus on these forms of graphs.

Construction of a rectangular graph of any form starts with the selection of the appropriate form of graph followed by the laying out of the coordinates (or axes). Even graphs which are going to encompass multivariate data (that is, more than two variables) generally have as their starting point two major coordinates. The vertical axis, or ordinate (also called the Y axis), is used to present a dependent variable. The horizontal axis (or abscissa, also called the X axis) is used to present an independent variable. Each of these axes is scaled in the units of measure which will most clearly present the trends of interest in the data. The range covered by the scale of each axis is selected to cover the entire region for which data are presented. The actual demarking of the measurement scale along an axis should allow for easy

TABLE 4

FORMS OF STATISTICAL GRAPHICS (By Function)

EXPLORATION

Data Summary	Two Variables	Three or More Variables
Box and whisker plot	Autocorrelation plot	Biplot*
Histogram*	Cross-correlation	Cluster trees*
Dot-array diagram	plot	Labeled scatter plot*
Fequency polygon	Scatter plot*	Glyphs and metro-
Ogive	Sequence plot	glyphs
Stem and leaf		Face plots
diagram		Fourier plot
		Similarity and prefer-
		ence maps
		Multidimensional
		scaling displays
		Weathervane plot

ANALYSIS

Distribution Assessment	Model Evaluation and Assumption Verification	Decision Making
Probability plot	Average versus	Control chart
Q-Q plot	standard deviation	Cusum chart
P-P plot	Component-plus-	Half-normal plot
Hanging histogram	residual plot	Ridge trace
Rootogram	Partial-residual plot	Youden plot
Poissonness plot	Residual plots	

COMMUNICATION AND DISPLAY OF DATA

Quantitative Graphics	Summary of Statistical Analyses
Line chart*	Means plots
Pictogram	Sliding reference distribution
Pie chart*	Notched box plot
Contour plot*	Factor space/response
Stereogram	Interaction plot
Color map	Contour plot
Histogram*	Predicted response plot
	Confidence region plot

GRAPHICAL AIDS

Confidence limits
Graph paper
Power curves
Nomographs
Sample-size curves
Trilinear coordinates

---

*Reviewed in text of this book.

and accurate assessment of the coordinates of any data point, yet should not be cluttered.

Actual data points should be presented by symbols which present the appropriate indicators of location and if they represent a summarization of population data, variability. For example, for summaries of data from a normal data population, it would be appropriate to present a symbol for the mean and some indication of the variability (or error) associated with that population, commonly by using "error bars" which present the standard deviation (or standard error) from the mean. If, however, the data are not normal or continuous it would be more appropriate to indicate location by the median and present the range or semiquartile distance for variability estimates. The symbols which are used to present data points can also be used to present a significant amount of additional information. At the simplest level a set of clearly distinct symbols (circles, triangles, squares, etc.) are very commonly used to provide a third dimension of data (most commonly treatment group). But by clever use of symbols, all sorts of additional information can be presented. Using a method such as Chernoff's faces (Chernoff, 1973), in which faces are used as symbols of the data points (and various aspects of the faces present additional data, such as the presence or absence of eyes denoting the presence or absence of a secondary pathological condition), it is possible to present a large number of different variables on a single graph.

Already presented in this book are the basics of constructing and using simple line (or curve) plots and scatterplots. Separate parts of this chapter will address biplots and cluster analysis. There are three other forms of graphs that are commonly used in toxicology which we will now look at. These are histograms, pie charts and contour plots.

Histograms are graphs of simple fequency distribution. Commonly, the abscissa is the variable of interest (such as life span or litter size), and is generally shown as classes or intervals of measurements (such as age ranges of 0 to 10, 10 to 20, etc. weeks). The ordinate, meanwhile, is the incidence or frequency of observations. The result is a set of vertical bars, each of which represents the incidence of a particular set of observations. Measures of error or variability about each incidence are reflected by some form of error bar on top of, or in the frequency bars, as shown in figure 8. The size of class intervals may be unequal (in effect, one can combine or pool several small class intervals), but it is proper in such cases to vary the width of the bars to indicate differences in interval size.

Pie charts are the only common form of quantitative graphic technique which is not rectangular. Rather, the figure is presented as a circle out of which several "slices" are delimited. The only major use of the pie chart is in presenting a breakdown of the components of a group. Typically the entire set of data under consideration (such as total body weight), constitutes the pie while each slice represents a percentage of the whole (such as the percentages represented by each of several organs). The total number of slices in a pie should be small for the presentation to be effective. Variability or error can be readily presented by having a subslice of each sector shaded and labelled accordingly.

Finally, there is the contour plot, which is used to depict the relationships in a three variable, continuous data system. That is, a contour plot visually portrays each contour as a locus of the values of two variables associated with a constant value of the third variable. An example would be a relief map that gives both latitude and longitude of constant altitude using contour lines.

Just as with tables, there are a number of practical guidelines for the construction and use of graphs.

1. Graphs should be used to present or communicate data when there are pronounced or interesting trends or data relationships. If these are not present, the data should be presented in the text or in a table.
2. The most common misuse of graphs is to either conceal or exaggerate the extent of a difference by using inappropriately scaled and ranged axes. Tufte (1983) has termed a statistic for evaluating the appropriateness of scale size, the lie factor, defined as:

$$\text{Lie factor} = \frac{\text{Size of effect shown in graph}}{\text{Size of effect in data}}$$

An acceptable range for the lie factor is from 0.95 to 1.05. Less means the size of an effect is being understated, more that the effect is being exaggerated.
3. There is rarely a reason for both graphs and tables of the same data to be presented. However, in some instances it is important to both present exact values and demonstrate a trend in the data which is not apparent from an inspection of the tabular data.
4. The axes should be clearly labeled with the names of the variables and the units of measurement.
5. Scale breaks should be used when there are large gaps between data points. The breaks should be clearly visible.
6. Visual comparison of related graphs should be made as easy as possible. This can be done by such actions as using identical scales of measurement and placing the graphs next to each other.
7. The legends should make the graphs as freestanding as possible. All the guidelines presented earlier for footnotes and headings for tables should also be followed for graphs.

There are a number of excellent references available for those who would like to pursue statistical graphics more. Anscombe (1973) presents an excellent short overview, while the books by Schmid (1983) and Tufte (1983) provide a wealth of information. A final reference that is very worthwhile is Crave's *Graph Paper From Your Copier*, which will provide the investigator with master forms to make over two hundred different kinds of graphs.

FIGURE 8
Acquisitions of Post-Natal Development Landmarks in Rats
(N = 10 Litters)

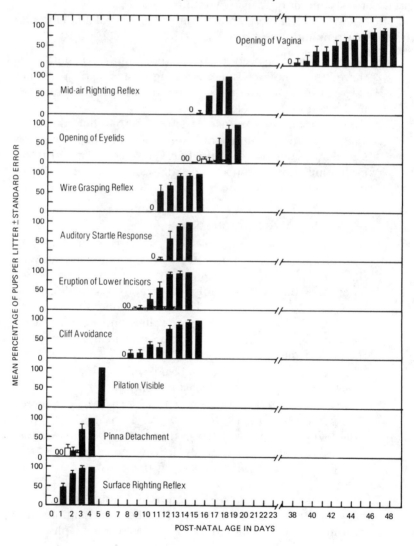

Multidimensional and Nonmetric Scaling

Multidimensional scaling (MDS) is a collection of analysis methods for data sets which have three or more variables making up each data point. MDS displays the relationships of 3 or more dimensional scalar data as a geometric graph and as such is a quantitative extension of the methods of statistical graphics.

MDS presents the structure of a set of objects from data that approximate the distances between pairs of the objects. The data, called similarities, dissimilarities, distances, or proximities, must be in such a form that the degree of similarities and differences between pairs of the objects (each of which represents a real-life data point) can be measured and handled as a distance (remember the discussion of measures of distance under classifications). Similarity is a matter of degree-small differences between objects cause them to be similar (a high degree of similarity) while large differences cause them to be considered dissimilar (a small degree of similarity).

In addition to the traditional human conceptual or subjective judgments of similarity, data can be an "objective" similarity measure (the difference in weight between a pair of animals) or an index calculated from multivariate data (the proportion of agreement in the results of a number of carcinogenicity studies). However, the data must always represent the degree of similarity of pairs of objects.

Each object or data point is represented by a point in a multidimensional space. These plotted or projected points are arranged in this space so that the distances between pairs of points have the strongest possible relation to the degree of similarity among the pairs of objects. That is, two similar objects are represented by two points that are close together, and two dissimilar objects are represented by a pair of points that are far apart. The space is usually a two or three dimensional Euclidean space, but may be non-Euclidean and may have more dimensions.

MDS is a general term which includes a number of different types of techniques. However, all seek to allow geometric analysis of multivariate data. The forms of MDS can be classified (Young, 1985) according to the nature of the similarities in the data. It can be qualitative (nonmetric) or quantitative (metric MDS). The types can also be classified by the number of variables involved and by the nature of the model used; for example, classical MDS (there is only one data matrix, and no weighting factors are used on the data), replicated MDS (more than one matrix and no weighting) and weighted MDS (more than one matrix and at least some of the data has been weighted).

MDS can be used in toxicology to analyze the similarities and differences between effects produced by different agents, in an attempt to use an understanding of the mechanism underlying the actions of one agent to determine the mechanisms of the other agents. Actual algorithms and a good intermediate level presentation of MDS can be found in Davison (1983).

Nonmetric scaling is a set of graphic techniques closely related to MDS, and definitely useful for the reduction of dimensionality. Its major objective is to arrange a set of objects (each object, for our purposes, consisting of a number of related observations) graphically in a few dimensions, while retaining the maximum possible fidelity to the original relationships between members (that is, values which are most different are portrayed as most distant). It is not a linear technique, it does not preserve linear relationships (i.e., A is not shown as twice as far from C as B, even though its "value difference" may be twice as much). The spacings (interpoint distances) are kept such that if the distance of the original scale between members A and B is greater than that between C and D, the distances on the model scale shall likewise be greater between A and B than between C and D. Figure 5, presented earlier, uses a form of this technique in adding a third dimension by using letters to present degrees of effect on the skin.

This technique functions by taking observed measures of similarity or dissimilarity between every pair of M objects, then finding a representation of the objects as points in Euclidean space such that the interpoint distances in some sense "match" the observed similarities or dissimilarities by means of weighting constants.

Cluster Analysis

Cluster analysis in a quantitative form of classification. It serves to help develop decision rules and then use these rules to assign a heterogeneous collection of objects to a series of sets. This is almost entirely an applied methodology (as opposed to theoretical). The final result of a cluster analysis is one of several forms of graphic displays and a methodology (set of decision classifying rules) for the assignment of new members into the classifications.

The classification procedures used are based on either density of population or distance between members. These methods can serve to generate a basis for the classification of large numbers of dissimilar variables such as behavorial observations and compounds with distinct but related structures and mechanisms (Gad *et al.*, 1984; Gad *et al.*, 1985), or to separate tumor patterns caused by treatment from those caused by old age (Salsburg, 1979).

There are five types of clustering technique (Everitt, 1980)

    a. Hierarchical techniques: Classes are subclassified into groups, with the process being repeated at several levels to produce a tree which gives sufficient definition of groups.

b. Optimization techniques: Clusters are formed by optimization of a clustering criterion. The resulting classes are mutually exclusive, the objects are partitioned clearly into sets.

c. Density or mode-seeking techniques: Clusters are identified and formed by locating regions in a graphic representation which contains concentrations of data points.

d. Clumping techniques: A variation of density-seeking techniques in which assignment to a cluster is weighted on some variables, so that clusters may overlap in graphic projections.

e. Others: Methods which do not clearly fall into classes a - d.

Romesburg (1984) provides an excellent step-by-step guide to cluster analysis.

Fourier Or Time Series Analysis

Fourier analysis (Bloomfield, 1975) is most frequently a univariate method used for either simplifying data (which is the basis for its inclusion in this chapter) or for modeling. It can, however, also be a multivariate technique for data analysis.

In a sense, it is like trend analysis; it looks at the relationship of sets of data from a different perspective. In the case of Fourier analysis, the approach is by resolving the time dimension variable in a data set. At the most simple level, it assumes that many events are periodic in nature, and if we can remove the variation in other variables because of this periodicity (by using Fourier transforms), we can better analyze the remaining variation from other variables. The complications to this are (a) there may be several overlying cyclic time-based periodicities, and (b) we may be interested in the time cycle events for their own sake.

Fourier analysis allows one to identify, quantitate, and (if we wish) remove the time-based cycles in data (with their amplitudes, phases, and frequencies) by use of the Fourier transform:

$$nJ_i = x_i \exp(-iw_i t)$$

where n = length

J = The discrete Fourier transform for that case
x = actual data
i = increment in the series
w = frequency
and t = time

A graphic example of the use of Fourier analysis in toxicology is provided in Figure 9.

FIGURE 9

Use Of Time Series Analysis

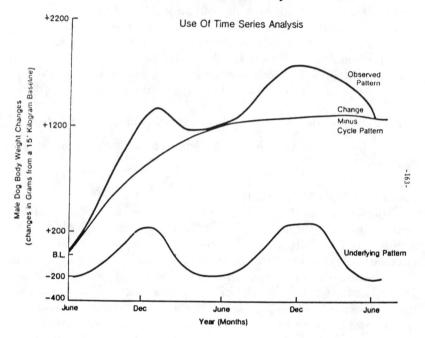

Use Of Time Series Analysis

Male Dog Body Weight Changes (changes in Grams from a 15' Kilogram Baseline)

Observed Pattern

Change Minus Cycle Pattern

Underlying Pattern

Year (Months)

-163-

Life Tables

Chronic *in vivo* toxicity studies are generally the most complex and expensive studies conducted by a toxicologist. Answers to a number of questions are sought in such a study - notably if a material results in a significant increase in mortality or in the incidence of tumors in those animals exposed to it. But we are also interested in the time course of these adverse effects (or risks). The classic approach to assessing these age-specific hazard rates is by the use of life tables (also called survivorship tables).

It may readily be seen that during any selected period of time (t_i) we have a number of risks competing to affect an animal. There are the risks of (a) "natural death," (b) death induced by a direct or indirect action of the test compound, and (c) death due to such occurrences of interest as tumors (Hammond et al. 1978). And we are indeed interested in determining if (and when) the last two of these risks become significantly different from the "natural" risks (defined as what is seen to happen in the control group). Life table methods enable us to make such determinations as the duration of survival (or time until tumors develop) and the probability of survival (or of developing a tumor) during any period of time.

We start by deciding the interval length (t_i) we wish to examine within the study. The information we gain becomes more exact as the interval is shortened. But as interval length is decreased, the number of intervals increases and calculations become more cumbersome and less indicative of time-related trends because random fluctuations become more apparent. For a two-year or lifetime rodent study, an interval length of a month is commonly employed. Some life table methods, such as the Kaplan-Meyer, have each new event (such as a death) define the start of a new interval.

Having established the interval length we can tabulate our data (Cutler and Ederer, 1958). We start by establishing the following columns in each table (a separate table being established for each group of animals—i.e., by sex and dose level):

(a) The interval of time selected (t_i);
(b) the number of animals in the group that entered that interval of the study alive (l_i);
(c) the number of animals withdrawn from study during the interval (such as those taken for an interim sacrifice or that may have been killed by a technician error) (ω_i);
(d) the number of animals that died during the interval (d_i);
(e) the number of animals at risk during the interval, $l_i = l_i - \frac{1}{2} \omega_i$, or the number on study at the start of the interval minus one half of the number withdrawn during the interval;
(f) the proportion of animals that died $= D_i = d_i / l_i$;
(g) the cumulative probability of an animal surviving until the end of that interval of study, $P_i = 1 - D_i$, or one minus the number of animals that died during that interval divided by the number of animals at risk;
(h) the number of animals dying until that interval (M_i);
(i) animals found to have died during the interval (m_i);
(j) the probability of dying during the interval of the study $c_i = 1 - (M_i + m_i / l_i)$, or the total number of animals dead until that interval plus the animals discovered to have died during that interval divided by the number of animals at risk through the end of that interval;
(k) the cumulative proportion surviving, p_i, is equivalent to the cumulative product of the interval probabilities of survival (i.e., $p_i = p_1 \cdot p_2 \cdot p_3 \cdots p_x$); and
(l) the cumulative probability of dying, C_i, equal to the cumulative product of the interval probabilities to that point (i.e., $C_i = c_1 \cdot c_2 \cdot c_3 \cdots c_x$).

With such tables established for each group in a study (as shown in Example 29), we may now proceed to test the hypotheses that each of the treated groups has a significantly shorter duration of survival,

EXAMPLE 29

Test level 1

Interval (months) l_i	Alive at beginning of interval l_i	Animals withdrawn w_i	Died during interval d_i	Animals at risk l_i	Proportion of animals dead D_i	Probability of survival P_i	Cumulative proportion surviving P_i	Standard error of survival S_i
8- 9	109	0	0	109	0	1.0000	1.0000	0.0000
9-10	109	0	2	109	0.0184	0.9816	0.9816	0.0129
10-11	107	0	0	107	0	1.0000	0.9816	0.0128
11-12	107	10	0	102	0	1.0000	0816	0.0128
12-13	97	0	1	97	0.0103	0.9897	0.9713	0.0162
13-14	96	0	1	96	0.0104	0.9896	0.9614	0.0190
14-15	95	0	12	95	0.1263	0.8737	0.8400	0.0367
15-16	83	0	2	83	0.0241	0.9759	0.8198	0.0385
16-17	81	0	3	81	0.0370	0.9630	0.7894	0.0409
17-18	78	20	1	68	0.0147	0.9853	0.7778	0.0419
18-19	57	0	2	57	0.0351	0.6949	0.7505	0.0446

Control level

Interval (months) l_i	Alive at beginning of interval l_i	Animals withdrawn w_i	Died during interval d_i	Animals at risk l_i	Proportion of animals dead D_i	Probability of survival P_i	Cumulative proportion surviving P_i	Standard error of survival S_i
11-12	99	0	1	99	0.0101	0.9899	0.9899	0.0100
12-13	98	0	0	98	0	1.0000	0.9899	0.0100
13-14	98	0	0	98	0	1.0000	0.9899	0.0100
14-15	98	0	2	98	0.0204	0.9796	0.9697	0.0172

Interval (months) l_i	Alive at beginning of interval l_i	Animals withdrawn w_i	Died during interval d_i	Animals at risk l_i	Proportion of animals dead D_i	Probability of survival P_i	Cumulative proportion surviving P_i	Standard error of survival S_i
15-16	96	0	1	96	0.0104	0.9896	0.9596	0.0198
16-17	95	0	0	95	0	1.0000	0.9596	0.0198
17-18	95	20	2	85	0.0235	0.8765	0.9370	0.0249
18-19	73	0	2	73	0.0274	0.9726	0.9113	0.0302

Now, for these two groups, we wish to determine effective sample size and to compare survival probabilities in the interval months 14-15.

For the exposure group we compute sample size as

$$I_{g14-15} = \frac{0.8400(1 - 0.8400)}{(0.0367)^2} = 99.7854$$

Likewise we get a sample size of 98.1720 for the control group.
The standard error of difference for the two groups here is

$$SD = \sqrt{0.0367^2 + 0.0173^2} = 0.040573$$

The probability of survival differences is $P_D = 0.9697 - 0.8400 = 0.1297$. Our test statistic is then $0.1297/0.040573 = 3.196$. From our z value table we see that the critical values are

$$p \leqslant 0.05 = 1.960$$
$$p \leqslant 0.01 = 2.575$$
$$p \leqslant 0.001 = 3.270$$

As our calculated value is larger than all but the last of these, we find our groups to be significantly different at the 0.01 level ($0.01 > p > 0.001$).

or that each of the treated groups died more quickly (note that plots of total animals dead and total animals surviving will give one an appreciation of the data, but can lead to no statistical conclusions).

There are a multiplicity of methods for testing significance in life tables, with (as is often the case) the power of the tests increasing as does the difficulty of computation (Breslow, 1975; Cox, 1972; Haseman, 1977; Tarone, 1975)

We begin our method of statistical comparison of survival at any point in the study by determining the standard error of the K interval survival rate as (Garrett, 1947).

$$S_K = P_k \sqrt{\sum_1^k \left(\frac{D_i}{I'_x - d_x} \right)}$$

We may also determine the effective sample size (l_1) in accordance with

$$l_1 = \frac{P(1-P)}{S^2}$$

We may now compute the standard error of difference for any two groups (1 and 2) as

$$S_D = \sqrt{S_1^2 + S_2^2}$$

The difference in survival probabilities for the two groups is then calculated as

$$P_D = P_1 - P_2$$

We can then calculate a test statistic as

$$t' = \frac{P_D}{S_D}$$

This is then compared to the z distribution table. If $t' > z$ at the desired probability level, it is significant at that level. Example 29 illustrates the life table technique for mortality data. With increasing recognition of the effects of time (both as age and length of exposure to unmeasured background risks), life table analysis has become a mainstay in chronic toxicology. An example is the reassessment of the ED_{01} study (SOP ED_{01} Task Force, 1981) which radically changed interpretation of the results and understanding of underlying methods when adjustment for time on study was made.

The increased importance and interest in the analysis of survival data has not been restricted to toxicology, but rather has encompassed all the life sciences. Those with further interest should consult Lee (1980) or Elandt-Johnson and Johnson (1980), both general in their approach to the subject.

REFERENCES

Anderson E. (1960): A Semigraphical Method for the Analysis of Complex Problems. *Technomet*, 2, 387–391.

Anscombe, F.J. (1973): Graphs in Statistical Analysis *Amer Stat.*, 27: 17–21.

Bloomfield, P. (1976): *Fourier Analysis of Time Series: An Introduction*. John Wiley, New York.

Breslow, N.E. (1975): Analysis of survival data under the proportional hazards model. *Int. Stat. Rev.*, 43: 45–58.

Chernoff H. (1973): The Use of Faces to Represent Points in K-Dimensional Space Graphically *J. Amer Stat Assoc.*, 68: 361–368.

Cox, D.R. (1972): Regression models and life-tables. *J. Roy. Stat. Soc.*, 34B: 187–220.

Craver, J.S. (1980): *Graph Paper From Your Copies*. H.P. Books, Tucson.

Cutler, S.J., and Ederer, F. (1958): Maximum utilization of the life table method in analyzing survival. *J. Chron. Dis.*, 8: 699–712.

Davison, M.L. (1983): *Multidimensional Scaling*. John Wiley, New York.

Elandt-Johnson, R.C. and Johnson, N.L. (1980): *Survival Models and Data Analysis*. John Wiley, New York.

Everitt, B. (1980): *Cluster Analysis*. Halsted Press, New York.

Garrett, H.E. (1947): *Statistics in Psychology and Education*, pp. 215–218. Longmans, Green, New York.

Gad, S.C., Gavigan, F.A., Siino, K.M. and Reilly, C. (1984): The Toxicology of Eight Ionophores: Neurobehavioral and Membrane and Acute Effects and Their Structure Activity Relationships (SAR's). *Toxicologist*, 4:702

Gad, S.C.; Reilly, C.; Siino, K.M. and Gavigan, F.A. (1985): Thirteen Cationic Ionoores: Neurobehavioral and Membrane Effects. *Drug and Chemical Toxicology*, 8: (6) 451-468.

Glass, L. (1975): Classification of Biological Networks by their Qualitative Dynamics. *J Theor. Bio.*, 54: 85–107

Gordon, A.D. (1981) *Classification* Chapman and Hall, New York.

Hammond, F C., Garfinkel, L. and Lew, E.A. (1978): Longevity, selective mortality, and competitive risks in relation to chemical carcinogenesis. *Environ. Res.*, 16: 153–173.

Hartigan, J.A. (1983): Classification. In: Katz, S. and Johnson, N.L. (Eds) *Encyclopedia of Statistical Sciences*, Vol 2. John Wiley, New York.

Haseman, J.K. (1977): Response to use of statistics when examining life time studies in rodents to detect carcinogenicity. *J. Toxicol. Environ. Health.*, 3:633–636.

Kowalski, B.R. and Bender, C.F. (1972): Pattern Recognition. A Powerful Approach to Interpreting Chemical Data. *J. Amer Chem Soc.*, 94: 5632–5639.

Lee, E.T. (1980): *Statistical Methods for Survival Data Analysis*, Lifetime Learning Publications, Belmont.

Litchfield, J.T. and Wilcoxon, F. (1949): A simplified method of evaluating dose effect experiments. *J. Pharmacol. Exp. Ther.*, 96:99–113.

Romesburg, H.C. (1984): *Cluster Analysis for Researchers* Lifetime Learning Publications, Belmont.

Salsburg, D. (1979): The Effects of Life-Time Feeding Studies on Patterns of Senile Lesions In Mice and Rats (unpublished manuscript).

Schaper, M.; Thompson, R.D. and Alarie, Y. (1985): A Method to Classify Airborne Chemicals Which Alter the Normal Ventilatory Response Induced by CO_2 *Toxicol Appl Pharmacol.*, 79: 332–341

Schmid, C.F. (1983): *Statistical Graphics* John Wiley, New York.

SOT ED_{01} Task Force (1981) Reexamination of the ED_{01} Study-Adjusting for Time on Study. *Fundam. Appl. Toxicol.*, 1:8–123.

Tarone, R.E. (1975): Tests for trend in life table analysis. *Biometrika.*, 62:679–682.

Tufte, E.R. (1983): *The Visual Display of Quantitative Information* Graphics Press, Cheshire.

Young F.W. (1985): Multidimensional Scaling In Katz, S. and Johnson, N.L. (Eds) *Encyclopedia of Statistical Sciences* Vol. 5. pp 649–659 John Wiley, New York.

CHAPTER 10

MULTIVARIATE METHODS

In a book of this kind, an in-depth explanation of the available multivariate statistical techniques is an impossibility. However, as the complexity of problems in toxicology increases, we can expect to confront more frequently data that are not unvariate but rather multivariate (or multidimensional). For example, a multidimensional study might be one in which the animals are being dosed with two materials that interact. Suppose we measure body weight, tumor incidence, and two clinical chemistry values for test material effects and interaction. Our dimensions - or variables - are now: A = dose "x", B = dose "y", W = body weight, C = tumor incidence, D and E = levels of clinical chemistry parameters, and possibnly also t(length of dosing).

These situations are particularly common in chronic studies (Schaffer, *et al.* 1967). Though we can continue to use multiple sets of univariate techniques as we have in the past, there are significant losses of power, efficiency, and information when this is done, as well as an increased possibility of error (Davidson, 1972).

In this chapter we will try to communicate an understanding of the nature of multivariate data, its distributions and descriptive parameters, how to collect and prepare these data. We will also look briefly at the workings and uses of each of the most commonly employed multivariate techniques, together with several examples from the literature of their employment in toxicology and the other biological sciences. We shall group the methods according to their primary function: hypothesis testing (are these significant or not?), model fitting (what is the relationship between these variables, or what would happen if a population would exposed to x?), and reduction of dimensionality (which variables are most meaningful?). It should be noted (and will soon be obvious), however, that most multivariate techniques actually combine several of these functions.

The most fundamental concept in multivariate analysis is that of a multivariate population distribution. By this point it is assumed that the reader is familiar with the univariate random variable and with such standard distributions as the normal distribution. This chapter extends these univariate ideas to the multivariate case. We will discuss the general properties of multivariate distributions and consider the particular example of the multivariate normal distribution.

We will denote an n-dimensional random variable, sometimes called a random vector, by X where

$$X^t = [X_1,.....,X_n]$$

and $X_1,.....,X_n$ are univariate random variables, where $X_1,.....,X$ are matrices.

We are primarily concerned with the case where the variables are continuous, but it is probably easier to understand the ideas if we start by considering the case where the components of X are discrete random variables. In this case, the (joint) distribution of X is described by the joint probability function $P(x_1,....x_n)$, where

$$P(x_1,.....,X_n) = Prob(X_1 = x_1,.....,X_n = x_n)$$

We will abbreviate $P(x_1,.....,x_n)$ as $P(x)$. Note that lowercase letters indicate particular values of the corresponding random variables.

The function $P(x)$ must satisfy two conditions similar to those required in the univariate case, namely that

$$P(x) \geqslant 0 \text{ for every } x$$
$$\text{and } \Sigma P(x) = 1$$

where the summation is over all possible values of X.

From the joint distribution, it is often useful to calculate two other types of distribution-the marginal distributions and the conditional distributions.

Suppose we are interested in the distribution of one component of X, say X_1, without regard to the values of the other variables. The probability distribution of X_i can then be obtained from the joint distribution by summing over all the other variables. Thus

$$Prob (X_i = x_i) = \Sigma P (x_1,.....,x_n)$$

where the summation is for all x such that the ith component is fixed to be x_i, in other words over $x_i,.....,x_{i-1}, x_{i+1},.....,x_n$.

When the distribution of a single variable is obtained from a joint distribution by summing over all other variables, then it is usually called a marginal distribution. If the joint distribution is equal to the product of all the marginal distributions for every x, so that

$$P(x) = \prod_{i=i}^{n} P_i(x_i)$$

where $P_i(X_i)$ denotes the marginal distribution of X_i, then the random variables are said to be independent.

Also note that marginal joint distributions are possible by summing over less than $(p - 1)$ variables. For example, the marginal joint distribution of X_i and X_2 is obtained by summing the joint distribution for all variables from X_3 to X_n.

If some of the variables are set equal to specified constant values, then the distribution of the remaining variables is called a conditional distribution. For a conditional probability, we should note that for two events, A and B,

$$\text{Prob}(A \mid B) = \text{probability of event A given that B has occurred}$$
$$= P(A \, \Omega \, B)/P(B),$$

where $A \, \Omega \, B$ denotes the intersection of events A and B, meaning that both events occur. By analogy, we find that the conditional distribution of a random variable is given by the ratio of the joint distribution to the appropriate marginal distribution.

In the case $p = 2$, the conditional distribution of X_1, given that X_2 take the particular value x_2, is given by

$$P(x_1 \mid x_2) = \text{Prob}(X_1 = x_1 \mid X_2 = x_2)$$
$$= P(x_1, x_2)/P_2(x_2)$$

where $P_2(x_2)$ is the marginal distribution of X_2. More generally,

$$P(x_1,....,x_k \mid x_{k + 1},....,x_n) = P(x)/P_M (x_{k + 1},....,x_n)$$

where $P_M(x_k + 1,....,x_n)$ denotes the marginal joint distribution of

$X_k + 1,....,X_n$

These concepts are demonstrated in example 30.

EXAMPLE 30

Groups of four rats are each dosed one at a time, with a new chemical. If we let

X_1 = number of deaths in first two animals dosed
X_2 = number of deaths in last three animals dosed

we can then find the joint distribution of X_1 and X_2, the marginal distribution of X_1, and the conditional distribution of X_1 given that $X_2 = 2$.

The joint distribution

X_2	X_1			Marginal distribution of X_2
	0	1	2	
0	1/16	1/16	0	1/8
1	1/8	2/16	1/16	2/8
2	1/16	2/16	1/8	2/8
3	0	1/16	1/16	1/8
Marginal distribution of X_1	1/2	1/2	1/2	

Note that the sum of the joint probabilities is 1. The marginal distributions of X_1 and X_2 can be found by summing the column and row joint probabilities respectively. Of course, in this simple case we could write down the (marginal) distribution of X_1 (and of X_2) directly. The conditional distribution of X_1, given that $X_2 = 2$, is obtained by looking at the row of joint probabilities where $X_2 = 2$ and normalizing them so that they sum to 1. This is done by dividing by the row total, which is the appropriate marginal probability. Thus

$$\text{Prob}(X_1 = 0 | X_2 = 2) = \frac{1/16}{3/8} = 1/6$$

$$\text{Prob}(X_1 = 1 | X_2 = 2) = 1/2$$

$$\text{Prob}(X_1 = 2 | X_2 = 2) = 1/3$$

Note that these three conditional probabilities sum to unity (that is, 1.0).

In the two-variable case, the distribution of a continuous random variable may be described by the cumulative distribution function (abbreviated c.d.f.) or by its derivative, called the probability density function (abbreviated p.d.f.). For continuous multivariate distributions, we may define suitable multivariate analogues of these functions. The joint c.d.f., which we will denote by $F(x_1...,x_n)$, is defined by

$$F(x_1,....,x_n) = \text{Prob}\,(x_1 \leqslant x_{1....},x_n \leqslant x_n).$$

The joint p.d.f., which we denoted by $f(x_1,....,x_n)$ or $f(x)$, is then given by the nth partial derivative

$$f(x) = \frac{\delta^p F(x_1,...,x_n)}{\delta x_1\, \delta x_2...\delta x_n}$$

assuming that $F(x)$ is absolutely continuous. This joint p.d.f. satisfies the assumptions:

(a) $f(x) \geqslant 0$ for every x;

(b) $\int_{-\infty}^{\infty} \cdots \int_{-\infty}^{\infty} f(x)dx_1 \ldots dx_n = 1.$

As in the univariate case, the joint p.d.f. is not a single probability, but rather the probabilities which can be found by integrating over the required subset of n-space. The above definitions can be related to the bivariate case where n = 2, and one can think of the two variables as being defined along perpendicular axes in a plane. For any point (x_1, y_2) in this plane, the joint p.d.f. gives the height of a surface above this plane. The total volume under this three dimensional surface is defined to be 1 and is the total probability. For any area in the plane the corresponding volume underneath the surface gives the probability of having a bivariate observation in the given area.

Marginal and conditional distributions are easily defined in the continuous case. The marginal p.d.f. of one component of X, say X_i, may be found from the joint p.d.f. by integrating out all the other variables. Thus

$$f_i(s_i) = \int_{-\infty}^{\infty} \cdots \int_{-\infty}^{\infty} f(x)dx_1...dx_{i-1}\,dx_{i+1}...dx_n$$

The random variables are independent if the joint p.d.f. is equal to the product of all the marginal p.d.f.s for every x. We also note that marginal joint distributions are possible by integrating out less than $(n - 1)$ variables.

The density functions of conditional continuous distributions can be found by dividing the joint p.d.f. by the appropriate marginal p.d.f., which is clearly analogous to the discrete case. Thus, in the case n = 2, the conditional p.d.f. of X_1, given that X_2 takes the particular value x_2, will be denoted by $h(x_1 \mid x_2)$ and is given by

$$h(x_1 \mid x_2) = f(x_1, x_2) / f_2(x_2)$$

More generally, the conditional joint p.d.f. of $X_1,...X_1$ given $X_{k+1} = $ - $x_{k+1},..., X_n = x_n$ is given by

$$h(x_1,...,x_k \mid x_{k+1},...,x_n) = f(x)/f_M(x_{k+1},...,x_n)$$

where $f_M(x_K + 1,...,x_n)$ denotes the marginal joint p.d.f. of $X_k - 1,...X_n$.

In the two-variable (or univariate) case, it is common to summarize a probability distributions's characteristics by giving two parameters, the mean and standard deviation. To summarize multivariate distributions, we need to find the mean and variance (the square of the standard deviation) of each of the n variables, together with a measure of the way each pair of variables is related. The latter target is achieved by calculating a set of quantities called covariances, or their standarized counterparts called correlations. These quantities are defined as below.

Means. The mean vector T = [1,..., n] is such that

$$T = E(x_i) = \int_{-\infty}^{\infty} x \; f_i(x)dx$$

is the mean of the ith component of X. This definition is given for the case where X_i is continuous. If X_i is discrete, then $E(X_i)$ is given by $\Sigma \, xP_i(x)$, where $P_i(x)$ is the (marginal) probability distribution of X_i.

Variances. The variance of the ith component of X is given by

$$Var(X_i) = E[(X_i - \mu_i)^2]$$
$$= E(X_i^2) - \mu_i^2$$

This is usually denoted by σ_i^2 in the univariate case, but in order to fit in with the covariance notation provided below, we will usually denote it by σ_{ii} in the multivariate case.

Covariances. The covariance of two variables X_i and X_j is defined by

$$Cov(X_i \; X_j) = E[(X_i - \mu_i)(X_j - \mu_j)]$$

Thus, it is the product moment of the two variables about their respective means. In particular, if i = j, we note that the covariance of a variable with itself is simply the variance of the variable. Thus, there is really no need to define variance separately in the multivariate case, as it is a special case of covariance.

The covariance of X_i and X_j is usually denoted by σ_{ij}. Thus, if i = j, the variance of X_i is denoted by σ_{ii}, as noted above.

The equation given above for the covariance is often presented as

$$\sigma_{ij} = E[X_i \; X_j] - \mu_i \, \mu_j$$

The covariance matrix. With n variables, there are n variances and ½ n (n − 1) covariances, and these quantities are all second moments. It is often useful to present these quantities in a (n x n) matrix, denoted by ε, whose (i, j)th element is σ_{ij}. Thus,

$$\Sigma = \begin{bmatrix} \sigma_{11} & \sigma_{12} & \cdots \sigma_{1n} \\ \sigma_{21} & \sigma_{22} & \cdots \sigma_{2n} \\ \vdots & & \\ \sigma_n{}^1 & \sigma_n{}^1 & \cdots \sigma_{nn} \end{bmatrix}$$

This matrix is called the dispersion matrix, or the covariance matrix, and we will use the latter term. The diagonal terms are the variances, while the off diagonal terms, the covariances, are such that ij = ji. Thus the matrix is symmetric.

Using the two covariance equations, we can express the matrix in two alternative and useful forms, namely.

$$\Sigma = E[X - \mu)(X - \mu)^{\tau}]$$
$$= E[XX^{\tau}] - \mu\mu^{\tau}$$

Linear compounds. Perhaps the main use of covariances is as a stepping stone to the calculation of correlations (see below), but they are also useful for a variety of other purposes. Here we illustrate their use in finding the variance of any linear combination of the components of X. Such combinations arise in a variety of situations. Consider the general linear compound

$$Y = a^{T}X$$

where $a^{T} = (a_1,...,a_n]$ is a vector of constants. Then Y is a univariate random variable. Its mean is clearly given by

$$E(Y) = a^{T}\mu$$

while its variance is given by

$$Var(Y) = E[a^{T}(X - \mu)]^2$$

As $a^{T}(X - \mu)$ is a scalar and therefore equal to its transpose, we can express Var (Y) in terms of Σ, using the formula above, as

$$Var(Y) = E[a^{\tau}(X - \mu)(X - \mu)^{\tau}a]$$
$$= a^{\tau}E[(X - \mu)(X - \mu)^{\tau}]a$$
$$= a^{\tau}\Sigma a$$

Correlation. Although covariances are useful for many mathematical purposes, they are rarely used as descriptive statistics. If two variables are related in a linear way, then the covariance will be positive or negative depending on whether the relationship has a positive or negative slope. But the size of the coefficient is difficult to interpret because it depends on the units in which the two variables are measured. Thus the covariance is often standardized by dividing by the product of the standard deviations of the two variables to give a quantity called the correlation coefficient. The correlation between variables X_i and X_j will be denoted by r_{ij}, and is given by

$$r_{ij} = \sigma_{ij}/\sigma_i \sigma_j$$

where σ_i denotes the standard deviation of X_i.

It can be shown that ρ_{ij} must lie between -1 and $+1$, using the fact that Var $(aX_i + bX_j) \geq 0$ for every a,b, and putting $a = Var(X_j)$ and $b = \pm Var(X_i)$.

The correlation coefficient provides a measure of the linear association between two variables. The coefficient is positive if the relationship between the two variables has a positive slope so that "high" values of one variable tend to go with "high" values of the other variable.

Conversely, the coefficient is negative if the relationship has a negative slope.

If two variables are indpendent then their covariance, and hence their correlation, will be zero. But it is important to note that the converse of this statement is not true. It is possible to construct examples where two variables have zero correlation and yet are dependent on one another, often in a nonlinear way. This emphasizes the fact that the correlation coefficient is of no real use as a descriptive statistic (and may be positively misleading) if the relationship between two variables is of a non-linear form. However, if the two variables follow a bivariate normal distribution, then a zero correlation implies independence (or no correlation).

The correlation matrix. With n variables, there are $p(p - 1)/2$ distinct correlations. It is often useful to present them in a ($p \times p$) matrix whose (i,j)th element is defined to be r_{ij}. This matrix, called the correlation matrix, will be denoted by P which is the Greek letter for capital rho. The diagonal terms of P are unity, and the off-diagonal terms are such that P is symmetric.

In order to relate the covariance and correlation matrices, let us define a ($p \times p$) diagonal matrix, D, whose diagonal terms are the standard deviations of the components of X, so that

$$D = \begin{bmatrix} \sigma_1 & 0 & \cdots & 0 \\ 0 & \sigma_2 & \cdots & 0 \\ \vdots & & & \\ 0 & 0 & \cdots & \sigma_p \end{bmatrix}$$

Then the covariance and correlation matrices are related by

$$\Sigma = DPD$$

or

$$P = D^{-1} \Sigma D^{-1}$$

where the diagonal terms of the matrix D^{-1} are the reciprocals of the respective standard deviations.

We can now complete this section with a slightly more advanced discussion of the matrix properties of Σ and P, and in particular of their rank.

Firstly, we show that both Σ and P are positive and semidefinite. As any variance must be non-negative, we have that

$$\text{Var } (a^T X) \geq 0 \text{ for every a}$$

But Var $(a^T X) = a^T \Sigma a$, and so Σ must be positive semidefinite. We also note that Σ is related to P, where D is non-singular, and so it follows that P is also positive semidefinite.

Because D is non-singular, we may also show that the rank of P is the same as the rank of Σ. This rank must be less than or equal to n.

If Σ (and hence P) is of full rank n, then Σ (and hence P) will be positive definite. In this case, Var $(a^TX) = a^T \Sigma a$ is strictly greater than zero for every $a \neq 0$. But if rank $(\Sigma) < p$, then Σ (and hence P) will be singular, and this indicates a linear constraint on the components of X. This means that there exists a vector $a \neq 0$ such that a^TX is identically equal to a constant. The most commonly assumed and used multivariate distribution is the multivariate normal distribution.

First we should remember that a univariate normal random variable X, with mean $\bar{X}$ and variance σ^2, has density function

$$f(x) = \frac{1}{\sqrt{(2_\pi)}\sigma} \exp[-(x-\bar{x})^2/2\sigma^2]$$

and we write $X \sim N(\bar{X}, \sigma^2)$.

In the multivariate case, we say that an n-dimensional random variable X follows the multivariate normal distribution if its joint p.d.f. is of the form

$$f(x) = \frac{1}{(2\pi)_n^{2}|\Sigma|^{1/2}} \exp[-\tfrac{1}{2}(x-\bar{x})]^T \Sigma^{-1}(x-\bar{x})]$$

where Σ is any (n x n) symmetric positive definite matrix. If $X_1...,X_p$ are independent random variables where $X_i \approx N(\mu_i, \sigma^2 i)$, then their joint p.d.f. is simply the product of the appropriate (marginal) density functions, so that

$$f(x_1,...,x_n^{1} = \frac{1}{(2\pi)_n^{2}\prod_{i=i} \sigma_i} \exp\left[-\tfrac{1}{2}\sum_{i=i}^{n}\left(\frac{x_i - \bar{x}_1}{\sigma_i}\right)^2\right]$$

In this case $X^T = [X_1....,X_n]$ has mean $\bar{X}^T = [\bar{X}_1....,\bar{X}_p]$ and covariance matrix

$$\Sigma = \begin{bmatrix} \sigma_1^2 & 0 & \cdots & 0 \\ 0 & \sigma_2^2 & \cdots & 0 \\ \vdots & & & \\ 0 & 0 & \cdots & \sigma_n^2 \end{bmatrix}$$

There are other important multivariate distributions - the multivariate discrete distribution (where the data are rank - order and not continuous) and the multivariate continuous distribution (where the data are continuous but not normally distributed).

Multivariate data are virtually never processed and analyzed other than by computer. One must first set up an appropriate data base file, then enter the data, coding some of them to meet the requirements of the software being utilized (for example, if only numerical data are analyzed, sex may have to be coded as 1 for male and 2 for females).

Having recorded the data, it is then essential to review for suspect values and errors of various kinds. There are many different types of suspect values and it is helpful to distinguish among them.

(a) Outliers. These are defined to be observations which appear to be inconsistent with the rest of the data. They may be caused by gross recording or entering errors. But it is important to realize that an apparent outlier may occasionally be genuine and indicate a non-normal distribution or valuable data point.

(b) Inversions. A common type of error occurs when two consecutive digits are interchanged at the recording, coding or entering stage. The error may be trivial if, for example, 56.74 appears as 56.47, but it may generate an outlier if 56.74 appears as 65.74.

(c) Repetitions. At the coding or entering stage, it is quite easy to repeat an entire number in two successive rows or columns of a table, thereby omitting one number completely.

(d) Values in the wrong column. It is also easy to get numbers into the wrong columns.

(e) Other errors and suspect values. There are many other types of error including possible misrecording of data of a minor nature.

The general term used to denote procedures for detecting and correcting errors is data editing. This includes checks for completeness, consistency and credibility. Some editing can be done at the end of the data entry stage. In addition, many routine checks can be made by the computer itself, particularly those for gross outliers. An important class of such checks are range tests. For each variable an allowable range of possible values is specified, and the computer checks that all observed values lie within the given range. Bivariate and multivariate checks are also possible. For example, one may specify an allowable range for some function of two or more variables. A set of checks called "if-then" checks are also possible. For example if both age and date of birth are recorded for each animal, then one can check that the answers are consistent. If the date of birth is given, then one can deduce the corresponding age. In fact, in this example the age observation is redundant. It is sometimes a good idea to include one or two redundant variables as a check on accuracy. Various other general procedures for detecting outliers are described by Barnett and Lewis (1978) as were briefly discussed earlier.

In addition to the above procedure, another simple but very useful check is to get a printout of the data and examine them visually.

Although it may be impractical to check every digit visually, the eye is very efficient at picking out many types of obvious error, particularly repetitions and gross outliers.

When a questionable value or error has been detected, the toxicologist must decide what to do about it. One may be able to go back to the original data source and check the observation. Inversions, repetitions and values in the wrong column can often be corrected in this way. Outliers are more difficult to handle, particularly when they are impossible to check or have been misrecorded in the first place. It may be sensible to treat them as missing values and try to insert a value "guessed" in an appropriate way (e.g., by interpolation or by prediction from other variables). Alternatively, the value may have to be left as unrecorded and then either all observations for the given individual will have to be discarded or one will have to accept unequal numbers of observations for the different variables. With a univariate set of observations, the analysis usually begins with the calculation of two summary statistics, namely the mean and standard deviation. In the multivariate case, the analysis usually begins with the calculation of the mean and standard deviation for each variable and, in addition, the correlation coefficient for each pair of variables is usually calculated. There summary statistics are vital in having a preliminary look at the data.

The sample mean of the jth variable is given by

$$\bar{x}_j = \sum_{r=1}^{n} x_{rj}/n$$

and the sample mean vector, x, is given by $x^T = [x_1, x_2,...,x_n]$. If the observations are a random sample from a population with mean $\bar{x}$, then the sample mean vector x is usually the point estimate of x, and this estimate can easily be shown to be unbiased.

The standard deviation of the jth variable is given by

$$s_j = \sqrt{\left[\sum_{r=1}^{n} (x_{rj} - \bar{x}_j{}^2/(n-1)\right]}$$

The correlation coefficient of variables i and j is given by

$$r_{ij} = \sum_{r=1}^{n} (x_{ri} - \bar{x}_j)(x_{rj} - \bar{x}_j)/(n-1)s_i s_j$$

These coefficients can be conveniently assembled in the sample correlation matrix, R, which is given by

$$R = \begin{bmatrix} 1 & r_{12} & \cdots & r_{1n} \\ r_{21} & 1 & \cdots & r_{2n} \\ \vdots & & & \\ r_n{}^1 & r_n{}^2 & \cdots & 1 \end{bmatrix}$$

Note that the diagonal terms are all unity. This matrix provides an estimate of the corresponding population correlation matrix, P, which was defined earlier in this section. We note in passing that this estimate is generally not unbiased, but the bias is generally small and does not stop us from using the estimate. The virtues of lack of bias are sometimes overstressed.

The interpretation of means and standard deviations is straightforward. It is worth looking to see if, for example, some variables have much higher scatter than others. It is also worth looking at the form of the distribution of each variable, and considering whether any of the variables need to be transformed. For example, the logarithmic transformation is often used to reduce positive skewness and produce a distribution which is closer to normal. One may also consider the removal of outliers at this stage.

There are three significant multivariate techniques which have hypothesis testing as their primary function - MANOVA, MANCOVA and factor analysis.

MANOVA (multivariate analysis of variance) is the multidimensional extension of the ANOVA process we explored before. It can be shown to have grown out of Hotelling's T^2 (Hotelling, 1931), which provides a means of testing the overall null hypothesis that two groups do not differ in their means on any of p measures. MANOVA accomplishes its comparison of two (or more) groups by reducing the set of p measures on each group to a simple number applying the linear combining rule $W_i = w_j X_{ij}$ (where w_j is a weighting factor) and then computing a univariate F-ratio on the combined variables. New sets of weights (w_j) are selected in turn until that set which maximizes the F-ratio is found. The final resulting maximum F-ratio (based on the multiple discriminant functions) is then the basis of the significance test. As with ANOVA, MANOVA can be one-way or higher order, and MANOVA has as a basic assumption a multivariate normal distribution.

Gray and Laskey (1980) used MANOVA to analyze the reproductive effects of manganese in the mouse, allowing identification of significant effects at multiple sites. Witten et al. (1981) utilized MANOVA to determine the significance of the effects of dose, time, and cell division in the action of abrin on the lymphocytes.

Multivariate analysis of covariance (MANCOVA) is the multivariate analog of analysis of covariance. As with MANOVA, it is based on the assumption that the data being analyzed are from a multivariate normal population. The MANCOVA test utilizes the two residual matrices using the statistic, and is an extension of ANCOVA with two or more uncontrolled variables (or covariates). A detailed discussion can be found in Tatsuoka (1971).

Factor analysis is not just a technique for hypothesis testing, it can also serve a reduction of dimensionality function. It seeks to separate the variance unique to particular sets of values from that common to all members in that variable system, and is based on the assumption that the intercorrelations among the n original variables are the result of there being some smaller number of variables ("factors") which explain the bulk of variation seen in the variables. There are several approaches to achieving the end results, but they all seek a determination of what percentage of the variance of each variable is explained by each factor (a factor being one variable or a combination of variables). The model in factor analysis is $y = A + z$, where:

y = n dimensional vector of observable responses;
A = factor loadings an n x q matrix of unknown parameters;
f = q dimensional vector of common factor;
z = n dimensional vector of unique factor.

Used for the reduction of dimensionality, factor analysis is said to be a linear technique because it does not change the linear relationships between the variables being examined.

Joung *et al.* (1979) used factor analysis to develop a generalized water quality index that promises suitability across the U.S., with appropriate weightings for ten parameters.

Factor analysis promises great utility as a tool for developing models in risk analysis where a number of parameters act and interact.

Now we move on to multivariate modeling techniques. We shall briefly discuss two of these: multiple regression and discriminant analysis.

Multiple regression and correlation seeks to predict one (or a few) variable from several others. It assumes that the available variables can be logically divided into two (or more) sets and serves to establish maximal linear (or some other scale) relationships among the sets;

The linear model for the regression is simply

$$Y = b_0 + b_1X_1 + b_2X_2 + ... + b_pX_p$$
where Y = the predicted value
b = values set to maximize correlations between X and Y and X and Y = the actual observations

(with X's being independent of predictor variables and Y's being dependent variables or outcome measures). One of the outputs from the process will be the coefficient of multiple correlation, which is simply the multivariate equivalent of the correlation coefficient (r).

Schaeffer *et al.* (1982) have neatly demonstrated the utilization of multiple regression in studying the contribution of two components of a mixture to its toxicologic action, using quantitative results from an Ames test as an end point. Paintz *et al.* (1982) similarly used multiple regression to model the quantitative structure-activity relationships of a series of fourteen 1-benzoyl-3-methyl-pyrazole derivatives.

Discriminant analysis has for its main purpose finding linear combinations of variables which maximize the differences between the populations being studied, with the objective of establishing a model to sort objects into their appropriate populations with minimal error. At least four major questions are, in a sense, being asked of the data:

1. Are there significant differences among the K groups?
2. If the groups do exhibit statistical differences, how do the central masses (or centroids, the multivariate equivalent of means) of the populations differ?
3. What are the relative distances among the K groups?
4. How are new (or at this point unknown) members allocated to *establish* groups? How do you predict the set of responses of characteristics of an as yet untried exposure case?

The discriminant functions used to produce the linear combinations are of the form:

$$D_i = d_{i1}Z_1 + d_{i2}Z_2 \ldots + d_{ip}Z_p$$

where D_i = the score on the discriminant function i
d's = weighing coefficients
Z's = standardized values of the discriminating
variables used in the analysis

It should be noted that discriminant analysis can also be used for the hypothesis testing function by the expedient of evaluating how well it correctly classifies members into proper groups (say control, treatment 1, treatment 2, etc.)

Taketomo *et al.* (1982) used discriminant analysis in a retrospective study of gentamycin nephrotoxicity to identify patient risk factors (that is, variables which contributed to a prediction of a patient being at risk).

Finally, we introduce four techniques whose primary function is the reduction of dimensionality - canonical correlation analysis, principal components analysis, biplot analysis and correspondence analysis.

Canonical correlation analysis provides the canonical R, an overall measure of the relationship between two sets of variables (one set consisting of several outcome measures, the other of several predictor variables). The canonical R is calculated on two numbers for each subject:

$$W_i = \Sigma w_j X_{ij} \text{ and } V_i = \Sigma v_i Y_{ij}$$

where X's = predictor variables
Y's = outcome measures
W_j and V_j = canonical coefficients

MANOVA can be considered a special case of canonical correlation analysis. Canonical can be used in hypothesis testing also for testing the association of pairs of sets of weights, each with a corresponding coefficient of canonical correlation, each uncorrelated with any of the preceding sets of weights, and each accounting for successively less of the variation shared by the two sets of variables. For example, Young and Matthews (1981) used canonical correlation analysis to evaluate the relationship between plant growth and environmental factors at 12 different sites.

The main purpose of principal components analysis is to describe as economically as possible, the total variance in a sample in a few dimensions; one wishes to reduce the dimensionality of the original data while minimizing the loss of information. It seeks to resolve the total variation of a set of variables into linearly independent composite variables which successively account for the maximum possible variability in the data. The fundamental equation is $Y = AZ$, where:

A = matrix of scales eigenvectors
Z = original data matrix
and Y = principal components

The concentration here, as in factor analysis, is on relationships within a single set of variables. Note that the results of principal components analysis are affected by linear transformations.

Cremer and Seville (1982) used principal components to compare the difference in blood parameters resulting from each of two separate pyrethroids. Henry and Hidy (1979), meanwhile, used principal components to identify the most significant contributors to air quality problems.

The biplot display (Gabriel, 1981) of multivariate data is a relatively new technique, but promises wide applicability to problems in toxicology. It is, in a sense, a form of exploratory data analysis, used for data summarization and description.

The biplot is a graphical display of a matrix Y_{nmx} of N rows and M columns by means of row and column marker. The display carries one marker for each row and each column. The "bi" in biplot refers to the joint display of rows and columns. Such plots are used primarily for inspection of data and for data diagnostics when such data are in the form of matrices.

Shy-Modjeska *et al.* (1984) illustrated this usage in the analysis of aminoglycoside renal data from beagle dogs, allowing the simultaneous display of relationships among different observed variables and presentation of the relationship of both individuals and treatment groups to these variables.

Correspondence analysis is a technique for displaying the rows and columns of a two-way contingency table as points in a corresponding low dimensional vector space. As such it is equivalent to simultaneous linear regression (for contingency table data, such as tumor incidences, which is a very common data form in toxicology). As such it can be considered a special case of canonical correlation analysis. The data are defined, described and analyzed in a geometric framework. This is particularly attractive to such sets of observations in toxicology as multiple end point behavioral scores and scored multiple tissue lesions.

There are a number of good surveys of multivariate techniques available (Atchely and Bryant, 1975; Bryant and Atchely, 1975; Seal, 1964) which are not excessively mathematical. More rigorous mathematical treatments on an introductory level are also available (eg Gnanadesikan, 1977). It should be noted that most of the techniques we have described are available in the better computer statistical packages.

REFERENCES

Atchely, W.R., and Bryant, E.H. (1975): *Multivariate Statistical Methods: Among Groups Covariation*. Dowden, Hutchinson and Ross, Stroudsburg.

Barnett, V., and Lewis, T. (1978): *Outliers in Statistical Data*. John Wiley, New York.

Bryant, E.H., and Atchely, W.R. (1975): *Multivariate Statistical Methods: Within-Groups Covariation*. Dowden, Hutchinson and Ross, Stroudsburg.

Cremer, J.E. and Seville, M.P. (1982): Comparative effects of two pyrethroids dietamethrin and cismethrin, on plasma catecholamines and on blood glucose and lactate. *Toxicol. Appl. Pharmacol.*, 66:124–133.

Davidson, M.L. (1972): Univariate versus multivariate tests in repeated-measures experiments. *Psych. Bull.*, 77:446–452.

Gabriel, K.R. (1981) Biplot Display of Multivariate Matrices for Inspection of Data and Diagnosis: *In: Interpreting Multivariate Data* pp. 147–173. (V. Barnett, Ed) John Wiley, New York.

Gnanadesikan, R. (1977): *Methods for Statistical Data Analysis of Multivariate Observations*. John Wiley, New York.

Gray, L.E. and Laskey, J.W. (1980): Multivariate Analysis of the Effects of Manganese on the Reproductive Physiology and Behavior of the Male House Mouse. *J. Toxicol. Environ. Health.*, 6:861–868.

Greenacre, M.J. (1981): Practical Correspondence Analysis in *Interpreting Multivariate Data* (V. Barnett, Ed.) John Wiley, New York.

Henry, R.D. and Hidy, G.M. (1979): Multivariate Analysis of Particulate Sulfate and Other Air Quality Variables by Principal Components. *Atmos. Environ.*, 13:1581–1596.

Hotelling, H. (1931): The generalization of Student's ratio. *Ann. Math. Stat.*, 2:360–378.

Joung, H.M., Miller, W.M., Mahannah, C.N., and Guitjens, J.C. (1979): A Generalized Water Quality Index Based on Multivariate Factor Analysis. *J. Environ. Qual.*, 8:95–100.

Paintz, M., Bekemeier, H., Metzner, J. and Wenzel, U. (1982): Pharmacological Activities of a Homologous Series of Pyrazole Derivatives including Qunatitative Structure - Activity Relationships (QSAR). *Agents Actions;* (Suppl) 10:47–58.

Schaeffer, D.J., Glave, W.R. and Janardan, K.G. (1982): Multivariate Statistical Methods in Toxicology. III. Specifying Joint Toxic Interaction Using Multiple Regression Analysis *J. Toxicol. Env. Health*, 9:705–718.

Schaffer, J.W., Forbes, J.A. and Defelice, E.A. (1967): Some sugggested approaches to the analysis of chronic toxicity and chronic drug administration data. *Toxicol. Appl. Pharmacol.*, 10:514–522.

Seal, H.L. (1964): *Multivariate Statistical Analysis for Biologists*. Methuen, London.

Shy-Modjeska, J.S., Riviere, J.E. and Rawldings, J.O. (1984): Application of Biplot Methods to the Multivariate Analysis of Toxicological and Pharmacokinetic Data. *Toxicol. Appl. Pharmacol.*, 72:91–101.

Taketomo, R.T., McGhan, W.F., Fushiki, M.R., Shimada, A. and Gumpert, N.F. (1982): Gentamycin nephrotoxicity application of multivariate analysis. *Clin. Pharm.*, 1: 554–549.

Tatsuoka, M.M. (1971) *Multivariate Analysis*, John Wiley, New York

Witten, M., Bennet, C.E. and Glassman, A. (1981): Studies on the toxicity and binding kinetics of abrin in normal and Epstein Barr virus - transformed lymphocyte culture - I: experimental results *Exp. Cell. Biol.*, 49–306–318.

Young, J.E. and Matthews, P. (1981): Pollution Injury in Southeast Northumberland, England UK; The Analysis of Field Data Using Economical Correlation Analysis. *Environ. Pollut. Sen. B. Chem. Phys.*, 2:353–366.

CHAPTER 11

DATA ANALYSIS APPLICATIONS IN TOXICOLOGY

Having reviewed basic principles and provided a set of methods for statistical handling of data, the remainder of this book will address the practical aspects and difficulties encountered in day-to-day toxicological work.

As a starting point, we present in Table 5 an overview of data types actually encountered in toxicology, classified by type (as presented at the beginning of this book). It should be stressed, however, that this classification is of the most frequent measure of each sort of observation (such as body weight) and will not always be an accurate classification.

TABLE 5

Classification of Data Commonly Encountered in Toxicology, by Type

Continuous Normal:	Body Weights
	Food Consumption
	Organ Weights: Absolute & Relative
	Mouse Ear Swelling Test (MEST) Measurements
	Pregnancy Rates
	Survival Rates
	Crown-Rump Lengths
	Hematology (Some)
	Clinical Chemistry (Some)
Continuous But Not Normal:	Hematology (Some-WBC)
	Clinical Chemistry (Some)
	Urinalysis

TABLE 5 (cont'd)

Scalar Data: Neurobehavioral Signs (Some)
                PDI Scores
                Histopathology (Some)

Count Data: Resorption Sites
                Implantation Sites
                Stillborns
                Hematology
                (Some-Reticulocyte counts//Howel-Jolly
                //WBC Differentials)

Categorical Data: Clinical Signs
                    Neurobehavioral Signs (Some)
                    Ocular Scores
                    GP Sensitization Scores
                    Mouse Ear Swelling Tests (MEST) Sensiti-
                    zation Counts
                    Fetal Abnormalities
                    Dose/Mortality Data
                    Sex Ratios
                    Histopathology Data (Most)

There are now common practices in the analysis of toxicology data, though they are not necessarily the best. These are discussed in the remainder of this chapter, which seeks to review statistical methods on a use-by-use basis and to provide a foundation for the selection of alternatives in specific situations.

Median Lethal and Effective Doses

For many years, the starting point for evaluating the toxicity of an agent was to determine its LD_{50} or LC_{50}, which are the dose or concentration of a material at which half of a population of animals would be expected to die. These figures are analogous to the ED_{50} (effective dose for half a population) used in pharmacologic activities, and are derived by the same means.

To calculate either of these figures we need, at each of several dosage (or exposure) levels, the number of animals dosed and the number that died. If we seek only to establish the median effective dose in a range-finding test, then 4 or 5 animals per dose level, using Thompson's method of moving averages, is the most efficient methodology and will give a sufficiently accurate solution. With two dose levels, if the ratio between the high and low dose is two or less, even total or no mortality at these two dose levels will yield an acceptably accurate median lethal dose, although a partial mortality is desirable. If, however, we wish to estimate a number of toxicity levels (LD_{10}, LD_{90}) and are interested in more precisely establishing the slope of the dose/lethality curve, the use of at least 10 animals per dosage level with the log/probit regresion technique described in the Chapter VIII section would be the most common approach. Note that in the equation $Y_i = a + bx_i$, b is the slope of the regression line, and that our method already allows us to calculate 95% confidence intervals about any point on this line. Note that the confidence interval at any one point will be different from the interval at other points, and must be calculated separately. Additionally, the nature of the probit transform is such that toward the extremes - LD_{10} and LD_{90}, for example - the confidence intervals will "balloon". That is, they become very wide. Because the slope of the fitted line in these assays has a very large uncertainty, in relation to the uncertainty of the LD_{50} itself (the midpoint of the distribution), much caution must be used with calculated LD_xs other than LD_{50}s. The imprecision of the LD_{35}, a value close to the LD_{50}, is discussed by Weil (1972), as is that of the slope of the log dose-probit line (Weil, 1975). Debanne and Haller (1985) recently reviewed the statistical aspects of different methodologies for estimating a median effective dose.

There have been questions for years as to the value of LD_{50} and the efficiency of the current study design (which uses large numbers of animals) in determining it. As long ago as 1953, Weil *et al.* presented forceful arguments that an estimate having only minimally reduced precision could be made using significantly fewer animals. More recently, the last few years have seen an increased level of concern over the numbers and uses of animals in research and testing, and have produced additional arguments against existing methodologies for determining the LD_{50}, or even the need to make the determination at all (Zbinden and Flury-Roversi, 1981). In response, a number of suggestions for alternative methodologies have been advanced (Depass *et al.*, 1984; Gad *et al.*, 1984; Bruce, 1985).

Body and Organ Weights

Among the sets of data commonly collected in studies where animals are dosed with (or exposed to) a chemical are body weight and the weights of selected organs. In fact, body weight is frequently the most sensitive indication of an adverse effect. How to best analyze this and in what form to analyze the organ weight data (as absolute weights, weight changes, or percentages of body weight) have been the subject of a number of articles (Jackson, 1962; Weil, 1962; Weil, 1970; Weil and Gad, 1980).

Both absolute body weights and rates of body weight change (calculated as changes from a baseline measurement value which is traditionally the animal's weight immediately prior to the first dosing with or exposure to test material) are almost universally best analyzed by ANOVA followed, if called for, by a *post hoc* test. Even if the groups were randomized properly at the beginning of a study (no group being significantly different in mean body weight from any other group, and all animals in all groups within two standard deviations of the overall mean body weight), there is an advantage to performing the computationally slightly more cumbersome (compared to absolute body weights) changes in body weight analysis. The advantage is an increase in sensitivity, because the adjustment of starting points (the setting of initial weights as a "zero" value) acts to reduce the amount of initial variability. In this case, Bartlett's test is performed first to ensure homogeneity of variance and the appropriate sequence of analysis follows.

With smaller sample sizes, the normality of the data becomes increasingly uncertain and nonparametric methods such as Kruskal-Wallis may be more appropriate (see Zar, 1974).

The analysis of relative (to body weight) organ weights is a valuable tool for identifying possible target organs (Gad *et al.*, 1984). How to perform this analysis is still a matter of some disagreement, however.

Weil (1962) presented evidence that organ weight data expressed as percentages of body weight should be analyzed separately for each sex. Furthermore, since the conclusions from organ weight data of males differed so often from those of females, data from animals of each sex should be used in this measurement. Also, Weil (1970, 1973) Boyd and Knight (1963), and Boyd (1972) have discussed in detail other factors which influence organ weights and must be taken into account.

The two competing approaches to analyzing relative organ weights call for either

(1) calculating organ weights as a percentage of total body weight (at the time of necropsy) and analyzing the results by ANOVA, or

(2) analyzing results by ANCOVA, with body weights as the covariates as discussed previously by the authors (Weil and Gad, 1980).

A number of considerations should be kept in mind when these questions are addressed. First, one must keep a firm grasp on the difference between biological significance and statistical significance. In this particular case, we are especially interested in examining organ weights when an organ weight change is not proportional to changes in whole body weights. Second, we are now required to detect smaller and smaller changes while still retaining a similar sensitivity (i.e., the $p < 0.05$ level).

There are several devices to attain the desired increase in power. One is to use larger and larger sample sizes (number of animals) and the other is to utilize the most powerful test we can. However, the use of even currently employed numbers of animals is being vigorously questioned and the power of statistical tests must, therefore, now assume an increased importance in our considerations.

The biological rationale behind analyzing both absolute body weight and the organ weight to body weight ratio (this latter as opposed to a covariance analysis of organ weights) is that in the majority of cases, except for the brain, the organs of interest in the body change weight (except in extreme cases of obesity or starvation) in proportion to total body weight. We are particularly interested in detecting cases where this is not so. Analysis of actual data from several hundred studies (unpublished data) has shown no significant difference in rates of weight change of target organs (other than the brain) compared to total body weight for healthy animals in those species commonly used for repeated dose studies (rats, mice, rabbits and dogs). Furthermore, it should be noted that analysis of covariance is of questionable validity in analyzing body weight and related organ weight changes, since a primary assumption is the independence of treatment - that the relationship of the two variables is the same for all treatments (Ridgeman, 1975). Plainly, in toxicology this is not true.

In cases where the differences between the error mean squares are much greater, the ratio of F ratios will diverge in precision from the result of the efficiency of covariance adjustment. These cases are where either sample sizes are much larger or where the differences between means themselves are much larger. This latter case is one which does not occur in the designs under discussion in any manner that would leave analysis of dovariance as a valid approach, because group means start out being very similar and cannot diverge markedly unless there is a treatment effect. As we have discussed earlier, a treatment effect invalidates a prime underpinning assumption of analysis of covariance.

Shirley and Newnham (1984) have argued the case for ANCOVA, but without providing answers to arguments presented above.

Clinical Chemistry

A number of clinical chemistry parameters are commonly determined on the blood and urine collected from animals in chronic, subchronic, and occasionally acute, toxicity studies. In the past (and still, in some places), the accepted practice has been to evaluate these data using univariate-parametric methods (primarily t-tests and/or

ANOVA). However, this can be shown to be not the best approach on a number of grounds.

First, such biochemical parameters are rarely independent of each other. Neither is our interest often focused on just one of the parameters. Rather, there are batteries of the parameters associated with toxic actions at particular target organs. For example, increases in creatinine phosphokinase (CPK), γ-hydroxybutyrate dehydrogenase (γ-HBDH), and lactate dehydrogenase (LDH), occurring together, are strongly indicative of myocardial damage. In such cases, we are not just interested in a significant increase in oen of these, but in all three. Table 6 gives a brief overview of the association of varios parameters with actions at particular target organs. A more detailed coverage of the interpretation of such clinical laboratory tests can be found in Wallach (1978).

Similarly, the serum electrolytes (sodium, potassium, and calcium) interact with each other; a decrease in one is frequently tied, for instance, to an increase in one of the others. Furthermore, the nature of the data (in the case of some parameters), either because of the biological nature of the parameter or the way in which it is measured, is frequently either not normally distributed (particularly because of being markedly skewed) or not continuous in nature. This can be seen in some of the reference data for experimental animals in Mitruka and Rawnsley, (1977) or Weil (1982) in, for example, creatinine, sodium, potassium, chloride, calcium and blood urea nitrogen. It should be remembered that both normal distribution and continuous data are underlying assumptions in the parametric statistical techniques described in this chapter.

In recent acute, subchronic and chronic studies we have been involved with, clinical chemistry statistical test methodologies were selected in accordance with the decision tree approach presented at the beginning of this volume. The methods this approach most frequently resulted in are outlined in Table 7. This may serve as a guide to the uninitiated. A more detailed discussion may be found in Martin *et al.* (1975) or Harris (1978).

Hematology

Much of what we said about clinical chemistry parameters is also true for the hematologic measurements made in toxicology studies. Which test to perform should be evaluated by use of a decision tree until one becomes confident as to the most appropriate methods. Keep in mind that sets of values and (in some cases) population distribution vary not only between species, but also between the commonly used strains of species and that "control" or "standard" values will "drift" over the course of only a few years.

TABLE 6

ASSOCIATION OF CHANGES IN BIOCHEMICAL PARAMETERS WITH ACTIONS AT PARTICULAR TARGET ORGANS

PARAMETER	ORGAN SYSTEM								NOTES
	BLOOD	HEART	LUNG	KIDNEY	LIVER	BONE	INTESTINE	PANCREAS	
Albumin				↓	↓				Produced by the liver. Very significant reductions indicate extensive liver damage.
AP (Alkaline phosphatase)					↑	↑	↑		Elevations usually associated with cholestasis. Bone alkaline phosphatase tends to be higher in young animals.
Bilirubin (Total)	↑				↑				Usually elevated due to cholestasis-either due to obstruction or hepatopathy

TABLE 6 (continued)

PARAMETER	ORGAN SYSTEM								NOTES
	BLOOD	HEART	LUNG	KIDNEY	LIVER	BONE	INTESTINE	PANCREAS	
BUN (Blood Urea Nitrogen)				↑	↓				Estimates blood filtering capacity of the kidneys. Doesn't become significantly elevated until kidney function is reduced 60-75%
Calcium				↑					Can be life threatening and result in acute death.
Cholinesterase				↑	↓				Found in plasma, brain and RBC
CPK (Creatinine Phosphokinase)		↑							Most often elevated due to skeletal muscle damage but can also be produced by cardiac muscle damage. Can be more sensitive

PARAMETER	BLOOD	HEART	LUNG	KIDNEY	LIVER	BONE	INTESTINE	PANCREAS	NOTES
									than histopathology
Creatinine				←					Also estimates blood filtering capacity of kidney as BUN does. More specific than BUN
Glucose					←			←	Alterations other than those associated with stress are uncommon and reflect an effect on the pancreatic islets or anorexia
GGT (Gamma glutamyl transferase)									Elevated in cholestasis. This is a microsomal enzyme and levels often increase in response to microsomal enzyme induction.

TABLE 6 (continued)

ORGAN SYSTEM

PARAMETER	BLOOD	HEART	LUNG	KIDNEY	LIVER	BONE	INTESTINE	PANCREAS	NOTES
HBDH (Hydroxybutyric dehyrogenase)		←			←				
LDH (Lactic dehydrogenase)		←	←	←	←				Increase usually due to skeletal muscle, cardiac muscle and liver damage. Not very specific.
Protein (Total)				←	←				Absolute alterations are usually associated with decreased production (liver) or increased loss (kidney).
SGOT (Serum glutamic-oxaloacetic transaminase)		←		←	←			←	Present in skeletal muscle and heart and most commonly associated

PARAMETER	BLOOD	HEART	LUNG	KIDNEY	LIVER	BONE	INTESTINE	PANCREAS	NOTES
									with damage to these.
SGPT (Serum glutamic-pyruvic transaminase)					↑				Elevations usually associated with hepatic damage or disease
Sorbitol dehydrogenase					↑				Liver enzyme which can be quite sensitive but is fairly unstable. Samples should be processed as soon as possible

Arrow indicates increase (↑) or decrease (↓)

TABLE 7

Tests often used in analysis of clinical chemistry data

Clinical chemistry parameters	Statistical test
Calcium	ANOVA, Bartlett's and/or F test, t-Test
Glucose	ANOVA, Bartlett's and/or F test, t-Test
Blood-urea-nitrogen	ANOVA, Bartlett's and/or F test, t-Test
Creatinine	ANOVA, Bartlett's and/or F test, t-Test
Cholinesterase	ANOVA, Bartlett's and/or F test, t-Test
Total bilirubin	Kruskal-Wallis nonparametric ANOVA
Total protein	ANOVA, Bartlett's and/or F test, t-Test
Albumin	ANOVA, Bartlett's and/or F test, t-Test
GGT	Kruskal-Wallis nonparametric ANOVA
HBDH	ANOVA, Bartlett's and/or F test, t-Test
AP	ANOVA, Bartlett's and/or F test, t-Test
CPK	ANOVA, Bartlett's and/or F test, t-Test
LDH	ANOVA, Bartlett's and/or F test, t-Test
SGOT	ANOVA, Bartlett's and/or F test, t-Test
SGPT	ANOVA, Bartlett's and/or F test, t-Test
Hgb	ANOVA, Bartlett's and/or F test, t-Test

Again, the majority of these parameters are interrelated and highly dependent on the method used to determine them. Red blood cell count (RBC), platelet counts, and mean corpuscular volume (MCV) may be determined using a device such as a Coulter counter to take direct measurements, and the resulting data are usually suitable for parametric methods. The hematocrit, however, may actually be a value calculated from the RBC and MCV values and, if so, is dependent on them. If the hematocrit is measured directly, instead of being calculated from the RBC and MCV, it may be compared by parametric methods.

Hemoglobin is directly measured and is an independent and continuous variable. However, and probably because at any one time a number of forms and conformations (oxyhemoglobin, deoxyhemoglobin, methemoglobin, etc.) of hemoglobin are actually present) the distribution seen is not typically a normal one, but rather may be a multimodal one. Here a nonparametric technique such as the Wilcoxon or multiple rank-sum test is called for.

Consideration of the white blood cell (WBC) and differential counts leads to another problem. The total WBC is, typically, a normal population amenable to parametric analysis, but differential counts are normally determined by counting, manually, one or more sets of one hundred cells each. The resulting relative percentages of neutrophils are then reported as either percentages or are multiplied by the total WBC count with the resulting "count" being reported as the "absolute" differential WBC. Such data, particularly in the case of eosinophils (where the distribution do not approach normality and should usually be analyzed by nonparametric methods. It is widely believed that "relative" (%) differential data should not be reported because they are likely to be misleading.

Lastly, it should always be kept in mind that it is rare for a change in any single hematologic parameter to be meaningful. Rather, because these parameters are so interrelated, patterns of changes in parameters should be expected if a real effect is present, and analysis and interpretation of results should focus on such patterns of changes. Classification analysis techniques often provide the basis for a useful approach to such problems.

Histopathologic Lesion Incidence

The last twenty years have seen increasing emphasis placed on histopathological examination of tissues collected from animals in subchronic and chronic toxicity studies. While it is not true that only those lesions which occur at a statistically significantly increased rate in treated/exposed animals are of concern (for there are the cases where a lesion may be of such a rare type that the occurrence of only one or a few such in treated animals "raises a flag"), it is true that, in most cases, a statistical evaluation is the only way to determine if what we see in treated animals is significantly worse than what has been seen in control animals. And although cancer is not our only concern, this category of lesions is that of greatest interest.

Typically, comparison of incidences of any one type of lesion between controls and treated animals are made using the multiple 2 x 2 chi square test or Fisher's exact test with a modification of the numbers of animals as the denominators. Too often, experimenters exclude from consideration all those animals (in both groups) which died prior to the first animals being found with a lesion at that site. The special case of carcinogenicity bioassays will be discussed in detail in the next chapter.

An option which should be kept in mind is that, frequently, a pathologist can not only identify a lesion as present, but also grade those present as to severity. This represents a significant increase in the information content of the data which should not be given up by performing an analysis based only on the perceived quantal nature (present/absent) of the data. Quantal data, analyzed by chi-square or Fisher's exact tests, are a subset (the 2 X 2 case) of categorical or contingency table data. In this case it also becomes ranked (or "ordinal") data - the categories are naturally ordered (for example, no effect > mild lesion > moderate lesion > severe lesion). This gives a 2 X R table if there are only one treatment and one control group, or an N X R ("multiway") table if there are three or more groups of animals.

The traditional method of analyzing multiple, cross-classified data has been to collapse the N X R contingency table over all but two of the variables, and to follow this with the computation of some measure of association between these variables. For an N-dimensional table this results in $N(N-1)/2$ separate analyses. The result is crude, "giving away" information and even (by inappropriate pooling of data) yielding a faulty understanding of the meaning of data. Though computationally more laborious, a multiway (N X R table) analysis should be utilized.

Reproduction

The reproductive implications of the toxic effects of chemicals are becoming increasingly important. Because of this, reproduction studies, together with other closely related types of studies (such as teratogenesis, dominant lethal, and mutagenesis studies, which are discussed later in this chapter), are now commonly companion to chronic toxicity studies.

One point that must be kept in mind with all reproduction-related studies is the nature of the appropriate sampling unit. What is the appropriate N in such a study; the number of individual pups, the number of litters, pregnant females? Fortunately, it is now fairly well accepted that the first case (using the number of offspring as the N) is inappropriate (Weil, 1970). The real effects in such studies actually occur in the female that was exposed to the chemical, or that is mated to a male which was exposed. What happens to her, and to the development of the litter she is carrying, is biologically independent of what happens to every other female/litter in the study. This cannot be said for each offspring in each litter; for example, the death of one member of a litter can and will be related to what happens to every other member. Or the effect on all of the offspring might be similar for all of those from one female and different or lacking for those from another.

As defined by Oser and Oser (1956), there are four primary variables of interest in a reproduction study. First, there is the fertility index (FI) which may be defined as the percentage of attempted matings (i.e., each female housed with a male) which resulted in pregnancy, pregnancy being determined by a method such as the presence of implantation sites in the female. Second, there is the gestation index (GI) which is defined as the percentage of mated females, as evidenced by a vaginal plug being dropped or a positive vaginal smear, which deliver viable litters (i.e., litters with at least one live pup). Two related variables which may also be studied are the mean number of pups born per litter and the percentage of total pups per litter that are stillborn. Third, there is the viability index (VI) which is defined as the percentage of offspring born that survive at least 4 days after birth. Finally (in this four variable system) there is the lactation index (LI), which is the percentage of animals per litter which survive 4 days and also survive to weaning. In rats and mice, this is classically taken to be 21 days after birth. An additional variable which may reasonably be included in such a study is the mean weight gain per pup per litter.

Given that our N is at least 10 (we will further explore proper sample size under the topic of teratology), we may test each of these variables for significance using a method such as the Wilcoxon-Mann-Whitney U test, or the Kruskal-Wallis nonparametric ANOVA. If N is less than 10, we cannot expect the central limit theorem to be operative and should use the Wilcoxon sum of ranks (for two groups) or the Kruskal-Wallis nonparametric ANOVA (for three or more groups) to compare groups.

Teratology

When the primary concern of a reproductive/developmental study is the occurrence of birth defects or deformations (terata, either structural or functional) in the offspring of exposed animals, the study is one of teratology. In the analysis of the data from such a study, we must consider several points.

First is sample size. Earlier in this book we reviewed this topic generally, and presented a method to estimate sufficient sample size. The difficulties with applying these methods here revolve around two points: (1) selecting a sufficient level of sensitivity for detecting an effect and (2) factoring in how many animals will be removed from study (without contributing a datum) by either not becoming pregnant or not surviving to a sufficiently late stage of pregnancy. Experience generally dictates that one should attempt to have twenty pregnant animals per study group if a pilot study has provided some confidence that the pregnant test animals will survive the dose levels selected. Again, it is essential to recognize that the litter, not the fetus, is the basic independent unit for each variable.

A more fundamental consideration, alluded to in the section on reproduction, is that as we use more animals, the mean of means (each variable will be such in a mathematical sense) will approach normality in its distribution. This is one of the implications of the Central Limit Theorem; even when the individual data are not normally distributed, their means will approach normality in their distribution. At a sample size of ten or greater, the approximation of normality is such that we may use a parametric test (such as a t-test or ANOVA) to evaluate results. At sample sizes less than ten, a nonparametric test (Wilcoxon rank-sum or Kruskal-Wallis nonparametric ANOVA) is more appropriate. Other methodologies have been suggested (Kupper and Haseman, 1978; Nelson and Holson, 1978) but do not offer any prospect of widespread usage. One nonparametric method that is widely used is the Mann-Whitney U test, which was described earlier. Williams and Buschbom (1982) further discuss some of the available statistical options and their consequences, and Rai and Ryzin (1985) have recommended a dose responsive model.

Dominant Lethal Assay

The dominant lethal study is essentially a reproduction study which seeks to study the end point of lethality to the fetuses after implantation and before delivery. The proper identification of the sampling unit (the pregnant female) and the design of an experiment so that a sufficiently large sample is available for analysis are the prime statistical considerations. The question of sampling unit has been adequately addressed in earlier sections. Sample size is of concern here because the hypothesis-testing techniques which are appropriate with small samples are of relatively low power, as the variability about the mean in such cases is relatively large. With sufficient sample size [e.g., from 30 to 50 pregnant females per dose level per week (Bateman, 1977)] variability about the mean and the nature of the distribution allow sensitive statistical techniques to be employed.

The variables that are typically recorded and included in analysis are (for each level/week): (a) the number of pregnant females, (b) live fetuses/pregnancy, (c) total implants/pregnancy, (d) early fetal deaths (early resorptions)/pregnancy, and (e) late fetal deaths/pregnancy.

A wide variety of techniques for analysis of these data have been (and are) used. Most common is the use of ANOVA after the data have been transformed by the arc sine transform (Mosteller and Youty, 1961).

Beta binomial (Aeschbacher *et al.*, 1977; Vuataz and Sotek, 1978) and Poisson distributions (Dean and Jonston, 1977) have also been attributed to these data, and transforms and appropriate tests have been proposed for use in each of these cases (in each case with the note that the transforms serve to "stabilize the variance" of the data). With sufficient sample size, as defined earlier in this section, the Mann-

Whitney U test is recommended for use here. Smaller sample sizes necessitate the use of the Wilcoxon rank-sum test.

Diet and Chamber Analysis

Earlier we presented the basic principles and methods for sampling. Sampling is important in many aspects of toxicology, and here we address its application to diet preparation and the analysis of atmospheres from inhalation chambers.

In feeding studies, we seek to deliver desired doses of a material to animals by mixing the material with their diet. Similarly, in an inhalation study we mix a material with the air the test animals breathe.

In both cases, we must then sample the medium (food or atmosphere) and analyze these samples to determine what levels or concentrations of material were actually present and to assure ourselves that the test material is homogeneously distributed. Having an accurate picture of these delivered concentrations, and how they varied over the course of time, is essential on a number of grounds:

1. The regulatory agencies and sound scientific practice require that analyzed diet and mean daily inhalation atmosphere levels be ± 10% of the target level.

2. Excessive peak concentrations, because of the overloading of metabolic repair systems, could result in extreme acute effects that would lead to results in a chronic study which are not truly indicative of the chronic low-level effects of the compound, but rather of periods of metabolic and physiologic overload. Such results could be misinterpreted if true exposure or diet levels were not maintained at a realtively constant level.

Sampling strategies are not just a matter of numbers (for statistical aspects), but of geometry, so that the contents of a container or the entire atmosphere in a chamber is truly sampled; and of time, in accordance with the stability of the test compound. The samples must be both randomly collected and representative of the entire mass of what one is trying to characterize. In the special case of sampling and characterizing the physical properties of aerosols in an inhalation study, some special considerations and terminology apply. Because of the physiologic characteristics of the respiration of humans and of test animals, our concern is very largely limited to those particles or droplets which are of a respirable size. Unfortunately, "respirable size" is a complex characteristic based on aerodynamic diameter, density, and physiological characteristics. Unfortunately, while those particles with an aerodynamic diameter of less than ten microns are generally agreed to be respirable in humans (that is, they can be drawn down to the deep portions of the lungs), three microns in aerodynamic diameter is a more realistically value. The one favorable factor is that there are now available a selection of instruments which accurately (and relatively easily) collect and measure particles or droplets. These measurements result in concentrations in a defined volume of gas, and can be expressed as either a number concentration or a mass concentration (the latter being more common). Such measurements generate categorical data - concentrations are measured in each of a series of aerodynamic size groups (such as > 100 microns, 100-25 microns, 25-10 microns, 10-3 microns, etc.). The appropriate descriptive statistics for this class of data are the geometric mean and its standard deviation. These aspects and the statistical interpretation of the data that are finally collected should be considered after sufficient interaction with the appropriate professionals. Typically, it then becomes a matter of the calculation of measures of central tendency and dispersion statistics, with the identification of those values which are beyond acceptable limits (Bliss, 1965).

Aerosol Statistics

An additional complication to characterizing atmospheres in inhalation chambers when the test material is delivered as an aerosol (either liquid or solid dispersed droplets or particles) is that the entire basis of descriptive statistics is different. Early in this book we introduced the geometric mean as the appropriate description of location for an aerosol population. A more rigorous and extensive discussion is necessary, however.

An aerosol atmosphere most commonly contains a wide range of particle sizes and cannot be defined adequately by an arithmetic average diameter. A knowledge of the size distribution and a mathematical expression to describe it are highly desirable, especially when it is necessary to estimate particulate characteristics that are not measured directly. Many mathematical relationships have been proposed to describe particle size distributions. Of these, the most widely used in aerosol work is the lognormal distribution, which is merely the normal distribution applied to the logarithms of the quantities actually measured. This discussion of the lognormal distribution, therefore, should be preceded by a review of the normal distribution.

If the quantity x = ln D is normally distributed, then the distribution of D (the particle diameter) is said to be lognormal. The lognormal distribution is particularly useful in particle size analysis because of the characteristics described in the following.

Consider a property of a particle that can be defined quantitatively by

$$Q_r(D) = \alpha_r D^r,$$

where Q_r is a constant (shape factor) for a given value of r. For a lognormal distribution, the relative number of particles having diameters whose logarithms fall in the interval x ± dx/2 is given by

$$f(x)\,dx = \frac{1}{\sigma(2\pi)^{1/2}} \cdot \exp[-(x\mu)^2/2\sigma^2]\cdot dx,$$

where μ is the true population mean, δ is the true population standard deviation, f(x) is the normal probability distribution function

$$\mu_0 = \ln \delta_{og},$$

and δ_{og} is the geometric mean diameter of the population.

The large amount of information available concerning the statistics of sampling from a normal distribution is directly applicable to particle size analysis when D is lognormally distributed. For a sample of N particles, the maximum likelihood statistics, m and s, are given by the following two equations: (Mercer, 1973)

$$m = \ln D_{og} = \sum_{1}^{N} \ln D_i / N,$$

and

$$s = \ln \sigma_g = \left[\sum_{1}^{N}(\ln D_i - \ln D_{og})^2/(N-1)\right]^{1/2}$$

In practice, D_{0g}, which estimates the population count median diameter $^\sigma og$, and $^\sigma g$, which estimates the population geometric standard deviation e^σ, are reported, rather than m and s. The mean logarithms of the D^r distributions are then estimated using the Hatch-Choate equation:

$$\ln D_{rg} = \ln D_{og} + rs^2,$$

or

$$D_{rg} = D_{0g} \cdot \exp(rs^2).$$

The diameter of the particle having the average amount of Qr is calculated from

$$\ln D_r = \ln D_{og} + rs^2/2,$$

or

$$\bar{D}_r = D_{0g} \cdot \exp(rs^2/2).$$

For samples of N particles, the sampling distribution of the mean logarithm of diameters m is normal and has a mean of μ_0 and a standard deviation equal to $\sigma \sqrt{N}$. For the values of N of interest in particle size work, the sampling distribution of the variance s^2 is also normal, having a mean of $\sigma 2$ and a standard deviation equal to $\sigma^2 (2/N)^{1/2}$. The sampling distribution of $\ln D_{rg}$ is normal, having a mean of μ_r and a standard deviation given by

$$\sigma(\ln D_{rg}) = (\sigma / \sqrt{N}) (1 + 2r^2 \sigma 2)^{1/2}.$$

The uncertainty in estimating μ_r (and, hence, D_{rg}) increases rapidly as $r\sigma$ increases.

The statistical relationships above are based on the assumptions that each particle diameter is measured independently and without error. In practice, however, it is common to sort the particles into a series of size intervals. The proper estimate of μ_o and σ then become quite complicated. The desired statistics can be approximated, however, by

$$\ln D_{og} = \left(\sum_{i=i}^{k} n_i \cdot \ln D_i \right) \Big/ \left(\sum_{i=1}^{k} n_i \right),$$

and

$$s = \ln \sigma_g = \left[\sum_{i=1}^{k} n_i \cdot (\ln D_i - \ln D_{og})^2 \Big/ \left(\sum_{i=1}^{k} n_i - 1 \right) \right]^{1/2},$$

where n_i is the number of particles in the ith size interval, D_i is an average diameter for that interval, and k is the total number of size intervals. Alternatively, the statistics can be approximated by plotting, on logarithmic-probability paper the cumulative percent

$$P_j = 100 \sum_{i=1}^{j} n_i \Big/ \sum_{i=1}^{k} n_i \quad (j < k)$$

against the upper limit of the jth size interval for a number of values of j and drawing the straight line which the resulting points appear to estimate. D_{og} is the diameter at which the line has the coordinate $P = 50\%$. Therefore,

$$\ln \sigma g = \ln D_{84} - \ln D_{og} = \ln(D_{84}/D_{og}),$$

and

$$\sigma g = D_{84}/D_{og},$$

where D_{84} is the diameter at which the line has the coordinate $P = 84\%$. The statistics can also be calculated from the cumulative distribution using the method of probit analysis described in an earlier chapter.

In the case,

$$\text{Probit } (P_j/100) = a' + b \ln D_j$$

For each value of $P_j/100$, the corresponding probit can be calculated and a' and b are calculated by the method of least squares. The desired statistics are

$$m = \ln D_{og} = (5 - a')/b,$$

and

$$s = \ln g = 1/b$$

Because a large value of N is encountered in most particulate samples, the confidence limits on the various median diameters are given by

$$D_{rg} \text{ (C.L.)} = D_{rg} \cdot \exp[\pm \tau_a \cdot \sigma (\ln D_{rg})],$$

The confidence limits on the population geometric standard deviation are found to be, approximately,

$$\sigma_g \text{ (C.L)} = \sigma_g{}^a,$$

where $a = [2 (N-1)]^{1/2}[\pm t_a + (2N-3)^{1/2}]$, the positive value of t_a giving the lower confidence limit. Here t_a is used in pace of z_a to relate it to the limits on the mean at the same level of confidence.

A goodness-of-fit test can be carried out if the transformation $X = \ln D$ is employed.

Excellent reviews of the field of aerosol measurement are now available (such as Mercer, 1973; Stockham and Fochtman, 1979; and Willeke, 1980).

Mutagenesis

In the last fifteen years a wide variety of tests (see Kilbey *et al* ., 1977 for an overview of those available) for mutagenicity have been developed and brought into use. These tests give us a quicker and cheaper (though not as conclusive) way of predicting whether a material of interest is a mutagen, and possibly a carcinogen, than do longer-term, whole-animal studies.

How to analyze the results of this multitude of tests (Ames, DNA repair, micronucleus, host-mediated, cell transformation, sister chromatid exchange, and *Drosophila* SLRL, to name just a few) is a new and extremely important question. Some workers in the field hold that it is not possible (or necessary) to perform statistical analysis, that the tests can simply be judged to be positive or not positive on the basis of whether or not they achieve a particular increase in the incidence of mutations in the test organism. This is plainly not an acceptable response, when societal needs are not limited to yes/no answers but rather include at least relative quantitation of potencies (particularly in mutagenesis, where we have come to recognize the existence of a nonzero background level of activity from naturally occurring factors and agents). Such quantitations of potency are complicated by the fact that we are dealing with a nonlinear phenomenon; although low dose of most mutagens produce a linear response curve with increasing does the curve will flatten out (and even turn into a declining curve) as the higher doses provoke an acute response.

Several concepts different from those we have previously discussed need to be examined, for our concern has now shifted from how a multicellular organism acts in response to one of a number of complex actions to how a mutational event is expressed, most frequently by a single cell. Given that we can handle much large numbers of experimental units in systems that use smaller test organisms, we can seek to detect both weak and strong mutagens.

Conducting the appropriate statistical analysis, and utilizing the results of such an analysis properly, must start with an understanding of the biological system involved and, from this understanding, developing the correct model and hypothesis. We start such a process by considering each of five interacting factors (Grafe and Vollmar, 1977, Vollmar, 1977).

1. α , which is the probability of our committing a type I error (saying an agent is mutagenic when it is not, equivalent to our p in such earlier considered designs as the Fisher's exact test); false positive;

2. β , which is the probability of our committing a type II error (saying an agent is not mutagenic when it is); false negative;

3. Δ , our desired sensitivity in an assay system (such as being able to detect an increase of 10% in mutations in a population);

4. σ , the variability of the biological system and the effects of chance errors; and

5.n, the necessary sample size to achieve each of these (we can, by our actions, change only this portion of the equation) as n is proportional to:

$$\frac{\sigma}{\alpha,\ \beta,\ \text{and } \Delta}$$

The implications of this are, therefore, that (a) the greater σ is, the larger n must be to achieve the desired levels of α, β, and Δ, (b) the smaller the desired levels of α, β, and/or Δ, if n is constant the larger our σ is.

What is the background mutation level and the variability in our technique? As any good genetic or general toxicologist will acknowledge, matched concurrent control groups are essential. Fortunately, with these test systems large n's are readily attainable, though there are other complications to this problem, which we shall consider later. An example of the confusion that would otherwise result is illustrated in the intralaboratory comparisons on some of these methods done to date, such as that reviewed by Weil (1978).

New statistical tests based on these assumptions and upon the underlying population distributions have been proposed, along with the necessary computational background to allow one to alter one of the input variables (α, β, or Δ). A set that shows particular promise is that proposed by Katz (1978 and 1979) in his two articles. He described two separate test statistics: ϕ for when we can accurately estimate the number of individuals in both the experimental and control groups, and Θ, for when we do not actually estimate the number of surviving individuals in each group, and we can assume that the test material is only mildly toxic in terms of killing the test organisms. Each of these two test statistics is also formulated on the basis of only a single exposure of the organisms to the test chemicals. Given this, then we may compute

$$\phi = \frac{\alpha(M_E - 0.5) - Kb(M_c + 0.5)}{\sqrt{K\alpha\beta(M_E + M_c)}}$$

where a and b are the number of groups of control (c) and experimental (e) organisms, respectively.

N_C and N_E are the numbers of surviving microorganisms.

$$[K = N_E/N_C]$$

M_E and M_C are the numbers of mutations in experimental and control groups.

μ_e and μ_c are the true (but unknown) mutation rates (as μ_c gets smaller, N's must increase).

We may compute the second case as

$$\theta = \frac{a(M_E - 0.5) + (M_c + 0.5)}{ab(M_E + M_c)}$$

with the same constituents.

In both cases, at a confidence level for α of 0.05, we accept that $\mu_c = \mu_e$ if the test statistic (either ϕ or θ) is less than 1.64. If it is equal to or greater than 1.64, we may conclude that we have a mutagenic effect (at $\alpha = 0.05$).

In the second case (θ, where we do not have separate estimates of population sizes for the control and experimental groups) if K deviates widely from 1.0 (if the material is markedly toxic), we should use more containers of control organisms (tables for the proportions of each to use given different survival frequencies may be found in Katz, 1979). If different levels are desired, tables for θ and φ may be found in Kastenbaum and Bowman (1970).

An outgrowth of this is that the mutation rate per surviving cells (μ_c and μ_e) can be determined. It must be remembered that if the control mutation rate is so high that a reduction in mutation rates can be achieved by the test compound, these test statistics must be adjusted to allow for a two-sided hypothesis (Ehrenberg, 1977). The α levels may likewise be adjusted in each case, or tested for, if we want to assure ourselves that a mutagenic effect exists at a certain level of confidence (note that this is different from disproving the null hypothesis).

It should be noted that there are numerous specific recommendations for statistical methods designed for individual mutagenicity techniques, such as that of Bernstein *et al.* (1982) for the Ames test. Exploring each of them is beyond the scope of this chapter, however.

Behavioral Toxicology

A brief review of the types of studies/experiments conducted in the area of behavioral toxicology, and a classification of these into groups is in order. Although there are a small number of studies which do not fit into the following classification, the great majority may be fitted into one of the following four groups. Many of these points were first covered by one of the authors in an earlier article (Gad, 1982).

Observational score-type studies are based on observing and grading the response of an animal to its normal environment or to a stimulus which is imprecisely controlled. This type of result is generated by one of two major sorts of studies. Open-field studies involve placing an animal in the center of a flat, open area and counting each occurrence of several types of activities (grooming, moving outside a designated central area, rearing, ...) or timing until the first occurrence of each type of activity. The data generated are scalar of either a continuous or discontinuous nature, but frequently are not of a normal distribution. Tilson, *et al.* (1980) presented some examples of this sort.

Observational screen studies involve a combination of observing behavior and evoking a response to a simple stimulus, the resulting observation being graded as normal or as deviating from normal on a graded scale. Most of the data so generated are rank in nature, with some portions being quantal or interval. Irwin (1968) and Gad (1982) have presented schemes for the conduct of such studies. Table 8 gives an example of the nature (and of one form of statistical analysis) of such data generated after exposure to one material.

TABLE 8

Irwin screen parameters showing significant differences between treated and control groups

Parameter	Rats (18-crown-6 animals given 40 mg/kg i.p.)				
	Control sum of ranks	N_c	18-crown-6 treated sum of ranks	N_T	Observed difference in treated animals (as compared to controls)
Twitches	55.0	10	270.0	15	Involuntary muscle twitches
Visual placing	55.0	10	270.0	15	Less aware of visual stimuli
Grip strength	120.0	10	205.0	15	Considerable loss of strength, especially in hind limbs
Respiration	55.0	10	270.0	15	Increased rate of respiration
Tremors	55.0	10	270.0	15	Marked tremors

All parameters above are significant at $p < 0.05$

The second type of study is one which generates rates of response as data. The studies are based on the number of responses to a discrete controlled stimulus or are free of direct connectic to a stimulus. The three most frequently measured parameters are licking of a liquid (milk, sugar water, ethanol, or a psychoactive agent in water), gross locomotor activity (measured by a photocell or electro-magnetic device), or lever pulling. Work presenting examples of such studies has been published by Annau (1972) and Norton (1973). The data generated are most often of a discontinuous or continuous scalar nature, and are often complicated by underlying patterns of biological rhythm (to be discussed more fully later).

The third type of study generates a variety of data which is classified as error rate. These are studies based on animals learning a response to a stimulus or memorizing a simple task (such as running a maze or a Skinner box-type shock avoidance system). These tests or trials are structured so that animals can pass or fail on each of a number of successive trials. The resulting data are quantal, though frequently expressed as a percentage.

The final major type of study is that which results in data which are measures of the time to an endpoint. They are based on animals being exposed to or dosed with a toxicant and the time taken for an effect to be observed is measured. The endpoint is usually failure to continue to be able to perform a task and can, therefore, be death, incapacitation, or the learning of a response to a discrete stimulus. Burt (1972) and Johnson et al. (1972) present data of this form. The data are always of a censored nature - that is, the period of observation is always artifically limited as in measuring time-to-incapacitation in combustion toxicology data, where animals are exposed to the thermal decomposition gases of test materials for a period of 30 minutes. If incapacitation is not observed during these 30 minutes, it is judged not to occur. The data generated by these studies are continuous, discontinuous, or rank in nature. They are discontinuous because the researcher may check, or may be restricted to checking for the occurrence of the endpoint only at certain discrete points in time. On the other hand, they are rank if the periods to check for occurrence of the endpoint are far enough apart, in which case one may actually only know that the endpoint occurred during a broad period of time - but not where in that period.

There is a special class of test which should also be considered at this point - the behavioral teratology or reproduction study. These studies are based on dosing or exposing either parental animals during selected periods in the mating and gestation process or pregnant females at selected periods during gestation. The resulting offspring are then tested for developmental defects of a neurological and behavioral nature. Analysis is complicated by a number of facts: (1) the parental animals are the actual targets for toxic effects, but observations are made on offspring; (2) the toxic effects in the parental generation may alter the performance of the mother in rearing its offspring, which in turn can lead to a confusion of prenatal and postnatal effects; (3) finally, different capabilities and behaviors develop at different times (discussed further below).

A researcher can, by varying the selection of the animal model (species, strain, sex), modify the nature of the data generated and the degree of dispersion of these data. In behavioral studies particulary, limiting the within-group variability of data is a significant problem and generally should be a highly desirable goal.

Most, if not all, behavioral toxicology studies depend on at least some instrumentation. Very frequently overlooked here (and, indeed, in most research) is that instrumentation, by its operating characteristics and limitations, goes a long way towards determining the nature of the data generated by it. An activity monitor measures motor activity in discrete segments. If it is a "jiggle cage" type monitor these segments are restricted so that only a distinctly limited number of counts can be achieved in a given period of time and then only if they are of the appropriate magnitude. Likewise, technique can also readily determine the nature of data. In measuring response to pain, for example, one could record it as a quantal measure (present or absent), a rank score (on a scale of 1-5 for from decreased to increased responsiveness, with 3 being "normal") or as scalar data (by using an analgesia meter which determines either how much pressure or heat is required to evoke a response).

Study design factors are probably the most widely recognized of the factors which influence the type of data resulting from a study. Number of animals used, frequency of measures, and length of period of observation are three obvious design factors which are readily under the control of the researcher and which directly help to determine the nature of the data.

Finally it is appropriate to review each of the types of studies presently seen in behavioral toxicology, according to the classification presented at the beginning of this section, in terms of which statistical methods are used now and what procedures should be recommended for use. The recommendations, of course, should be viewed with a critical eye. They are intended with current experimental design and technique in mind and can only claim to be the best when one is limited to addressing the most common problems from a library of readily and commonly available and understood tests.

Table 9 summarizes this review and recommendation process.

TABLE 9

Overview of statistical testing in behavioral toxicology - those tests commonly used[a] as opposed to those most frequently appropriate.

Type of observation	Most commonly used procedures[a]	Suggested procedures
Observational scores	Either Student's *t*-test or one-way ANOVA	Kruskal-Wallis non-parametric ANOVA or Wilcoxon Rank sum
Response rates	Either Student's *t*-test or one-way ANOVA	Kruskal-Wallis ANOVA or one way ANOVA
Error rates	ANOVA followed by a post-hoc test	Fisher's exact, or RXC Chi square, or Mann-Whitney U-test
Times to endpoint	Either Student's *t*-test or one-way ANOVA	ANOVA then a post-hoc test or Kruskal-Wallis ANOVA
Teratology and reproduction	ANOVA followed by a post-hoc test	Fisher's exact test, Kruskal-Wallis ANOVA, or Mann-Whitney U-test

[a]That these are the most commonly used procedures was established by an extensive literature review which is beyond the scope of this book. The reader need only, however, look at the example articles cited in the text of this chapter to verify this fact.

REFERENCES

Aeschbacher, H.U., Vautaz, L., Sotek, J., and Stalder, R. (1977): Use of the beta binomial distribution in dominant-lethal testing for "weak mutagenic activity," Part. 1. *Mutat. Res.*, 44:369–390.

Annau, Z. (1972): The comparative effects of hypoxia and carbon monoxide hypoxia on behavior. In: Weiss, B. and Laties, V.G. (eds) *Behavioral Toxicology* pp 105–127., Plenum Press, New York.

Bateman, A.T. (1977): The dominant lethal assay in the male mouse. In: Handbook of Mutagenicity Test Procedures, edited by B.J. Kilbey, M. Legator, W. Nichols, and C. Ramel, pp. 325–334. Elsevier, New York.

Bernstein, L., Kaldor, J., McCann, J. and Pike, M.C. (1982): An empirical approach to the statistical analysis of mutagenesis data from the Salmonella test. *Mutation Res.*, 97:267–281.

Bliss, C.I. (1965): Statistical relations in fertilizer inspection. *Bulletin* 674. Connecticut Agricultural Experiment Station, New Haven.

Boyd, E.M. (1972): *Predictive Toxicometrics*. Williams & Wilkins, Baltimore.

Boyd, E.M. and Knight, L.M. (1963): Postmortem shifts in the weight and water levels of body organs, *Tox. Appl. Pharm.*, 5, 119–128.

Bruce, R.D. (1985): An up-and-down procedure for acute toxicity testing. *Fund. Appl. Toxicol.*, 5, 151–157.

Burt, G.S. (1972) Use of behavioral techniques in the assessment of environmental contaminants. In: Weiss, B., Laties, V.G. (eds) *Behavioral Toxicology* pp. 241–263. Plenum Press, New York.

Dean, B.J., and Johnston, A. (1977): Dominant lethal assays in the male mice: evaluation of experimental design, statistical methods and the sensitivity of Charles River (CD1) mice. *Mutat. Res.*, 42:269–278.

Debanne, S.M. and Haller, H.S. (1985): Evaluation of statistical methodologies for estimation of median effective dose. *Tox. Appl. Pharm.*, 79:274–282.

DePass, L.R., Myers, R.C., Weaver, E.V. and Weil, C.S. (1984): An asessment of the importance of number of dosage levels, number of animals per dosage level, sex and method of LD_{50} and slope calculations in acute toxicity studies. *Alternate Methods in Toxicology, Vol. 2: Acute Toxicity Testing: Alternate Approaches*, Goldberg, A.M., ed., Mary Ann Liebert, Inc. New York.

Ehrenberg, L. (1977): Aspects of statistical inference in testing genetic toxicity. In: *Handbook of Mutagenicity Test Procedures*, edited by Kilbey, B.J., Legator, M., Nichols, W. and Ramel, C., pp. 419–459. Elsevier, New York.

Gad, S.C. (1982): A neuromuscular screen for use in industrial toxicology. *J. Toxicol. Env. Hlth.*, 9:691–704.

Gad. S.C. (1982): Statistical Analysis of Behavioral Toxicology Data and Studies. *Arch. Toxicol. Suppl.*, 5:256–266.

Gad, S.C.; Smith, A.C.; Cramp, A.L.; Gavigan, F.A. and Derelanko, M.J. (1984): Innovative designs and practices for acute systemic toxicity studies: *Drug Chem. Toxicol.*, 7:423–434.

Grafe, A. and Vollmar, J. (1977): Small numbers in mutagenicity tests. *Arch. Toxicol.*, 38:27–34.

Harris, E.K. (1978): Review of statistical methods of analysis of series of biochemical test results. *Ann. Biol. Clin.*, 36:194–197.

Irwin, S. (1968): Comprehensive observational assessment. Ia: Systematic, quantitative procedure for assessing the behavioral and physiologic state of the mouse. *Psychopharmaco-logia*. 13:222–257.

Jackson, B. (1962): Statistical analysis of body weight data. *Toxicol. Appl. Pharmacol.*, 4:432–443.

Johnson, B.L., Anger, W.K., Setzer, J.V., Xinytaras, C. (1972): The application of a computer controlled time discrimination performance to problems. In: Weiss, B., Laties, V.G. (eds) *Behavioral Toxicology.* pp. 129–153. Plenum Press, New York.

Kastenbaum, M.A. and Bowman, K.O. (1970): Tables for determining the statistical significance of mutation frequencies. *Mutat. Res.*, 9:527–549.

Katz, A.J. (1978): Design and analysis of experiments on mutagenicity. I. Minimal sample sizes. *Mutat. Res.*, 50:301–307.

Katz, A.J. (1979): Design and analysis of experiments on mutagenicity. II. Assays involving micro-oranisms. *Mutat. Res.*, 64:61–77.

Kilbey, B.J., Legator, M., Nicholas, W., Ramel, C. (1977): *Handbook of Mutagenicity Test Procedures*, pp. 425–433. Elsevier, New York.

Kupper, L.L., and Haseman, J.K. (1978): The use of a correlated binomial model for the analysis of certain toxicological experiments. *Biomet.*, 34:69–76.

Martin, H.F., Gudzinowicz, B.J. and Fanger, H. (1975): *Normal Values in Clinical Chemistry*. Marcel Dekker, New York.

Mercer, T.T. (1973) *Aerosol Technology in Hazard Evaluation*, Academic Press, New York.

Mitruka, B.M., and Rawnsley, H.M. (1977): *Clinical Biochemical and Hematological Reference Values in Normal Experimental Animals*. Masson, New York.

Mosteller, F., and Youtz, C. (1961): Tables of the Freeman-Tukey transformations for the binomial and Poisson distributions. *Biometrika*, 48:433–440.

Nelson, C.J., and Holson, J.F. (1978): Statistical: analysis of teratologic data: Problems and advancements. *J. Environ. Pathol. Toxicol.*, 2: 187–199.

Norton, S. (1973): Amphetamine as a model for hyperactivity in the rat. *Physiol. Behav.*, 11:181–186.

Oser, B.L., and Oser, M. (1956): Nutritional studies in rats on diets containing high levels of partial ester emulsifiers. II. Reproduction and lactation. *J. Nutr.*, 60:429.

Rai, K. and Ryzin, J.V. (1985): A dose-response model for teratological experiments involving quantal responses. *Biomet.*, 41:1–9.

Ridgemen, W.J. (1975): *Experimentation in Biology*. pp. 214–215. Wiley, New York.

Stockham, J.D. and Fochtman, E.G., (1979). *Particle Size Analysis* Ann Arbor Science, Ann Arbor.

Tilson, H.A., Cabe, P.A., Burne, T.A. (1980) Behavioral procedures for the assessment of neurotoxicity. In: Spencer P.S. Schaumburg, N.H. (eds) *Experimental and Clinical Neurotoxicology*. pp 758–766. Williams & Wilkins, Baltimore.

Vollmar, J. (1977): Statistical problems in mutagenicity tests. *Arch. Toxicol.*, 38–13–25.

Vuataz, L., and Sotek, J. (1978): Use of the beta-binomial distribution indominant-lethal testing for "Weak Mutagenic Activity," Part 2. *Mutat. Res.*, 52.211–230.

Wallach, J. (1978): *Interpretation of Diagnostic Tests* Little, Brown and Company; Boston.

Weil, C.S. (1962): Applications of methods of statistical analysis to efficient repeated-dose toxicological tests. I. General considerations and problems involved. Sex differences in rat liver and kidney weights. *Toxicol. Appl. Pharmacol.*, 4:561–571.

Weil, C.S. (1970): Selection of the valid number of sampling units and a consideration of their combination in toxicological studies involving reproduction, teratogenesis or carcinogenesis. *Food Cosmet. Toxicol.*, 8:177–182.

Weil, C.S. (1972): Statistics vs. safety factors and scientific judgement in the evaluation of safety for man. *Toxicol. Appl. Pharmacol.*, 21: 459–472

Weil, C.S. (1973). Experimental design and interpretation of data from prolonged toxicity studies, in *Proc. 5th Int. Congr. Pharmacol.*, Beacon Press San Francisco, Vol. 2, pp. 4–12.

Weil, C.S. (1975): Toxicology experimental design and conduct as measured by inter-laboratory collaboration studies. *J. Assoc. Off. Anal. Chem.*, 58:687–688.

Weil C.S. (1978): A critique of the collaborative cytogenetics study to measure and minimize interlaboratory variation. *Mutat. Res.*, 50:285–291.

Weil, C.S. (1982): Statistical analysis and normality of selected hematologic and clinical chemistry measurements used in toxicologic studies, *Arch. Toxicol.*, Suppl 5:237–253.

Weil, C.S., Carpenter, C.P., and Smith, H.I. (1953): Specifications for calculating the median effective dose. *Amer. Indust. Hyg. Assoc. Quart.*, 14:200–206.

Weil, C.S. and Gad, S.C. (1980): Applications of methods of statistical analysis to efficient repeated-dose toxicologic tests. 2. Methods for analysis of body, liver and kidney weight data. *Toxicol. Appl. Pharmacol.*, 52:214–226.

Willeke, K. (1980): *Generation of Aerosols and Facilities for Exposure Experiments*. Ann Arbor Science, Ann Arbor.

Williams, R. and Buschbom, R.L. (1982): Statistical Analysis of Litter Experiments in Teratology *Battelle PNL-4425*.

Zar, J.H. (1974): *Biostatistical Analysis*, p. 50. Prentice-Hall, Englewood.

Zbinden, G. and Flury-Roversi, M. (1981): Significance of the LD_{50}-Test for the Toxicological Evaluation of Chemical Substances *Arch. Tox-icol.*, 47:77–99.

CHAPTER 12

CARCINOGENESIS AND RISK ASSESSMENT

Both carcinogenesis and the broader realm of risk assessment (as it applies to toxicology) have in common that, based on experimental results in a nonhuman species at some relatively high dose or exposure level, an attempt is made to predict the level of impact in humans at much lower levels. In this chapter we will examine the assumptions involved in these undertakings, review the aspects of design and interpretation of animal carcinogenicity studies, take a critical look at low dose extrapolation models and methods, and present the framework on which risk assessment is based.

The reader should first understand that, contrary to popular belief, risk assessment in toxicology is not limited to carcinogenesis. Rather, it may be applied to all the possible deferred toxicologic consequences of exposure to chemicals or agents which are of a truly severe nature. That is, those things (such as carcinogenesis, teratogenesis, or reproductive impairment) that threaten life (either existing or prospective) at a time distant to the actual exposure to the chemical or agent. Because the consequences of these toxic events are extreme yet are distanced from the actual cause by time (unlike overexposure to an acutely lethal agent, such as carbon monoxide), society is willing to accept only a low level of risk while maintaining the benefits of use of the agent. Though the most familiar (and, to date, best developed) case is that of carcinogenesis, much of what is presented for risk assessment may also be applied to the other endpoints of concern.

Carcinogenicity Bioassays

At least in a general way, we now understand what appear to be most of the mechanisms underlying chemical and radiation induced carcinogenesis. A review of these mechanisms is not germane to this chapter (readers are referred to Miller and Miller, 1981 for a good short review), but it is now clear that cancer as seen in humans is the result of a multifocal set of causes. The single most important statistical consideration in the design of bioassays in the past was based on the point of view that what was being observed and evaluated was a simple quantal response (cancer occurred or it didn't), and that a sufficient number of animals needed to be used to have reasonable expectations of detecting such an effect. Though the single fact of whether or not the simple incidence of neoplastic tumors is increased due to an agent of concern is of interest, a much more complex model must now be considered. The time-to-tumor, patterns of tumor incidence, effects on survival rate, and age at first tumor all must now be included in a model.

Bioassay Design

As presented earlier in the section on experimental design, the first step which must be taken is to clearly state the objective of the study to be undertaken. Carcinogenicity bioassays have two possible objectives, though (as we shall see) the second is now more important and (as our understanding of carcinogenesis has increased) is increasingly crowding out the first.

The first objective is to detect possible carcinogens. Compounds are evaluated to determine if they can or cannot induce a statistically detectable increase if tumor rates over background levels, and only by happenstance is information generated which is useful in risk assessment. Most older studies have such detection as their objective. Current thought is that at least two species must be used for detection.

The second objective for a bioassay is to provide a range of dose response information (with tumor incidence being the response) so that a risk assessment may be performed. Unlike detection, which requires only one treatment group with adequate survival times (to allow expression of tumors), dose response requires at least three treatment groups with adequate survival. We will shortly look at the selection of dose levels for this case. However, given that the species is known to be responsive, only one species of animal need be used for this objective.

To address either or both of these objectives, three major types of study designs have evolved. First is the classical skin painting study, usually performed in mice. A single, easily detected endpoint (the formation of skin tumors) is evaluated during the course of the study. Though dose response can be evaluated in such a study (dose usually being varied by using different concentrations of test material in volatile solvent), most often detection is the objective of such a study. Though others have used different frequencies of application of test material to vary dose, there are data to suggest that this only serves to introduce an additional variable (Wilson and Holland, 1982). Traditionally, both test and control groups in such a test consist of 50 or 100 mice of one sex (males being preferred because of their very low spontaneous tumor rate). This design is also used in tumor initiation/promotion studies.

The second common type of design is the original National Cancer Institute (NCI) bioassay. The announced objective of these studies was detection of moderate to strong carcinogens, though the results have also been used in attempts at risk assessment. Both mice and rats were used in parallel studies. Each study used 50 males and 50 females at each of two dose levels (high and low) plus an equal-sized control group. The National Toxicology Program (NTP) has recently moved away from this design because of a recognition of its inherent limitations.

Finally, there is the standard industrial toxicology design, which uses at least two species (usually rats and mice) in groups of no fewer than 100 males and females each. Each study has three dose groups and at least one control. Frequently, additional numbers of animals are included to allow for interim terminations and histopathological evaluations. In both this and the NCI design, a long list of organs and tissues are collected, processed, and examined microscopically. This design seeks to address both the detection and dose response objectives with a moderate degree of success.

Selecting the number of animals to use for dose groups in a study requires consideration of both biological (expected survival rates, background tumor rates, etc.) and statistical factors. The prime statistical consideration is reflected in Table 10, below. It can be seen in this table that if, for example, we were studying a compound which caused liver tumors, and were using mice (with a background or control incidence of 30%), we would have to use 389 animals per sex per group to be able to demonstrate that an incidence rate of 40% in treatment animals was significant compared to the controls at the $p \leq 0.05$ level.

Perhaps the most difficult aspect of designing a good carcinogenicity study is the selection of the dose levels to be used. At the start, it is necessary to consider the first underlying assumption in the design and use of animal cancer bioassays - the need to test at the highest possible dose for the longest practical period.

The rationale behind this assumption is that though humans may be exposed at very low levels, detecting the resulting small increase (over background) in the incidence of tumors would require the use of an impractically large number of test animals per group. This point is illustrated by Table 11, where, for instance, while only forty-six animals (per group) are needed to show a 10% increase over a zero background (that is, a rarely occuring tumor type), 770,000 animals (per group) would be needed to detect a tenth of a percent increase

TABLE 10

Sample size required to obtain a specified sensitivity at p < 0.05
Treatment Group Incidence

Back-ground tumor incidence	P*	0.95	0.90	0.80	0.70	0.60	0.50	0.40	0.30	0.20	0.10
0.30	0.90	10	12	18	31	46	102	389			
	0.50	6	6	9	12	22	32	123			
0.20	0.90	8	10	12	18	30	42	88	320		
	0.50	5	5	6	9	12	19	28	101		
0.10	0.90	6	8	10	12	17	25	33	65	214	
	0.50	3	3	5	6	9	11	17	31	68	
0.05	0.90	5	6	8	10	13	18	25	35	76	464
	0.50	3	3	5	6	7	9	12	19	24	147
0.01	0.90	5	5	7	8	10	13	19	27	46	114
	0.50	3	3	5	5	6	8	10	13	25	56

*P = Power for each comparison of treatment group with background tumor incidence.

above a five percent background. As we increase dose, however, the incidence of tumors (the response) will also increase until it reaches the point where a modest increase (say 10% over a reasonably small background level (say 1%) could be detected using an acceptably small-sized group of test animals (in Table 11 we see that 51 animals would be needed for this example case). There are, however, at least two real limitations to the highest dose level. First, the test rodent population must have a survival rate after receiving a lifetime (or two years) of regular doses to allow for meaningful statistical analysis. Second, we really want the metabolism and mechanism of action of the chemical at the highest level tested to be the same as at the low levels where human exposure would occur. Unfortunately, we usually must select the high dose level based only on the information provided by a sub-chronic or range finding study, but selection of too low a dose will make the study invalid for detection of carcinogenicity, and may seriously impair the use of the results for risk assessment.

There are several solutions to this problem. One of these has been the rather simplistic approach of the NTP Bioassay Program, which is to conduct a 3 month range finding study with sufficient dose levels to establish a level which significantly (10%) decreases the rate of body weight gain. This dose is defined as the maximum tolerated dose (MTD) and is selected as the highest dose. Two other levels, generally one half MTD and one quarter MTD, are selected for testing as the intermediate and low dose levels. In many earlier NCI studies, only one other level was used.

The dose range-finding study is necessary in most cases, but the suppression of body weight gain is a scientifically questionable bench mark when dealing with establishment of safety factors. Physiologic, pharmacologic or metabolic markers generally serve as better indicators of systemic response than body weight. A series of well-defined acute and subchronic studies designed to determine the "chronicity factor" and to study onset of pathology can be more predictive for dose setting than body weight suppression.

Also, the NTP's MTD may well be at a level where the metabolic mechanisms for handling a compound at real-life exposure levels have been saturated or overwhelmed, bringing into play entirely artifactual metabolic and physiologic mechanisms (Gehring and Blau, 1977). The regulatory response to questioning the appropriateness of the MTD as a high dose level (exemplified by Haseman, 1985) has been to acknowledge that occasionally an excessively high dose is selected, but to counter by saying that using lower doses would seriously decrease the sensitivity of detection.

Selection of levels for the intermediate and lower doses for a study is easy only in comparison to the selection of the high dose. If an objective of the study is to generate dose response data, then the optimal placement of the doses below the high is such that they cover as much of the range of a response curve as possible and yet still have the lowest dose at a high enough level that one can detect and quantify a response. If the objective is detection, then having too great a distance between the highest and next-highest dose creates a risk to the validity of the study. If the survival in the high dose is too low, yet the next highest dose does not show non-neoplastic results (that is, cause other-than-neoplastic adverse biological effects) such as to support it being a high enough dose to have detected a strong or moderate carcinogen, the entire study may have to be rejected as inadequate to address its objective. Portier and Hoel (1984) have proposed statistical guidelines (for setting dose levels below the high) based on response surfaces. In so doing they suggest that the lowest dose be no less than 10% if the highest.

Though it is universally agreed that the appropriate animal model for testing a chemical for carcinogenicity would be that whose metabolism, pharmacokinetics and biological responses were most similar to humans, economic considerations have largely constrained practical choices to rats and mice. The use of both sexes of both species is preferred on the grounds that it provides for (in the face of a lack of understanding of which species would actually be most like humans for a particular agent) a greater likelihood of utilizing the more sensitive species. Use of the mouse is both advocated and defended on these grounds and because of the economic advantages and the species' historical utilization (Grasso and Crampton, 1972). There are those who believe that the use of the mouse is redundant and represents a diversion of resources while yielding little additional information (Wittenau and Estes, 1983), citing a "unique contribution" for mouse data in 273 bioassays of only 13.6% of the cases (that is, 37 cases). Others question the use of the mouse based on the belief that it gives artifactual liver carcinogenesis results. One suggestion for the interpretation of mouse bioassays is that in those cases where there is only an increase in liver tumors in mice (or lung tumors in strain A mice) and no supporting mutagenicity findings (a situation characteristic of some classes of chemicals), the test compound should not be considered an overt carcinogen (Ward et al., 1979). This last question, however, is even more strongly focused on the strain of mouse that is used than on the use of the species itself.

TABLE 11

Average number of animals needed to detect a significant increase in the incidence of an event (tumors, anomalies, etc.) over the background incidence (control) at several expected incidence levels using the Fisher exact probability test ($p \leqslant 0.05$)

Background Incidence, %	Expected Increase in Incidence, %					
	0.01	0.1	1	3	5	10
0	46,000,000[a]	460,000	4,600	511	164	46
0.01	46,000,000	460,000	4,600	511	164	46
0.1	47,000,000	470,000	4,700	520	168	47
1	51,000,000	510,000	5,100	570	204	51
5	77,000,000	770,000	7,700	856	304	77
10	100,000,000	1,000,000	10,000	1,100	400	100
20	148,000,000	1,480,000	14,800	1,644	592	148
25	160,000,000	1,600,000	16,000	1,840	664	166

[a]Number of animals needed in each group—controls as well as treated.

The NCI/NTP (National Toxicology Program) currently recommends an F1 hybrid cross between two inbred strains, the C57B1/6 female and the C3H male, the results being commonly designated as the B6C3F1. This mouse was found to be very successful in a large-scale pesticide testing program in the mid-1960s. It is a hardy animal with good survival, easy to breed, disease resistant, and has been reported to have a relatively low spontaneous tumor incidence. Usually at least 80% of the control mice are still alive at a 24 months termination.

Unfortunately, while it was originally believed (Page, 1977) that the spontaneous liver tumor incidence in male B6C3F1 mice was 15.7%, it actually appears to be closer to 32.1% (Nutrition Foundation, 1983). The issue of spontaneous tumor rates and their impact on the design and interpretation of studies will be discussed more fully later. Thus, use of a cross of two inbred mouse strains is also a point of controversy. Haseman and Hoel (1979) have presented data to support the idea that inbred strains have lower degrees of variability of biological functions and tumor rates, making them more sensitive detectors and quantitators. These authors also suggest that the use of a cross from two such inbred strains allows one to more readily detect tumor incidence increases. On the other hand, it has been argued that such genetically homogeneous strains do not properly reflect the diversity of metabolic functions (particularly ones which would serve to detoxify or act as defense mechanisms) which are present in the human population.

Study length and the frequency of treatment are design aspects which must also be considered. These are aspects where the objectives of detection and dose response definition conflict.

For the greatest confidence in a "negative" detection result, an agent should be administered continuously for the majority of an animal's lifespan. The NTP considers that 2 years is a practical treatment period in rats and mice, although the animals currently used in such studies may survive an additional 6 - 12 months. Study lengths of 15 - 18 months are considered adequate for shorter-lived species, such as hamsters. An acceptable exposure/observation period for dogs is considered to be 7 - 10 years, an age equivalent to about 45 - 60 yr in humans. For dietary treatments, continuous exposure is considered desirable and practical. With other routes, practical considerations may dictate interrupted treatments. For example, inhalation treatment for 6 - 8 hr per day on a 5 day/wk schedule is the usual practice. Regimens requiring special handling of animals, such as parenteral injections, are usually on a 5 day/wk basis. With some compounds intermittent exposures may be required because of toxicity. Various types of recovery can occur during exposure-free periods, which may either enhance or decrease chances of carcinogenicity. In view of the objective of assessing carcinogenicity as the initial step, intermittent exposure on a 3 - 5 day/wk basis is considered both practical and desirable for most compounds.

Following cessation of dosing or exposure, continued observation during a non-treatment period may be required before termination of the experiment. Such a period is considered desirable because (1) induced lesions may progress to more readily observable lesions, and (2) morphologically similar but noncarcinogenic proliferative lesions that are stress-related may regress. Neoplastic or "neoplastic-like" lesions that persist long after removal of the stimulus are considered of serious consequences, from the hazard viewpoint. Many expert anatomical pathologists, however, feel able to diagnose and determine the biological nature of tumorous lesions existing at the time of treatment without the added benefit of a treatment-free period.

In determining the length of an observation period, several factors must be considered: period of exposure, survival pattern of both treated and control animals, nature of lesions found in animals that have already died, tissue storage and retention of the chemical, and results of other studies that would suggest induction of late-occurring tumors. The usual length of a treatment-free observation period is 3 months in mice and hamsters and 6 months in rats. An alternative would be to terminate the experiment or an individual treatment group on the basis of survival (say at the point at which 50% of the group with the lowest survival has died).

The arguments against such prolonged treatment and maintenance on study revolve around the relationship between age and tumor incidence. As test animals (or humans) become older, the background ("naturally occurring") incidence of tumors increases (Dix and Cohen, 1980) and it becomes increasingly difficult to identify a treatment effect from the background effect. Salsburg (1980) has published an analysis of patterns of senile lesions in mice and rats, citing what he calls the principle of biological confounding. "If a particular lesion (e.g. pituitary tumor) is part of a larger syndrome induced by the treatment, it is impossible to determine whether the treatment has 'caused' that lesion."

This could lead to a situation where any real carcinogen would be nonidentifiable. If the usual pattern of old age lesions for a given species or strain of animals includes tumors, then almost every biologically active treatment can be expected to influence the incidence of tumors in a cluster of lesions at a sufficiently high dose.

Reconsidering our basic principles of experimental design, it is clear that we should try to design bioassays so that any carcinogenesis is a clear-cut, single event, unconfounded by the occurrence of significant numbers of lesions due to other causes (such as age). One answer to this problem is the use of interim termination groups. When an evaluation of tumor incidences in an interim sacrifice sample of animals indicates that background incidence is becoming a source of confounding data, termination plans for the study can be altered to minimize the loss of power. Several authors (such as Louis and Orva, 1985 and Ciminera, 1985) have presented such adaptive sacrifice plans.

A number of other possible confounding factors can enter into a bioassay unless design precludes them. These include (a) cage and litter effects (Lagakos and Mosteller, 1981) which can be avoided by proper prestudy randomization of animals and rotation of cage locations, (b) vehicle (corn oil, for example, has been found to be a promoter for liver carcinogens) and (c) the use of the potential hazard route for man, e.g. dietary inclusion instead of gastric intubation.

In the last chapter of this book we will discuss several controversial statistical issues which apply to carcinogenesis. Other general aspects of the design of carcinogenicity bioassay may be found in Robens *et al.* (1982) and Neal and Gibson (1984).

Bioassay Interpretation

The interpretation of the results of even the best designed carcinogenesis bioassay is a complex statistical and biological problem. In addressing the statistical aspects, we shall have to review some biological points which have statistical implications as we proceed.

First, all such bioassays are evaluated by comparison of the observed results in treatment groups with those in one or more control groups. These control groups always include at least one group that is concurrent, but because of concern about variability in background tumor rates, a historical control group is also considered in at least some manner.

The underlying problem in the use of concurrent controls alone is the belief that the selected populations of animals are subject both to an inordinate degree of variability in their spontaneous tumor incidence rates and that the strains maintained at separate breeding facilities are each subject to a slow but significant degree of genetic drift. The first problem raises concern that, by chance, the animals selected to be controls for any particular study will be either "too high" or "too low" in their tumor incidences, leading to either a false positive or false negative statistical test result when test animals are compared to these controls. The second problem leads to concern that, over the years, different laboratories will be using different standards (control groups) against which to compare the outcome of their tests, making any kind of relative comparison between compounds or laboratories impossible.

The last ten years has seen at least eight separate publications reporting 5 sets of background tumor incidences in test animals. These eight publications are summarized and compared in Tables 12 and 13 for B6C3F1 mice and Fischer 344 rats, respectively.

It should be kept in mind in considering these separate columns of numbers that there are some overlaps in the populations being reported. For example, it is almost certain that some NCI/NTP study control groups were incorporated in several separate publications. At the same time, the related survival and growth data on control animals (broken out by type of treatment and vehicle) has also been published (Cameron *et al.*, 1985) allowing for some assessment of comparability

TABLE 12
Reported Background Tumor Incidences In B6C3F1 Mice

ORGAN/TISSUE	Chu 1977 M	Chu 1977 F	Fears et al.1977; Page, 1977; Gart et al., 1979 M	Fears et al.1977; Page, 1977; Gart et al., 1979 F	Chu et al., 1981 M	Chu et al., 1981 F	Tarone et al., 1981 M (Ranges)	Tarone et al., 1981 F
Brain	.1	.1	<	0	<.1	.1		
Skin/Subcutaneous	1.9	1.6	1	<1.0	<.1	.1		
Mammary Gland	–	.8	–	<1.0	–	1.3		
Circulatory System	2.4	1.7		<1.0	2.9	2.4		
Lung/Trachea	11.7	4.4	9.2	3.5	13.7	5.2	10.6-21.9	3.6-7.1
Heart	.1	.1	<1.0	0				
Liver	21.9	4.0	15.6	2.5	24.6	4.7	25.0-40.1	4.6-9.7
Pancreas	.1	.1	<1.0	<1.0	2.1	<.1		
Stomach	.3	.3	1.1	<1.0	.4	.4		
Intestines	.4	.4	<1.0	<1.0	.5	.2		
Kidney	.2	.1	<1.0	<1.0	.3	<.1		
Urinary/Bladder	.1	.1	0	1.0	<.1	<.1		
Preputial Gland	–	–	–	–	–	–		
Testis	.5	NA	<1.0	NA	.4	NA		
Ovary	NA	.7	NA	<1.0	NA	.9		
Uterus	N	1.2	NA	1.9	NA	1.6		
Pituitary	.2	3.2	<1.0	3.5	.3	3.6		
Adrenal	.9	.7	<1.0	<1.0	1.4	.6		
Thyroid	1.0	1.3	1.1	<1.0	1.0	1.7		
Pancreatic Islets	.3	.1	<1.0	<1.0	.4	.2		
Body Cavities	.1	.3	<1.0	<1.0	.4	.3		
Leukemia/Lymphoma	5.6	12.7	1.6	6.8	10.3	20.6	7.2-12.2	1.7-30.4
N	2355	2365	1132	1176	3543	3617	?	?

TABLE 13
Reported Background Tumor Incidences In Fischer 344 Rats

ORGAN/TISSUE	Chu 1977		Fears et al 1977; Page, 1977; Gart et al., 1979		Goodman et al., 1979		Chu et al., 1981		Tarone et al., 1981	
	M	F	M	F	M	F	M	F	M	F
Brain	.9	.6	1.3	<0	8.1	.55	.8	.6		
Skin/Subcutaneous	6.6	3.2	5.7	2.5	6.4	3.0	7.8	3.2		
Mammary Gland	1.4	17.9	0	18.8	1.54	8.5	1.5	20.9		
Circulatory System	.4	.5	<1.0	<1.0	3.8	.27	.7	.4		
Lung/Trachea	3.1	1.8	2.4	<1.0	2.9	2.0	3.0	1.9		
Heart	.3	.1	<1.0	<1.0	.2	.05				
Liver	1.8	3.1	1.2	1.3	1.74	3.9	2.2	1.9	0.7-3.4	0.5-2.9
Pancreas	.2	—	<1.0	<0	.16	0	.2	—		
Stomach	.3	.2	<1.0	<1.0	.32	.2	.3	.2		
Intestines	.3	.5	<1.0	<1.0	.31	.36	.6	.3		
Kidney	.4	.2	<1.0	<1.0	.38	.16	.5	.2		
Urinary/Bladder	.1	.2	<1.0	<1.0	.1	.22	.1	.3		
Preputial Gland	1.4	1.2	—	—	1.4	1.2	2.4	1.8		
Testis	80.6	NA	76.2	NA	80.1	NA	2.3	NA		
Ovary	NA	.3	NA	<1.0	NA	.33	NA	.4		
Uterus	NA	15.6	NA	16.8	NA	5.55	NA	17		
Pituitary	11.5	30.5	10.2	29.5	11.4	0.3	4.7	34.9	7.5-31.2	31.0-58.6
Adrenal	10.0	4.6	8.7	4.0	9.95	4.58	2.4	5.2		
Thyroid	7.1	6.5	5.1	5.6	7.16	6.65	8.2	6.8	3.6-	4.7-
Pancreatic Islets	.8	1.0	3.2	1.3	3.89	1.05	3.9	.8		
Body Cavities	1.1	.3	<1.0	<1.0	2.51	.38	2.6	.4	2.8-9.0	1.0-1.9
Leukemia/Lymphoma	11.7	9.1	6.5	5.4	12.3	9.9	9.9	13.4	9.1-23.6	7.5-15.4
N	1806	1765	846	840	1794	1754	**			

*Gives detailed breakdown of neoplastic and nonneoplastic lesions in aged animals.
**Range of averages, 6 different laboratories.

of control animal populations based on grounds other than just tumor incidences. It is interesting that in these NCI/NTP bioassay program control populations, mean survival of B6C3F1 mice was greater than that of F344 rats.

Generally, historical control group data are used primarily as a check to ensure that the statistical evaluations used in comparing treatment groups to concurrent controls have a sound starting point (Chu et al., 1981)

Dempster et al. (1983) have, however, proposed a method for incorporating historical control data in the actual process of statistical analysis. A variable degree of pooling (combining) of historical with concurrent controls is performed based on the extent to which the historical data fit an assumed normal logistic (log transform) model.

Age (in either animals or humans) is clearly related to both "background" cancer incidence and chemically induced carcinogenesis. Indeed, one view of chemically induced carcinogenesis is that it serves in many (if not all) cases to accelerate the rate at which developing deficencies in the body's defense system allow cancers to be expressed. As either a carcinogen becomes more potent or a larger dose is used, neoplasms sucessfully overcome or evade defense mechanisms and are expressed as tumors. In some cases, the effect of a test chemical clearly results in the earlier appearance of tumors in a test animal population than in nontreated members of the same population. Unless a study is designed and conducted so that a reasonably accurate measurement of time-to-tumor can be made, one is left with only the incidence of tumors found at the end of the study and the variable incidence in animals that died on study, and cannot rule out the possibility that, though the terminal incidences were comparable, the test chemical resulted in an earlier development or expression of these same tumors. This is one of the strengths of the traditional skin painting studies, which allow easy detection of skin tumors as soon as they appear, and tracking of their progress.

If the target organ is not the skin, the only reasonably sensitive manner of evaluating time-to-tumor (unless the tumors are rapidly life threatening and there is an accordingly high early mortality rate leading to necropsy of spontaneous deaths in test animals) is to periodically, during the study, terminate, necropsy and histopathologically evaluate random samples of test and control animals. The traditional NCI bioassay had no such interim or serial sacrifices (Chu et al., 1981), and therefore could not address such issues.

Such serial sacrifices are usually conducted on at least twenty animals per sex per group starting at one year into the study. Several statistical methods other than life table procedures are available for analysis of such data (Bratcher, 1977, Dinse, 1985).

A related issue is the age at which to terminate the animals. We have already stressed that as a study progresses, the rise in the background level of tumors makes it more and more difficult to clearly partition treatment-effect tumors from age-effect tumors. Swenberg (Swenberg, 1985; Solleveld *et al.*, 1984) has made the point that the incidence of many tumor types has increased from 100 to 500% when control rat results from two year studies (rats 110 - 116 weeks of age) were compared to those from lifespan studies (140 to 146 weeks of age). If such an increase in age (25%) can result in such extreme increases in spontaneous tumors, what is the effect on interpretation of incidence rates seen in concurrent treatment groups? This is especially the case if, as Salsburg (1980) has suggested, any biologically active treatment will result in a shift in the patterns of neoplastic lesions occurring in aging animals. The current practice is to interpret tumor incidence on an independent site-by-site basis (on the assumption that what happens at each tissue site is independent of what happens elsewhere), and no allowance or factoring is made for the fact that what may be occurring in animals over their life span (as expressed by tumor incidence levels at an advanced age) is merely a shifting of patterns from one tumor site to another. In other words, commonly the "significantly" increased incidence of liver tumors is focused on, while the just as statistically significant decrease in kidney tumors compared to controls is ignored. Clearly, we should not be trying to analyze tumor data from animals that are advancing into senescence in the same manner that we do the data from those which lack these confounding factors. Where should a cut-off point be? This is a problem, but clearly Cameron's data (Cameron *et al.*, 1985) suggest that the growth curves of 9,385 B6C3F1 mice and 10,023 F344 rats from control groups in NCI/NTP studies show consistent patterns of decline in body weights from these animals starting at the following ages (in weeks).

	Males	Females
B6C3F1 Mice	96	101
Fischer 344 Rats	91	106

The existence of similar data for tumor incidences (unfortunately not available from NCI/NTP studies) would certainly improve our confidence in selecting cutoff points for age, but the above ages merit consideration as termination points.

Having reviewed the preceding biological factors, we may now begin to directly address the statistical interpretation of carcinogenesis bioassays. Such interpretation, once believed to be a simple problem of calculating the statistical significance of increases of tumor incidences in treatment groups at each of a number of tissue sites, is now clearly a more complex task. Assuming dose level and route were appropriate, at least four separate questions must still be addressed in such an interpretation of incidence.

1. Are the data resulting from the bioassay sufficient to warrant analysis and interpretation? Factors which may invalidate a bioassay include inadequate survival in test or control groups, extreme (high or low) control group tumor incidence levels, excessive loss of tissues from autolysis, infection during the study, and the use of contaminated diet or water.
2. Are there increases in tumor incidences in test groups compared to those in control groups? If so, then we must proceed to an incidence comparison on some form of contingency table arrangement of the data. Such comparisons are traditionally performed using a series of Fisher's Exact tests as presented in Chapter 6.
3. If there is a significant increase in tumor incidence, is there a trend (dose response) in the data for these sites which concurs with what we know about biological responses to toxicants? That is, as dose increases, response should increase. A significant increase occurring only in a low dose group (with the incidence levels in the higher dose groups being comparable to controls), would be of very questionable biological significance.
4. If significant incidence and trend are present, is there supporting evidence of the material being a carcinogen? An example of this was cited earlier in the case of mouse liver tumors where the presence of positive mutagenicity findings would support a belief of biological significance and concern about real-life exposure of humans.

Two major controversial questions are involved in such comparisons: (a) Should they be based on a one-tailed or a two-tailed distribution, and (b) what are the effects and implications of multiple comparisons? The one-or-two-tailed controversy revolves around the question of which hypothesis we are properly testing in a study such as a chronic carcinogenicity study. We might be asking whether the tumor incidence differs between the control and treated groups. In such cases, it is a bidirectional hypothesis and, therefore, a two-tailed distribution we are testing against. Or we might be asking whether the tumor incidence is greater in the treated group than in the control group? In the latter case, it is a unidirectional hypothesis and we are contemplating only the right hand tail of the distribution. The implications of the question we ask is of more than theoretical interest; significance is much greater (exactly double, in fact, for Fisher's Exact test) in the one-tailed case than in the two-tailed. For example, a set of data analyzed by Fisher's exact test which would have a two-tailed p level of 0.098 and one-tailed level of 0.049 would be flagged, therefore, as significantly different if the one tailed test were employed. Feinstein (1975) provides an excellent nonmathematical discussion. Determination of the correct approach must rest on a clear definition by the researcher, beforehand, of the objective of his study and of the possible outcomes (if a bidirectional outcome is possible, are we justified in using a one-tailed test statistic?).

The multiple comparisons problem is a much more lively one. In chronic studies, we test lesion/tumor incidence on each of a number of tissues, for each sex and species, with each result being flagged if it exceeds the fiducial limit of $p \leqslant 0.05$.

The point we must ponder here is the meaning of "$p \leqslant 0.05$." This is the level of the probability of our making a Type I error (incorrectly concluding we have an effect when, in fact, we do not). So we have accepted the fact that there is a 5% chance of our producing a false positive from this study. Our trade-off is a much lower chance (typically 1%) of a Type II error, that is, of our passing as safe a compound which is not safe. These two error levels are connected; to achieve a lower Type II level inflates our Type I level. The problem in this case is that when we make a large number of such comparisons, we are repeatedly taking the chance that we will "find" a false positive result. The set of lesions and/or tumor comparisons described above may number more than 70 tests for significance in a single study, which will result in a large inflation of our false positive level. The extent of this inflated false positive rate (and how to reduce its effects) has been discussed and estimated with a great degree of variability. Salsburg (1977) has estimated that the typical original National Cancer Institute (NCI) type cancer bioassay has a probability of Type I error ranging between 20 and 50%. Fears and colleagues (Fears and Tarone, 1977; Fears et al., 1977), however, have estimated it as being between 6 and 24%. Haseman (1985) has also reviewed some of Salsburg's calculations and concluded that, in correcting for multiple counting of individual animals and adjusting for survival differences, the false positive rate was markedly reduced. Without some form of correction factor, the "false positive" rate of a series of multiple tests can be calculated as being equal to $1-0..05^N$ where N is the number of tests and the selected alpha level is 0.05. Salsburg (1977) expressed the concern that such an exaggerated false positive result may cause a good compound to be banned. Though Haseman (1977) challenged this on the point that a much more mature decision process than this is used by the regulatory agencies, Salsburg has pointed out at least two cases, however, where the decision to ban was based purely on such a single statistical significance. What, then, is the proper use of such results? Or, conversely, how can we control for such an inflated error rate?

There are statistical methods available for dealing with this multiple comparisons problem. One such is the use of Bonferroni inequalities to correct for successive multiple comparisons (Wilks, 1962). This method has the drawback that there is some accompanying loss of power, expressed as an inability to identify true positives properly. A method proposed by McKnight and Crowley (1984) provides a reasonably sensitive yet unbiased means of evaluating such data, if information from frequent interim terminations is present. Similarly, Meng and Dempster (1985) have proposed a Bayesian approach to such analysis to solve the multiple comparisons problem. In this, a logistically distributed (or log transformed) model which accommodates the incidences of all tumor types or sites observed in the current experiment, as well as their historical control incidences, is developed. Exchangeable normal expected values are assumed for certain linear terms in the model. Posterior means, standard deviations, and Bayesian p-values are computed for an overall treatment effect as well as for the effects on individual tumor types or tissue sites. Model assumptions are then evaluated using probability plots and the sensitivity of the parameter estimates to alternative expected values is analyzed.

The third and fourth questions presented earlier are parts of what is evolving as a second set of approaches to the interpretation of bioassay results.

These new approaches use the information in a more mature decision-making process. First, the historical control incidence rates such as those given for the B6C3F1 mouse and the Fischer-344 rats in Tables 12 and 13 should be considered; as we have seen, some background incidences are so high that these tissues are "null and void" for making decisions. Second, we should look not just for a single significant incidence in a tissue, but rather for a trend. For example, we might have the following percentages of a liver tumor incidence in the female rats of a study: (a) control - 3%, (b) 10 mg/kg - 6%, (c) 50 mg/kg - 17%, and (d) 250 mg/kg - 54%. In this study only the incidence at the 250 mg/kg level might be statistically significant. However, the trend through each of the levels is suggestive of a dose-response. Looking for such a trend is an essential step in a scientific assessment of the results, and one of the available trend analysis techniques, such as presented in Chapter VIII, should be utilized. Another method for determining whether statistically significant incidences are merely random occurrences is to compare the results of the quantitative variables to two or more concurrently run control groups. Often the mean of one variable will differ from only one of these controls and be numerically within the range of this same variable of the two control means. If so, the statistical significance compared to the one control must be seriously questioned as to its being associated with a biological significance. Three different such stepwise interpretive procedures are common. These are the NCI method, the weight-of-evidence method, and the Peto method. The NCI approach is somewhat complex, involving each of the four steps outlined earlier in a process overviewed by Chu *et al.* (1981). The statistical aspects of this are outlined below.

NCI BIOASSAY METHOD

I. Survival analysis - by sex, species and organ. Exclude all animals dying prior to first incidence of tumor at that site. Do a life table analysis for survival at the same time.

II. Use Fisher-Exact test to obtain one tailed p at each site using the survival adjusted ratios obtained in I above.

III. Utilize the Bonferroni correction using r (where r = the number of dose levels; not k = the number of total comparisons). Multiply the computed p by r to maintain overall error rate. Significance is claimed only if p is less than α/r.

IV. Perform tests for linear trend using Cochran-Armitage test (dose response curve must be significantly different from zero, and positive).

NOTES: In a 100 animal bioassay, you need 5 or more animals to have tumors to achieve a one-tailed $p \geqslant 0.05$. With the Bonferroni correction, 7 or more are needed.

NCI believes and practices the rare tumor incidence flag mechanism.

REFERENCES: Bonferroni-Miller, R.G. (1966): *Simultaneous Statistical Interference*, pp 5–10: McGraw-Hill, New York

Trend - Tarone, R.E. (1975): Tests for trend in life table analysis, *Biometrika*, 62:679–682.

- Armitage, P. (1955): Tests for linear trends in proportions and frequencies. *Biomet.*, II, 375–386.

The nine possible interpretations of an analysis of tumor incidence and survival analysis, such as that presented in Chapter 9 (Cox, 1972; Byar, 1977 and Hammond *et al.*, 1978) are summarized in Table 14.

The weight-of-evidence approach consists primarily of the four steps of interpretation presented earlier, with emphasis on the last step (integration of related and supporting information into the evaluation process) as opposed to the NCI approach (which places emphasis

TABLE 14

INTERPRETATION OF THE ANALYSIS OF TUMOR INCIDENCE AND SURVIVAL ANALYSIS (Life Table)

OUTCOME TYPE	TUMOR ASSOCATION WITH TREATMENT*	MORTALITY ASSOCIATION WITH TREATMENT	INTREPRETATION**
A	+	+	Unadjusted test may underestimate tumorigenicity of treatment.
B	+	+	Unadjusted test gives valid picture of tumorigenicity of treatment.
C	+	−	Tumors found in treated groups may reflect longer survival of treated groups. Time adjusted analysis is indicated.
D	−	+	Apparent negative findings in tumors may be due to the shorter survival in treated groups. Time-adjusted analysis and/or a retest at lower doses is indicated.
E	−	0	Unadjusted test gives a valid picture of the possible tumor-preventive capacity of the treatment.
F	−	−	Unadjusted test may underestimate the possible tumor-preventive capacity of the treatment.
G	0	+	High mortality in treated groups may lead to unadjusted test missing a possible tumorigen. Adjusted analysis and/or retest at lower doses is indicated.
H	0	0	Unadjusted test gives valid picture of lack of association with treatment.
I	0	−	Longer survival in treated groups may mask tumor-preventive capacity of treatment.

* + = Yes, − = No and 0 = No bearing on discussion
**The unadjusted test referred to here is a contingency table type of analysis of incidence, such as a Fisher's Exact test.

on the two "statistical" steps). The weight-of-evidence approach poses difficulty in the regulatory and legal fields because it requires judgment and is not overtly quantitative. However, it does represent a scientifically valid approach for distinguishing important differences in the potential of chemicals to induce cancer. The greatest weight of evidence should be given to chemicals that induce dose-related increases in malignant tumors at multiple sites, in both sexes and in multiple species using appropriate routes of administration. At the other end of the spectrum, much less weight should be given to chemicals that induce only an increased incidence of a benign neoplasm, whose incidence is normally quite variable, in only the high dose group of one sex of a single species. One must also integrate a significant amount of additional information.

For example, the shape and extent of the dose-response curve should be known in relation to factors such as the chemical's pharmacokinetics, its overwhelming of host defenses or saturation of metabolic systems. Is the chemical genotoxic? How do the site and dose response for toxicity compare with those for carcinogenicity? This knowledge is highly relevant when attempting to understand the mechanisms involved in carcinogenesis for each specific chemical, and can and should be incorporated into both hazard identification and risk assessment to improve their accuracy. It is widely believed to be appropriate to test a chemical at the MTD in order to gain assurance that it has been adequately tested. However, if a chemical is not genotoxic, but induces frank cytotoxicity in the liver only at doses at which it also induces liver tumors, it should be considered differently than a chemical that is genotoxic and induces liver tumors over a large dose range, including noncytotoxic doses.

The Peto procedure is actually a collection of approaches arising from the central belief that it is possible to generate an additional vital set of data from a well-run bioassay, and that we should utilize these same pieces of data in interpreting results.

The data in question constitute an evaluation of the likelihood that each individual tumor would (or would not) be life threatening. The approach calls for the pathologist on a study to not only identify a mass or tumor as neoplastic or not, but also to categorize each neoplasm in one of several possible classes as to the risk it presents to the survival of the host organism. Such classification is generally in one of at least five different categories:

1. Tumor did or would definitely cause death of animal.
2. Tumor probably did or could cause death of animal.
3. Cannot be determined.
4. Tumor probably didn't or wouldn't cause death of animal.
5. Tumor didn't or wouldn't cause death of animal.

Such data can then be employed in a more precise interpretation of the meaning of the bioassay. An entire separate, sensitive set of significance tests based on such data have been proposed by Peto *et al.* (1980).

The last point to be addressed under the topic of the carcinogenicity bioassay is the use of the resulting data for the conduct of carcinogenic potency comparisons. Such a potency comparison would both be valuable in a scientific sense and provide a basis for prioritization of regulatory actions.

Potency and dose response of carcinogens for any single species of animals may be expressed in one of two manners - either as the incidence rate of tumors at the end of a set period of time or as the time lag from treatment to a specified incidence rate of tumors. This second manner has also been extended to determining time to death as a result of tumors produced by a carcinogen (Lijinsky *et al.* 1981).

Squire (1981) has proposed a ranking system for animal carcinogens based on data from NTP bioassays (that is, in the absence of time-to-tumor information). The major considerations are:

1. Number of species affected.
2. Number of different types of neoplasms induced in one or more species.
3. A negative correction for the spontaneous incidence in control groups of induced neoplasms.
4. Cumulative dose or exposure per kilogram body weight in affected groups.
5. The proportion of induced neoplasms which were malignant.
6. The degree of supporting genotoxicity (mutagenicity) data.

Of course, our real interest in the potency of carcinogens is in humans, which means an interspecies comparison. Crouch and Wilson (1979), using the results of some 70 NCI/NTP bioassays where carcinogenicity was established in both rats and mice, reported that a comparison demonstrated empirically that good correlations exist between these two species for suitably defined carcinogenic potencies for various chemicals. Such a correlation would allow sufficient accuracy in extrapolating from animal data to human risk to support a logical scheme for the evaluation of such risks. More recently, however, Bernstein *et al.* (1985) examined a larger NCI/NTP Bioassay Program data base. They observed that there is a very high correlation between the maximum doses tested (max-d) for rats and mice on a milligram per kilogram body weight per day basis. Calculating the carcinogenic potency (b-defined in their paper), they found it to be restricted to an approximately 30-fold range surrounding $\log(2)/\text{max-d}$, which has a biological as well as a statistical basis. Since the max-d's for the set of NCI/NTP test chemicals varied over many orders of magnitude, it necessarily follows statistically that the carcinogenic potencies will be highly correlated. This "artifact" of potency estimation does not imply that there is no basis for extrapolating animal results to man. They concluded that "it does suggest, however, that the interpretation of correlation studies of carcinogenic potency needs much further thought".

On an intermediate level, DuMouchel and Harris (1983) have suggested a class of Bayesian statistical methods for the interspecies extrapolation of potency functions that allows for the combining of data from different substances and species of animals, using the results as one constructs the model to estimate inter-experimental error between the different sources of data being combined.

Low Dose Extrapolation

Risk assessment, in the sense in which we will consider it in this book, and as it is performed by toxicologists, involves a number of separate steps, each of which involves some form of mathematical model to bridge gaps in biological knowledge. In a very crude sense, these steps can be categorized as answers to one of three problems:

1. Given knowledge of what happens at relatively high doses in one or more animal species, we must predict what would happen in the same species at much lower dose levels.
2. We must estimate what actual human exposures are. This means identifying groups or classes of exposed people and estimating "lifetime exposure".
3. Given the dose response estimation made (for animals from step 1) and exposure estimates for classes of people (from step 2), we must finally couple the two by some model which translates "mice-to-men". That is, we must perform a species-to-species extrapolation.

The second and third steps will be separately addressed in the final section of this chapter. The first step, known as low-dose extrapolation, will be addressed here.

Threshold

The process of low dose extrapolation, no matter which method is used, consists of three distinct steps. First, the actual dose-response data points available (which, for reasons discussed earlier, are invariably in the high dose and/or high response region) are identified, providing us with a starting point. Second, a mathematical method is selected and employed to extend the dose response relationship from the region we know to the regions we are interested in or concerned about. Third, we make a basic assumption about the nature of the dose response relationship in the extreme low dose and/or response region, then proceed to develop a model specific to the compound of interest.

This basic assumption about the extreme low-dose region is the question of threshold. For all biological phenomena except carcinogenesis and mutagenesis, it is a basic principle of biology that there is a dose level (threshold) below which no response is evolved. But there is an ongoing controversy as to applicability of the concept of a threshold for these two phenomena. Regulatory bodies in the U.S. have based much of their risk assessment work on the belief (which cannot, of course, be either proved or disproved) that a single molecule of any agent found to be a carcinogen or mutagen at high dose levels will involve some increase in the incidence of that response. Epstein (1973), in quoting Umberto Saffiotti, presented one major argument against the concept of the use of threshold.

"Certain approaches to the problem of identifying a 'safe threshold' for carcinogens are scientifically and economically unsound. I have in mind some proposals to test graded doses of one carcinogen down to extremely low levels, such as those to which a human population may be exposed through, say, residues in food. In order to detect possible low incidences of tumors, such a study would use large numbers of mice, of the order of magnitude of 100,000 mice per experiment. This approach seems to assume that such a study would reveal that there is a threshold dose below which the carcinogen is no longer effective, and, therefore, that a 'safe dose' can be identified in this manner. Now, there is presently no scientific basis for assuming that such a threshold would appear. Chances are that such a 'megamouse experiment' would actually confirm that no threshold can be determined. But let us assume that the results showed a lack of measurable tumor response below a certain dose level in the selected set of experimental conditions and for the single carcinogen under test. In order to base any generalization for safety extrapolations on such a hypothetical finding, one would have to confirm it and extend it to include other carcinogens and other experimental conditions such as variations in diet, in the vehicle used, in the age of the animals, their sex, etc. Each of these tests would then imply other "megamouse experiments." The task would be formidable: suffice it to say that an experiment on 100,000 mice would cost about 15 million dollars; if one did 20 such experiments, it would cost 300 million dollars. All this to try and estimate the possible shape of a dose response curve which would still leave most of our problems in the evaluation of carcinogenesis hazards unsolved. This effort would also block the nation's resources for long-term bioassays for years to come and actually prevent the use of such resources for the detection of potent carcinogenic hazards from yet untested environmental chemicals. If two million mice are made available as resources, they can be used effectively to test 4,000 new compounds, each on 500 mice, thereby detecting among them those that are highly carcinogenic in the test conditions."

The argument against the existence of a threshold for carcinogens continues with the following points:

1. *In vitro* a single molecule of a chemical can achieve an alteration of the genetic elements of a cell, mutating it. Such mutations can be to neoplastic forms, therefore including the process which (in the end) would produce a cancer *in vivo*. Albert *et al. (1979)* have presented a variation on this theme with initiation/promotion in mouse skin as a model.

2. Even if there is a biological threshold for any individual agent of concern due to various defense mechanisms, we cannot rule out the possibility of the presence of other agents in the environment which may either act as promoters for our agent of concern or saturate the existing defense mechanisms, effectively "jumping over" the threshold. Mantel presented this argument in his 1963 review of the concept of threshold in carcinogenesis.

3. The presence of a threshold would preclude the possibility of linear dose response. Mantel and Schneiderman (1975) presented this point of view, which is a variation on point one. Of course, the existence of a threshold would actually only mean that a linear (or any other dose-response relationship) would start at some point above zero, being discontinuous only in the extreme lowest dose range.

4. The presence of a background exposure of carcinogens and promoters, and of spontaneously occurring cancers in a population at risk as large and diverse as that of human beings, implies that even if there are thresholds for some or most individuals, there will still remain others who have been "jumped over" their individual thresholds by background events. Crump *et al. (1976)* termed this the existence of a "random threshold" such that there could be no exposure that was absolutely safe for absolutely everyone who might be exposed. Interestingly, Gross and Fitzhugh (1970) presented a similar argument for "absolute safety" in addressing reproductive toxicity data for a food additive.

5. Existing methods of low-dose risk extrapolation implicitly account for the increase in time-to-tumor statistics insofar as they accord for the decrease in tumor incidence, invalidating

the pro-threshold argument (to be reviewed later) that at very low doses time-to-tumor would become so long that it would exceed lifespan. Guess and Hoel (1977) proposed this argument against thresholds.

All five of these arguments against the existence of a threshold center on the belief that without proof of aboslute safety, we must proceed in the most conservative manner possible. Calabrese (1983) summarized the essence of this approach as lack of belief in threshold together with six other principles.

1. Use of upper confidence limits on the estimated VSD (Virtually Safe Dose) instead of on the VSD themselves.
2. Use of the most sensitive animal species.
3. Use of the most sensitive sex of that species.
4. Use of the most sensitive strain within a species.
5. Expression of dosage given on a dietary concentration basis rather than on a body weight basis when extrapolating from animals to humans; this will result in about a 15-fold lower acceptable exposure for humans as compared to the mouse.
6. The slope of unity by Mantel-Bryan (a model for low-dose extrapolation to be discussed later) is almost always less than the observed data, thereby resulting in lower acceptable exposure.

The arguments for the existence of the threshold are as numerous and tend to be more mechanistic. These are summarized as follows:

1. Most (if not all) carcinogens and mutagens exhibit a dose response relationship, resulting in an apparent or effective threshold for at least some agents. This is the classical toxicology argument, coming from the general case of all other toxic actions and finding no reason or data to support these actions being different (Klaassen and Doull, 1980). Theoretical analysis of the process of carcinogenesis as understood for radiation (the case in which we have the most human data) likewise suggests a lack of linearity at very low doses (Arley, 1961).
2. Toxicity, including carcinogenesis, is a dynamic process which includes absorption of an agent into the body, distribution to various tissues, reversible or irreversible reactions with cellular commponents, adaptation and repair by molecular and cellular components of the body, and ultimately clearance from the body by metabolism and/or excretion. Such pharmacokinetic processes are generally linear only within prescribed ranges. Gehring et al. (1977) have proposed that such pharmacokinetic processes provide a conceptual basis for understanding how

metabolic thresholds may lead to a disproportionate increase in toxicity, including carcinogenesis, above certain dose levels. They have also conducted and presented work on vinyl chloride carcinogenesis and pharmacokinetic data to support this proposal.

3. Because an organism as large as either a mouse or a man has a tremendous number of cells, a large number of defense mechanisms of high efficiency, and a low probability of a "hit" by a carcinogen being effective in initiating or promoting a neoplasm, there is a biological threshold based on just stochastic or probabilistic grounds. The last aspect (low probability of a "meaningful" reaction) arises from consideration of the fact that the vast majority of molecules that a carcinogen comes in contact with (and reacts with) in a multicellular organism cannot then contribute to the development of a neoplasm - they are, in effect, a multitude of "dummies", acting to block the assassin's shot.

Dinman (1972) originally proposed this concept with the following six elements:

a. A cell is estimated to be composed of approximately 10^{14} molecules and atoms with which a xenobiotic sustance may interact.

b. A major factor influencing activity is molecular specificity, as compared to the mere presence of an atom or molecule in a cell.

c. There are lower concentration limits for the occurrence of biologically significant intracellular molecular reactivity. Numerous examples of *in vitro* studies of specific inhibitors have demonstrated that a lower concentration limit for such inhibition is 10^{-8} M.

d. Binding or interaction with proteins or other molecules at sites where there is no resulting functional effect may not happen frequently.

e. All chemical components of the cells and cells themselves are in a dynamic flux. The major consideration is that the rate of loss exceeds the rate of normal replacement.

f. Cells of different types of tissues have the capacity to induce normal DNA repair mechanisms to repair genetic damage caused by environmental mutagens. In fact, the absence of DNA repair mechanisms in persons with xeroderma pigmentosum clearly demonstrates the life-saving functional capacity of this process in normal individuals.

Based on these elements and the estimate that 10^4 molecules per cell is the lower limit for a material to be biologically active,

Friedman (1973) has calculated threshold levels for a number of materials. The calculations were also based on the assumption that there are 6×10^{13} cells in a 70 kg "average man", therefore requiring a minimum effective dose of 8.6×10^{15} molecules per kilogram of cells. Some of these results are presented in Table 15.

Several such calculated values (vitamin A, estradiol and diethylstilbestrol) were also shown to be conservative—below experimentally established effect levels.

4. As dose or exposure to a carcinogenic agent decreases, it is well established that the time it takes for tumors to be expressed gets longer and longer. At some point in the dose time-to-tumor curve, the time necessary for a tumor to develop will exceed the life span of the exposed members of a population. Doll (1977) has presented human (cigarette smoker) data to support this dose time to tumor hypothesis, along with an excellent compilation of human age-related tumor incidences at a large number of sites. Yanysheva and Antomonov (1976) have reported on the dose-time-effect relationship with respect to the carcinogen benzo-(a)-pyrene. They found that the number of animals with tumors decreases as exposure to benzo-(a)-pyrene decreases. Furthermore, the latency period varies inversely with the dose. Based on their results, Yanysheva and Antomonov (1976) developed a dose-time-effect relationship as shown in Table 16.

Based on the information in Table 16, Yanysheva and Antomonov suggested a dose of benzo-(a)-pyrene that they believed would lead to a carcinogenic effect only after the normal life-span of the exposed individual. Kraybill (1977) combined arguments in 3 (above) and those for a time-to-tumor threshold in suggesting that "the fallacy of considering just singular insults in a biomedical assessment, the traditional approach, can thus be appreciated".

5. There are directly demonstrable physicochemical factors which cause some agents to be carcinogens above certain dose levels and, conversely, cause these particular materials not to be carcinogens (at least by the mechanism operative at the higher levels) at lower levels. Two examples of such mechanisms of threshold are xylitol and hexavalent chromium.

Elizabeth Miller used and presented the case of xylitol as part of her 1977 presidential address to the American Association for Cancer Research (Miller, 1978):

"The recent report on the development of tumors of the urinary bladder in male mice fed the sweetener xylitol as 10 to 20% of their

TABLE 15

Estimated No-Effect Quantities of Some Potent Carcinogens and Toxic Agents

Agent	Molecular Weight	Calculated No-Effect Level (g/kg Body Weight)	Molarity	Molecules per Kilogram Body Weight
Aflatoxin	312	5×10^{-9}	1.6×10^{-11}	9.6×10^{12}
1,2,5,6-diben-zanthracene (subcutaneous)	278	2.5×10^{-4}	9×10^{-7}	5.4×10^{17}
1,2,5,6-diben-zanthracene (subcutaneous)	278	2.5×10^{-5}	9×10^{-8}	5.4×10^{16}
3-Methylcholan-threne (subcutaneous)	268	2.5×10^{-4}	9.3×10^{-8}	5.6×10^{16}
3,4-Benz-a-pyrene (subcutaneous)	252	2.5×10^{-4}	1×10^{-6}	6×10^{17}
3,4-Benz-a pyrene (skin)	252	2.5×10^{-6}	1×10^{-8}	6×10^{16}
Aramite	335	1×10^{-1}	3×10^{-4}	1.8×10^{20}
Tetrachlorodi-benzodioxin	320	6×10^{-8}	1.9×10^{-10}	1.1×10^{14}
Botulinum toxin (mouse)	900,000	6.5×10^{-11}	7×10^{-17}	4.2×10^{7}

Source: Friedman (1973)

TABLE 16

Calulated Time for Appearance of the First Lung Tumor Following Administration of Various Total Benzo-a-pyrene Doses in 10 Portions, Intratracheally

Benzo-(a)-pyrene Dose (mg)	Time of Tumor Occurrence (months)
0.1	27.0
0.05	38.0
0.02	67.9
0.01	118.9
0.005	221.0
0.002	527.3

diets in 2-year tests and its possible implications for the use of xylitol in human foods provide an example of the problems to be resolved. These tumors apparently developed only in urinary bladders that contained stones (oxalates), a condition long known to predispose rodents to the development of bladder tumors. Neither bladder stones nor bladder tumors were reported in female mice fed the high levels of xylitol or in male mice fed 2% of the sweetener. Since xylitol is a normal intermediate in the metabolism of D-glucuronate, has not shown mutagenic activity, and would not be expected to yield strong electrophilic reactants on metabolism, there seems to be little reason for concern of hazard to humans ingesting low levels of xylitol in foods. Yet, strict interpretation of the Delaney amendment to the Pure Food and Drug Act would prohibit the use of xylitol, since the act does not permit addition to food of any chemical that has caused tumors in either humans or animals".

Hexavalent chromium is a somewhat more complex case which has only now come to completion. This is presented below as a case history.

CASE HISTORY

Evidence Supportive of a Threshold for Hexavalent Chromium Carcinogenicity

In animal studies chromates produce cancers only at the site of contact (lung carcinomas from intratracheal implantation or instillation and muscle sarcomas from intramuscular injection). No tumors have been found at distant sites. It is believed that the explanation for this observation is that hexavalent chromium is rapidly converted to trivalent chromium and that only the hexavalent form is capable of causing cancer. Carefully performed epidemiology studies have also failed to identify any excess risk of cancer in organ systems other than the respiratory tract.

The rat intratracheal instillation study (detailed below) found lung tumors in 20 of 80 rats exposed to 1..25 mg/Kg of sodium dichromate once a week. There were no tumors in 80 rats exposed to the same lifetime dose but at 0.25 mg/kg of sodium dichromate 5 days per week. One obvious explanation is that the animals were unable to detoxify the once a week dose and hence some tumors developed.

Several studies on the metabolism and/or detoxification of chromates have been published. These studies (Petrilli and De

Flora, 1978a and 1978b; De Flora 1978; Petrilli and De Flora 1980; De Flora, *et al.*, 1982; Petrilli and De Flora, 1982; Bennicelli *et al.*, 1983; De Flora *et al.*, 1984) have demonstrated that:

1. Hexavalent chromium (Cr^{+6}) is converted to trivalent chromium (Cr^{+3}) by saliva and gastric juice.
2. Cr^{+6} is converted to Cr^{+3} in red blood cells.
3. Cr^{+6} is converted in cytoplasm to Cr^{+3} by endogenous glutathione and other reducing compounds.
4. Cr^{+6} is metabolized to Cr^{+3} in certain cells, probably by DT diaphorase. This reduction, very potent in liver cells, is weaker in lung tissue but appears to be quite potent in human lung macrophages.
5. Cr^{+6} is mutagenic while Cr^{+3} is not. Trivalent chromium is an essential mineral which is incorporated into glucose tolerance factor.
6. While some scientists have suggested Cr^{+3} is the ultimate carcinogen binding to DNA (perhaps following reduction from Cr^{+6} in the immediate vicinity of DNA), there is some evidence that the ultimate carcinogen may be the more reactive Cr^{+5} ion (Jennette 1982). In any event, whether Cr^{+3} or Cr^{+5} is the ultimate carcinogen, reduction of Cr^{+6} to Cr^{+3} results in the practical elimination of carcinogenic risk as demonstrated by mutagenicity studies and the lack of tumors at distant sites following Cr^{+6} administration in animals.

A lifetime intratracheal instillation study was performed to specifically address the question of physicochemical defense system overload. Thirteen separate dose groups were included, as detailed below (Steinhoff *et al.*).

	5 X per week	1 X per week
$Na_2Cr_2O_7 \cdot 2H_2O$	0.25 mg/kg(40 ♂, 50 ♀)*	1.25 mg/kg(40♂, 40 ♀)
$Na_2Cr_2O_7 \cdot 2H_2O$	0.05 mg/kg(40 ♂, 45 ♀)**	0.25 mg/kg(40 ♂, 40 ♀)
$Na_2Cr_2O_7 \cdot 2H_2O$	0.01 mg/kg(40 ♂, 45 ♀)**	0.05 mg/kg(40 ♂, 40 ♀)
$CaCrO_4$	0.25 mg/kg(40 ♂, 50 ♀)*	1.25 mg/kg(40 ♂, 40 ♀)
Benzo(a)pyrene		5.00 mg/kg(−, 10 ♀)
Dimethylcarbamyl chloride		1.00 mg/kg(10 ♂, 10 ♀)
Physiolog- ical saline solution	1.00 ml/kg(40 ♂, 50 ♀)*	1.00 ml/kg(40 ♂, 40 ♀)

Untreated (40 ♂, 50 ♀)*

*   10 additional rats for intermediate sacrifice after 12 months of treatment, to decide whether further treatment would be possible.

**   5 additional rats for assessment under the electron microscope as well as some rats indicated by* being so assessed.

For the groups receiving sodium dichromate and calcium chromate (each as solutions), what the above design achieved was to give the same total lifetime doses, but in one set of cases (the 5 x per week) the total dose was spread over five smaller increments (which were each hopefully within the range of possible detoxification by defense mechanisms) and in the other set of cases delivered these as weekly "bolus" doses which overwhelmed defense mechanisms.

The survival in dosed test and negative control animals through two years of treatment was almost complete. The only increase in tumor incidence was in the lungs, as shown below.

		lung tumors benign	malignant
Untreated		–	–
phys. NaCl	5 x / week	–	–
phys. NaCl	1 x / week	–	–
$Na_2Cr_2O_7 \cdot 2H_2O$	5 x 0.01 mg/kg/week	–	–
$Na_2Cr_2O_7 \cdot 2H_2O$	5 x 0.05 mg/kg/week	–	–
$Na_2Cr_2O_7 \cdot 2H_2O$	5 x 0.25 mg/kg/week	–	–
$Na_2Cr_2O_7 \cdot 2H_2O$	1 x 0.05 mg/kg/week	–	–
$Na_2Cr_2O_7 \cdot 2H_2O$	1 x 0.25 mg/kg/week	1 (1♂)	–
$Na_2Cr_2O_7 \cdot 2H_2O$	1 x 1.25 mg/kg/week	12 (6♂, 6♀)	8 (5♂, ♀)
$CaCrO_4$	5 x 0.25 mg/kg/week	5 (5♂)	1 (1♀) .
$CaCrO_4$	1 x 1.25 mg/kg/week	11 (9♂,2♀)	3 (2♂,1♀)

There are numerous other cases of data which support the concept of a threshold. As early as 1943 Bryan and Shimkin reported skin painting data for three carcinogenic hydrocarbons which at least suggested thresholds.

In 1977, Wolfe reported a similar case for radiation exposure and Stokinger presented evidence for the existence of thresholds for seven chemical carcinogens (Table 17).

TABLE 17
Evidence for Thresholds in Carcinogenesis (Stokinger, 1977)

Test Substance	Route	Species	Dose Levels Eliciting Tumors	Dose Levels Not Eliciting Tumors	Duration
Bis-chloro-methyl ether	Inhalation	Rat	$100 \, \mu g/M^3$	$10 \, \mu g/liter$ $1 \, \mu g/liter$	6 months/ daily
1,4-Dioxane	Oral	Rat	1% in H_2O	0.1% in H_2O 0.01% in H_2O	2 years
	Inhalation	Rat	>1000 ppm	111 ppm	2 yrs./daily
Coal tar	Topical	Mouse	6400 mg 640 mg 64 mg	<0.64 mg weekly	64 weeks twice
β-Napthy-lamine	Inhalation Topical	Human	>5% in form	<0.5% in	22 years
Hexamethyl-phosphora-mide	Inhalation	Rat	4000 ppm 400 ppm	50 ppm	8 months
Vinyl chloride	Inhalation	Rat	2500 ppm 200 ppm 50 ppm	<50 ppm >10 ppm	7 months
Vinylidene chloride	Inhalation	Human	>200 ppm	1950-1955, 160 ppm average; 30-170 ppm	25 years
range				1960, <50 ppm decreasing to 10 ppm	

The ultimate empirical answer to the question of whether or not there are thresholds for carcinogens and mutagens in multicellular organisms would be a massive study with sufficient animals to allow for establishing a dose response curve across the broad dose range. Such a study is both logistically and economically unfeasible, but NCTR conducted a "megamouse" study which was designed to go part way towards this goal. In the Ed_{01} study, 24, 192 BALB/c female mice were fed 2-acetylaminofluorene (2-AAF), a carcinogen which results in tumors in two different organs (bladder and liver) by unrelated mechanisms. The spontaneous incidence rates for either of these two tumors in any one BALB/c female control was below 0.1% (Cairns, 1980). The entire study was initially reported as a complete issue of a journal (Staffa and Mehlman, 1980).

The data resulting from this study (Littlefield *et al.*, 1980) strongly suggest a threshold, but also emphasize the importance of time-to-tumor in the interpretation of results.

Models

There are at least eight different models for extrapolating a line or curve from a high-dose region to a low-dose region. In this section we will examine each of these models, and compare them in terms of characteristics and outcome. Not discussed here (but later, under risk assessment,) is the safety factor approach. Some of these models are such that they handle only quantal (also called dichotomous) data, while others will also accommodate time-to-tumor information.

In the models below, certain standard symbols are used. Most of these models express the probability of a response P, as a function, f, of dosage, D, so that $P = f(D)$ and the models differ only with respect to choice of function, f. The non-threshold models assume that if proportion p of control animals respond to a dose that $f(D) = p$ only for D equal to zero, and that for any nonzero D, $f(D) \blacktriangleright p$ (that is, there is a response). Threshold models assume the existence of a D_o such that for all $D < D_o$, $f(D) = p$ (that is, that there is some dose below which there is no response). If safety is defined as zero increase over control response, then a nonthreshold model would require that any nonzero dosage be associated with some finite risk.

One hit: The one-hit model is based on the assumption that cancer initiates from a single cell as a result of a random occurrence or "hit" that causes an irreversible alteration in the DNA of a susceptible cell type. It is also assumed that the likelihood of this hit is proportional to the level of carcinogen exposure. This suggests a direct linear dose response such that if one is to diminish the risk from 10^{-2} to 10^{-8}, then the dose should be divided by 10^6.

Accordingly, the one-hit model is also called the linear model, though a number of the other models also behave in a linear manner at lower doses. Based on the concept that a single receptor molecule of some form responds after an animal has been exposed to some single unit of an agent, the probability of tumor induction by exposure to the agent is then

$$P(D) = 1 - \exp(-1\lambda) D$$

where $\quad D \geq 0, 0 \leq P(D) \leq 1,$

λ is an unknown rate constant (or slope) and D is the expected number of hits at dose level D. "Dose" is used in a very general sense. It may mean the total accumulated dose or the dosage rate in terms of body weight, surface area approximations, or concentration in the diet. Computing the one-hit model in terms of the exponential series gives

$$P(D) = \frac{\lambda D}{1} \quad \frac{(\lambda D)^2}{1 \cdot 2} + \frac{(\lambda D)^3}{1 \cdot 2 \cdot 3} \cdots$$

which, for small values of $P(D)$, is well approximated by

$$P(D) = \lambda D$$

Though Hoel, Taylor, Kirchstein, Saffiotti and Schneiderman (1975) have argued that this model is consistent with reasonable biological assumptions, there is now almost universal agreement that the model is excessively conservative. The concept of a hit is a metaphor for a variety of possible elementary biochemical events and the model must be considered phenomenologic rather than molecular. This model is essentially equivalent to assuming that the dose-response curve is linear in the low-dose region. Thus, the slope of the one-hit curve at dose D is $\lambda [1 - P(D)]$, and for dose levels at which $P(D) < .05$ varies by less than 5%, i.e. is essentially constant and equal to λ. The linear model is one of two models, the other being the probit model, specified by the Environmental Protection Agency (1976) in its interim guidelines for assessment of the health risk of suspected carcinogens. The assumption of low-dose linearity will generally lead to a very low, virtually safe dose (VSD), so low as to lead the Food and Drug Administration Advisory Committee (1971) to remark that assuming linearity "...would lead to few conflicts with the results of applying the Delaney clause". The one-hit model, having only one disposable parameter, λ, will often fail to provide a satisfactory fit to dose-response data in the observable range. Other models described below, by introducing additional parameters, often lead to reasonable fits in the observable range.

An additional degree of conservatism is introduced by extrapolating back to zero from the upper confidence limit (UCL) for the net excess tumor rate (treated minus control rate). The linear model assumes that the tumor rate is proportional to dose, or that $P(D) = \lambda D$. The upper confidence limit for the slope is UCL divided by experimental dosage. Thus an estimate of an upper limit for the proportion of tumor bearing animals, P_u, for a given dose D is

$$P_u = \frac{UCL\, D}{D_e}$$

where D_e is the experimental dosage. Conversely, the dose D for a given P_u is

$$D = \frac{P_u D_e}{UCL}$$

The linear model may serve as a conservative upper boundary for probit dose-response curves. This upper boundary on the proportion of tumor-bearing animals may not be as conservative as one might imagine. Crump *et al.* (1976), Peto (1978), and Guess, Crump, and Peto (1977) have shown that the curvilinear dose-response curve resulting from the multistage model is well approximated by the linear model at low dose levels. Gross, Fitzhugh, and Mantel (1970) discussed the statistical aspects of a linear model for extrapolation.

Example 31 illustrates the linear extrapolation model.

EXAMPLE 31

A compound is administered as 5% (50,000 ppm) in diet for two years to a group of 100 animals. Twenty-two of these test animals and six of 100 control animals are found to have developed liver tumors at the end of the study.

Thus upper confidence limit on the excess tumor rate is approximately

$$(p_t - p_c) + Z \sqrt{\frac{p_t(1 - p_t)}{n_t} + \frac{p_c(1 - p_c)}{n_c}}$$

where p_t is the proportion of animals with tumors in n_t treated animals, p_c is the proportion of animals with tumors in n_c control animals, and Z is the normal deviate corresponding to the level of confidence desired.

The upper 99% confidence level for this example is thus

$$(0.22 - 0.06) + 2.33 \sqrt{\frac{0.22 \times 0.78}{100} + \frac{0.06 \times 0.94}{100}}$$

$$= (0.16) + 2.33\sqrt{.001716 + .000564}$$

$$= 0.16 + 2.33 (0.0477493)$$

$$= 0.271256$$

If it is then desired to estimate an upper limit of risk associated with exposure to 10 ppm of the material in diet this would be

$$= \frac{0.271256}{50,000} \times 10 = 5.43 \times 10^{-5}$$

The Probit Model: This model assumes that the log tolerances have a normal distribution with mean μ and standard deviation σ. The proportion of individuals responding to dose D, say P(D), is then simply

$$P(D) = \Phi [(\log D - \mu)/\sigma] = \Phi (\alpha + \beta \log D),$$

where $\Phi(x)$ is the standard normal integral froom $-\propto$ to X, $\alpha = -\mu/\sigma$ and $\beta = 1/\sigma$. This dose-response curve has P(D) near zero if D is near zero and P(D) increasing to unity as dose increases. A plot of a typical probit dose-response is given by an S-shaped (sigmoid) curve. The quantity above is referred to as the slope of the probit line, where

$$Y = \Phi^{-1}[P(D)] = \alpha + \beta \log D$$
and $\quad$ Y + 5 is the probit of P.

This is the same model we presented earlier in this book for linearizing a special case of quantal response, the data for LD_{50}'s. Despite its nonthreshold assumption it is a characteristic of the probit curve that as dose decreases, zero response is approached very rapidly, more rapidly than any power of dose. Other curves to be considered approach zero response more slowly than the probit.

An alternative derivation of the probit model which relates it to time-to-response has been given by Chand and Hoel (1974) using the Druckrey observation that median time to tumor, T, is related to dose, D, by the equation $DT^n = C$, where n and C are constants unrelated to D (Druckrey, 1967). Combining this relation with an assumed lognormal distribution of response time then gives the P(D) as probability of response to any given time, T_o, where α and β are simple functions of n, C, T_o and the standard deviation of the distribution of response times.

The actual method which has the probit model as its basis is the Mantel - Bryan procedure. As originally proposed, this procedure used the probit model but with a preassigned slope of unity. The rationale for this slope was that all observed probit slopes at the time of the proposal exceeded that value, the procedure therefore being considered conservative. An additional conservative feature involves use of the upper 99% confidence limit of the proportion responding at a dose level, rather than the observed proportion. The procedure then extrapolates downward to a response level of 10^{-8}, using each separate dose level in the experiment, or combinations, taking as the virtually safe dose (VSD) the highest of the values obtained. A conservative method of taking account of the response of the control group was also given. An improved version of the procedure, which included several sets of independent data and better methods of handling background response rates and responses at multiple doses has since been published (Mantel, Bohidar, Brown, Ciminera and Tukey, 1975).

A dosage D_o is said to be virtually safe if $f(D_o) < p + (1-p)P_o$, where P_o is some near-zero lifetime risk, such as 10^{-8}, the value proposed by Mantel and Bryan or 10^{-6}, the value adopted by the FDA. The virtually safe-dose (VSD) is then calculated as $f^{-1}[p + (1-p)P_o]$. The calculation thus requires choosing a model, f, determining the value of its disposable constants from observations in the observable range and extrapolating down to the unobservable elevation in response, P_o, to determine the VSD. This is illustrated in example 32.

EXAMPLE 32

From the data in example 31, we have already calculated an upper 99% confidence interval of 0.271, corresponding to a normal deviate of -0.61. If it is desired to determine the level corresponding to a tumor probability of less than one in a million (which has a normal deviate of -4.753), the extrapolation proceeds along the probit-log dosage line with a slope of 1 from the normal deviate of the upper 99% confidence limit on the observed result to the normal deviate for the selected probability or -0.61 − (-4.753) = 4.143 standard deviations.

The dose level corresponding to this risk is then

$$\frac{50,000 \, ppm}{10^{4.143}}$$

$$= \frac{5 \times 10^4}{1.39 \times 10^4}$$

$$= 3.597 \, ppm.$$

One of the advantages of the Mantel-Bryan procedure is that it rewards a larger experiment by reducing the upper confidence limit, which results in a larger dose for a selected proportion of tumor-bearing animals. Table 18 shows some dosages for a series of sample sizes; all yield observed tumor rates of 4%, with no tumors in the controls for a predicted tumor probability of less than one in a million.

TABLE 18

Mantel-Bryan Dosages for Various Sample Sizes with the Same Proportion of Experimental Animals with Tumors*

Sample size	No. of animals with tumors	Upper 99% confidence limit	Dosage (fraction of experimental dosage)
50	2	0.158	1/5630
100	4	0.112	1/3430
200	8	0.085	1/2400
400	16	0.069	1/1860

*Predicted tumor probability $< 10^{-6}$

Some situations, such as cigarette smoking in man and diethylstil-bestrol in mice, have indicated slopes on the order of 1. Thus one must be careful to establish that the slope of the dose-response is sufficiently large before applying the Mantel-Bryan procedure, indicating the desirability of multiple-dose experiments.

According to Mantel and Schneiderman (1975), the Mantel-Bryan methodology has several advantages:

a. It does not need an experimental estimate of the slope.
b. Statistical significance is not needed.
c. It takes into account a nonzero spontaneous background tumor incidence.
d. It considers multiple-dose studies.
e. Any arbitrary acceptable risk can be calculated.
f. It avoids categorizing a substance in absolute terms.
g. It permits the investigator flexibility in study design.

Mantel and Bryan (1961) provided an example of an actual study in which the carcinogen 3-methylcholanthrene was given to mice as a single injection, with 12 different dose levels used. Table 19 provides the methodology and findings of the Mantel-Bryan procedure.

Some criticisms of the Mantel-Bryan procedure are:

a. The normal distribution may not offer as accurate a description in the tails of the distribution as it does in the central parts, especially if one proceeds out to 10^{-6} or 10^{-8}.
b. The use of the arbitrarily low slope of unity for downward extrapolation has been criticized because of the lack of observational support.
c. The argument does not incorporate any of the present understandings of the process of carcinogenesis.
d. The model is insufficiently conservative, because the extrapolated probability approaches zero with decreasing dose more rapidly than any polynomial function of dose, and, in particular, more rapidly than a linear function of dose and hence may underestimate probability at low dose. (Crump, 1977).
e. The model is excessively conservative, because it does not postulate a threshold or accommodate time to tumor data.

Multistage: The multistage model (Armitage and Doll, 1961; Crump *et al.*, 1976) represents a generalization of the one-hit model and assumes that the carcinogenic process is composed of an unknown number of stages that are needed for cancer expression. Inherent in this model is the additional assumption that the effect of the carcinogenic agent in question is additive to a carcinogenic effect produced by external stimuli at the same stages. Such an assumption

TABLE 19

Illustration of Methodology for Determining the "Safe" Dose From Results at Several Dose Levels (Mantel and Bryan, 1961)

Dose per Mouse (mg)	Log Dose	Result	Combined Result			Calculated "safe" (1/100 Million)
		No. of Tumors No. of Mice	No. of Tumors No. of Mice	Maximum P Value 99% Assurance	Corresponding Normal Deviate	Log Dose (2) - (6) −5.612
(1)	(2)	(3)	(4)	(5)	(6)	(7)
0.000244	6.388−10	0/79	0/158	0.0288	−1.899	2.675−10
0.000975	6.990−10	0/41	0/79	0.0566	−1.584	2.962−10
0.00195	7.291−10	0/19	0/38	0.1141	−1.205	2.884−10
0.0039	7.592−10	0/19	0/19	0.2152	−0.789	2.769−10
0.0078	7.893−10	3/17	3/17	0.480	−0.050	2.331−10
0.0156	8.194−10	6/18	6/18	0.729	+0.610	1.972−10
0.0312	8.495−10	13/20	13/20	0.871	+1.131	1.752−10
0.0625	8.796−10	17/21	17/21	0.958	+1.728	1.456−10
0.125	9.097−10	21/21	—	—	—	—
0.25	9.398−10	21/21	—	—	—	—
0.50	9.699−10	21/21	—	—	—	—
1.0	10.000−10	20/20	—	—	—	—

generally leads one to expect a linear dose-response curve at low exposure levels.

This assumes that carcinogenesis occurs in a single cell as a point of origin and, according to the multistage model, is the result of several stages that can include somatic mutation. The transitional events are individually assumed to depend linearly on dose rate. This then leads in general to a model in which the probability of tumor approximates a low-order polynomial in dose rate. In the low dose region, which would relate to environmental levels, one finds that the responses are well approximated by a linear function of dose rate. The characteristic in which the low dose probability is proportional to the kth power of dose, where k is the number of stages, was considered by Armitage and Doll (1961) to be quite inconsistent with observation. They derived a multistage model, which by assuming that the effect of the agent at some stages was additive to an effect induced by external stimuli at those stages, led to a lower power than k for D. Crump, Hoel, Langley and Peto (1976) discussed this model and, by assuming additivity at all stages, have obtained as an expression for the required probability

$$P(D) = 1 - \exp\left\{ - \sum_{i=0}^{\infty} \alpha_i D^i \right\} \quad \alpha_i \geq 0.$$

Where $\alpha = -\mu / \sigma$. Hartley and Sielken (1977) combined this model with time to response, obtaining a more general result. For $\alpha_1 > 0$ these models also imply low dose linearity since

$$\lim_{D \downarrow 0} P'(D) = \alpha_1 \exp(-\alpha_0)$$

Armitage and Doll cited data relating lung cancer mortality to previous smoking habits as indicating to a linear dose-response curve, but errors in reporting the amount smoked would lead to such a curve even if the true curve were convex. This supports the view that the apparent low-dose linearity in many epidemiologic studies is an artifact of errors in the reporting of dose. Crump, et al. (1976) stress the crucial nature of the additivity assumption, pointing out that it can make orders of magnitude differences in the estimated risk associated with the low dose exposure.

A recent paper by Crump et al. (1977) describes a procedure for low-dose extrapolation in the presence of background which, although based on the generalized model above, reduces, (when upper confidence limits are used) to extrapolation using low-dose linearity. This is because the use of upper confidence limits on α_1 on the model is equivalent to admitting the possibility of a positive value of α_1, which at lose doses dominates the expression. Once upper confidence limits on the VSD or risk at a given dose are used, there may be little practical difference, therefore, between use of the one-hit model and the generalization given by the Crump et al. equation above.

Hartley and Sielken (1977) have developed a procedure based on maximum likelihood for the Armitage-Doll model. Their program is very general and allows for the inclusion of the effect of the time to a tumor.

In practice, these two approaches result in fitting a polynomial model to the dose response curve such that (where t is time):

$$\frac{p(D,t)}{1 - P(D,t)} = gDh(t)$$

where $P(D,t)$ is the probability of the observance of a tumor in an animal by time t at a dosage D,

$$p(D,t) = \frac{DP(D,t)}{Dt}$$

where g (D) is a function of dose such that

$$\begin{aligned}
g(dose) &= (a_1 + b_1\, dose)(a_2 + b_2\, dose)... \\
&\quad (a_n + b_n\, dose) \\
&= c_0 + c_1\, dose + c_2\, dose^2 + ... \\
&\quad + c_n\, dose^n,
\end{aligned}$$

where a_i, b_i, $c_i \geq 0$ are parameters that vary from chemical to chemical and h(t) is a function of time. The probability of a tumor by time t and dosage D is

$$P(D,t) = 1 - exp\,[-g(D)\,H(t)]$$

$$\text{where} \quad H(t) = \int_o^t h(t)\, Dt$$

This function generally fits well in the experimental dose range but has limited applicability to the estimation of potential risk at low doses. The limitations arise, first, because the model cannot reflect changes in kinetics, metabolism, and mechanisms at low doses and, second, because low dose estimates are highly sensitive to a change of even a few observed tumors at the lowest experimental dose.

A logical statistical approach to account for the random variation in tumor frequencies is to express the results in terms of best estimates and measures of uncertainty.

Important biological mechanisms of activation and detoxification are not usually specifically considered. However, a steady-state kinetic model that incorporates the process of deactivation as well as other pharmacokinetic considerations has been offered by Cornfield (1977). He noted that whenever the detoxification response is irreversible, low exposure levels are predicted to be harmless. However, the presence of a reversible response suggests linearity at low-dose exposures. He additionally predicted that when multiple protective responses are sequentially operational, the dose-response relationship will look like a hockey stick "with the striking part flat or nearly flat and the handle rising steeply once the protective mechanisms are saturated." Despite its seemingly greater biological veracity, the Food Safety Council (1978) challenged the multistage model general assumption of low-dose linearity on the basis of (1) the general absence of support for dosewise additivity seen in many studies in which additivity has been evaluated and (2) studies that showed the effects of one carcinogenic agent offset or prevented the carcinogenic effects of another.

Crump (1979) has noted that biostatistical models such as the multistage model assume that the quantity of carcinogen finding its way to the critical sites is proportional to the total body exposure, which is clearly not the case across the entire dose range covered by the model.

Criticisms of these models are summarized below.

a. These models do not consider the variation in susceptibility of the members of the population when deriving their dose-response relationships.
b. Low-dose linearity is not consistently found in experimental systems.
c. Low-dose linearity is assumed to occur by a mechanism of additivity to background levels, however, there is a lack of data supporting the additivity hypothesis.
d. They do not sufficiently recognize pharmacokinetic considerations including rates of absorption, tissue distribution, detoxification processes, repair, and excretion. (This would apply to the Mantel-Bryan model as well.)

Multi-hit: This model is also called the K-hit or gamma multi-hit model. It is a generalization of the one-hit model.

If k hits of a receptor are required to induce cancer, the probability of a tumor as a function of exposure to a dose (D) is given by

$$P(D) = 1 - \sum_{t=0}^{k-1} \frac{(\lambda D)^i e^{-\lambda D}}{i!} \approx \frac{(\lambda D)^k}{k!}$$

For small values of D, the k-hit model may be approximated by

$$P(D) = \gamma D^k$$

or $$\log P(D) = \log \gamma + k \log D$$

Thus k represents the slope of log P(D) versus log D. By the same reasoning, if at least k hits are required for a response, then

$$P(D) = P(X \geqslant k) = \int_{\bullet}^{\lambda D} \frac{u^{k-1} e^{-u} du}{(k-1)!}$$

Because this equation contains an additional parameter, k, it will ordinarily provide a better description of dose-response data than the one-parameter curve. This can be further generalized by allowing k to be any positive number, not necessarily an integer. In this case the above formula can be described as that dose-response curve which assumes a gamma distribution of tolerances with shape parameter k. We note

$$\lim_{D \downarrow 0} [P(D) / D^k] = \text{constant}.$$

Thus, in the low-dose region, the equation is linear for k = 1, concave for k < 1 and convex for k > 1. At higher doses the gamma and the lognormal distributions are hard to distinguish so that the model provides a blend of the probit model at high dose levels and the logit at low ones.

Procedures for estimating the parameters of the k-hit model by nonlinear maximum likelihood estimation have been developed by Rai and Van Ryzin (1979). This method has the advantage of permitting the data to determine the number of hits needed to describe the results without introducing more than two parameters. When only one dose level gives responses greater than zero and less than 100%, unique values of the two parameters can no longer be estimated. The background effect in this model is taken care of using Abbott's correction.

The multi-hit model is discussed in some detail in the Food Safety Council Report (1980). One derivation of this model follows from the assumption that k hits or molecular interactions are necessary to induce the formation of a tumor and the distribution of these molecular events over time follows a Poisson process. In practice the model appears to fit some data sets reasonably well and to give low-dose predictions that are similar to the other models. There are cases, however, in which the predicted values are inconsistent with the predictions of other models by many orders of magnitude. For instance, the virtually safe dose as predicted by the multi-hit model appears to be too high for nitrilotriacetic acid and far too low for vinyl chloride (Food Safety Council Report 1980).

Pharmacokinetic Models: Pharmacokinetic models have often been used to predict the concentration of the parent compound and metabolites in the blood and at reactive sites, if identifiable. Cornfield (1977), Gehring and Blau (1977), and Anderson, Hoel, and Kaplan (1980) have extended this concept to include rates for macromolecular events (e.g., DNA damage and repair) involved in the carcinogenic process. The addition of statistical distributions for the rate parameters and a stochastic component representing the probabilistic nature of molecular events and selection processes may represent a useful conceptual framework for describing the tumorigenic mechanism of many chemicals. Pharmacokinetic data are presently useful only in specific parts of the risk assessment process. A more complete understanding of the mechanism of chemically induced carcinogenesis would allow a more complete utilization of pharmacokinetic data. Pharmacokinetic comparisons between animals and humans are presently most useful for making species conversions and for understanding qualitative and quantitative species differences. The modeling of blood concentrations and metabolite concentrations identifies the existence of saturated pathways and adds to an understanding of the mechanism of toxicity in many cases.

Taking advantage of the similarity of the probit and pharmacokinetic models in the 5% to 95% range, Cornfield (1977) developed an approximate method of estimating its parameters, particularly the value of T, the saturation dose. Risks at dosages below T are crucially dependent on K*, the relative speed of the reverse, deactivation reaction and this cannot be well estimated from responses at dosages above T, so that low-dose assessment using this model may be more dependent on further pharmacokinetic experimentation than on further statistical developments.

This model considers an agent subjected to simultaneous activation and deactivation reactions, both reversible, with the probability of a response being proportional (linearly related) to the amount of activated complex. Denoting total amount of substrate in the system by S and deactivating agent by T and the ratios of the rate constants governing the back and forward reactions by K for the activation step and K* for the deactivation step, the model is, for

$$D > T \quad P(D) = \frac{D - S[P(D)] - y}{D - S[P(D)] - y + K}$$

where $y = K[P(D)] \, T \, / \, \{ K \, [P(D)] + K^* \, [1 - P(D)] \}$

$$D < T \quad P(D) \cong \frac{D}{S + K \left(1 + \dfrac{T}{K^*} \right)}$$

These equations follow from standard steady state mass action equations. Thus, at low dose levels, $D < T$, the dose-response curve is nearly linear, but for deactivating reactions in which the rate of the back reaction is small compared to that of the forward reaction, $K^* =$ will be quite small and the slope will be near zero. In fact, in the limiting case in which K* = 0 the dose-response curve has a threshold at D = T, but since the model is steady state and does not depend on the time course of the reaction, it cannot be considered to have established the existence of a threshold. For K* > 0, the dose-response curve is shaped like a hockey stick with the striking part nearly flat and rising sharply once the administered dose exceeds the dose, T, which saturated the system. Because of the great sensitivity of the slope at low doses to the value of K*/K, and insensitivity at high doses, responses at dose levels above D = T probably cannot be used to predict those below T. This can be considered a limitation of the model, but it can equally well be considered a limitation of high dose experimentation in the absence of detailed pharmacokinetic knowledge of metabolic pathways. The model can be generalized to cover a chain of simultaneous activating and deactivating reactions intervening between the introduction of D and the formation of activated complex, but this does not appear to change its qualitative characteristics. The kinetic constants, S, T, K and K* are presumably subject to animal-to-animal variation. This variation is not formally incorporated in the model, so that the possibility of negative estimates of one or more of these constants cannot be excluded.

Weibull: Another generalization of the one-hit model is the Weibull model:

$$P(D) = 1 - \exp(-\beta D^m),$$

where m and β are parameters. Note that

$$\lim_{D \downarrow 0} [P(D) / D^m =] = \text{constant}.$$

Thus, in the low-dose region, this last equation is linear for m = 1, concave for m < 1, and convex for m > 1. With a typical set of data, the Weibull model tends to give an estimated risk at a low dose which lies between the estimates for the gamma multi-hit and the Armitage-Doll models. The Weibull distribution for time-to-tumors has been suggested by human cancers (Cook, Doll, and Fellingham, 1969 and Lee and O'Neill, 1971);

$$I = bd^m (t-w)^k,$$

where I is the incidence rate of tumors at time t, b is a constant depending on experimental conditions, D is dosage, w the minimum time to the occurrence of an observable tumor, m, and k are parameters to be estimated. Also, Day (1967), Peto, Lee, and Paige (1972), and Peto and Lee (1973) have considered the Weibull distribution for time-to-tumor occurrence. Theoretical models of carcinogenesis also predict the Weibull distribution (Pike, 1966). Theoretical arguments and some experimental data suggest the Weibull distribution where tumor incidence is a polynomial in dose multiplied by a function of age. Hartley and Sielken (1977) adopted the form

$$H(t) = \sum_{i \geq 1} \xi_i t^i$$

where $\xi_i \geq 0$. They noted that this function can be regarded as a weighted average of Weibull hazard rates with positive weight coefficients, ξ_i. The conventional statistical procedure of weighted least-squares provides one method of fitting the Weibull model to a set of data. With a background response measured by the parameter p, the model, using Abbott's correction is:

$$P = p + (1 - p)(1 - \exp(-\beta D^m)) =$$
$$1 - \exp(-(\alpha + \beta D^m)),$$

where $\alpha = -\ln(1 - p)$. With the transformation $Y = -\ln(1 - P)$, the model becomes

$$Y = \alpha + \beta D^m$$

With a nonlinear weighted least-squares regression program, one can estimate the three parameters (m, α, β) directly. With only a linear weighted least-squares regression program, one can use trial and error on m to find the values of the three parameters which produce a minimum error sum of squares. A program for one electronic calculator (the TI-59, discussed earlier) which conveniently handles up to nine data points, is available from the Food Safety Council.

A nonlinear maximum likelihood method to obtain estimates of the parameters in the Weibull model can also be used. The use of the Weibull distribution for time-to-tumor leads to an extreme value distribution relating tumor response to dosage (Chand and Hoel, 1974). Hoel (1972) gives techniques for cases in which adjustments must be made for competing causes of death.

Logit: This model, like the probit model, leads to an S-shaped dose-response curve, symmetric about the 50% response point. Its equation (Berkson, 1944) is:

$$P(D) = 1/[1 + \exp\{-(\alpha + \beta \log D)\}]$$

It approaches zero response as D decreases more slowly than the probit curve, since

$$\lim_{D \to 0} |\, [P(D)/D^\beta] = K$$

where K is a constant.

The practical implication of this characteristic is that the logit model leads to lower VSD than the probit model, 1/25th as much in calculations reported by Cornfield, Carlborg and Van Ryzin (1978), even when both models are equally descriptive of the data in the observable range.

Albert and Altshuler (1973) have developed a related model for predicting tumor incidence and life shortening based on the work of Blum (1959) on skin tumor response and on Druckrey (1967) for a variety of chemical carcinogens in rodents. They had investigated cancer in mice exposed to radium. The basic relationship used was $Dt^n = c$, where D is dosage, t is the median time to occurrence of tumors, n is a parameter greater than 1, and c is a constant depending on the given experimental conditions. It is of interest to determine the time it takes for a small proportion of the population to develop tumors. With this formulation, as the dosage is increased, the time to tumor occurrence is shortened. Albert and Altshuler (1973) used the log normal distribution to represent time-to-tumor occurrence, assuming the standard deviation to be independent of dosage.

The log normal distribution of tumor times corresponds closely to the probit transformation as employed in the Mantel-Bryan procedure.

Log-Probit: The log-probit model assumes that the individual tolerances follow a lognormal distribution. Specific steps in the complex chain of events that lead to carcinogenesis are likely to have lognormal distributions. For example, it is reasonable to assume that the distribution of a population of kinetic rate constants for detoxification, metabolism, elimination, in addition to the distribution of immuno-suppression surveillance capacity and DNA repair capacity, can be adequately approximated by normal or lognormal distributions.

Tolerance distribution models have been found to adequately model many types of biological dose-response data, but it is an overly simplistic expectation to represent the entire carcinogenic process by one tolerance distribution. A tolerance distribution model may give a good description of the observed data, but from a mechanistic point of view there is no reason to expect extrapolation to be valid. The probit model extrapolation has, however, fit well in some instances (Gehring, Watanabe, and Park 1979).

The log-probit model has been used extensively in the bioassay of dichotomouse responses (see Finney, 1952). A distinguishing feature of this model is that it assumes that each animal has its own threshold dose below which no response occurs and above which a tumor is produced by exposure to a chemical. An animal population has a range of thresholds encompassing the individual thresholds. The log-probit model assumes that the distribution of log dose thresholds is normal. This model states that there are relatively few extremely sensitive ore extremely resistant animals in a population. For the log-probit model, the probability of a tumor induced by an exposure to a dose D of a chemical is given by

$$P(D) = \phi (\alpha + \beta \log_{10} D)$$

where ϕ denotes the standard cumulative Gaussian (normal) distribution. Chand and Hoel (1974) showed that the log-probit dose response is obtained when the time-to-tumor distribution is log normal under certain conditions.

Miscellaneous: There are a large number of other proposed models for low dose extrapolation, through these others have not gained any large following. Two examples of these are the extreme value and no-effect-level models.

Chand and Hoel (1974) showed that if the time-to-tumor distribution is a Weibull distribution, the dose-response model follows an extreme value model under certain conditions, with

$$P(D) = 1 - \exp [- \exp (\alpha + \beta \log D)]$$

Park and Snee (1983) made the observation that many biological responses vary linearly with the logarithm of dose, and that practical thresholds exist, and therefore the responses can be represented by the following model:

$$\text{Response} = B_1 \qquad\qquad \text{if dose} < D^*$$
$$\text{Response} = B_1 + B_2 \log (\text{dose}/D^*) \quad \text{if dose} \geq D^*$$

This model incorporates a parameter D^* that represents a threshold below which no dose-related response occurs. In this model, B_1 is the constant response level at doses less than D^*, and B_2 is the slope of the log-dose response curve at doses $\geq D^*$. It has been empirically found that many quantiative toxicological end points can be adequately described by the no-effect-level model. This model may, therefore, be useful for establishing thresholds for end points related to the carcinogenic process in situations where information other than the simple presence or absence of a tumor is available. Both the model and predicted threshold are of value when carcinogenicity is a secondary event.

Critique and Comparison of Models

None of the models presented here (or any others) can be "proved" on the basis of biological arguments or available experimental data, but some are more attractive than others on these grounds. The multistage model appears to be the most general model according to the values of the parameters. Unfortunately, most of these models fit experimental data equally well for the observable response rates at experimental dosage levels, but they give quite different estimated responses when extrapolated to low dosage levels. There are now numerous sets of data which have been used to compare two or more of the models against each other. The comparisons presented below are examples from the literature.

Case 1: In 1971, the FDA Advisory Committee on Protocols for Safety Evaluation compared three models (probit, logit, and one-hit) using the data presented in Table 20.

Table 20 Experimentally Determined (Actual) Incidences (%) of Animals with Tumor of Interest

Dose	Probit	Logit	One-hit
2	69	70	75
1	50	50	50
0.5	31	30	29
0.25	16	16	16
0.125	7	8	8
0.0625	2	4	4

It should be clear that with any adequately designed and executed study, these three sets of results are indistinguishable. But in Table 21 the extrapolated doses needed to achieve certain incidences of response in a population are presented. They are seen to give values varying by as much as four orders of magnitude.

Table 21 Extrapolated Doses for Low Incidences of Tumors

Incidence of animals with tumors	Probit	Units of dose Logit	One-hit
10^{-3}	1.5×10^{-2}	3.1×10^{-3}	1.4×10^{-3}
10^{-6}	1.4×10^{-3}	9.8×10^{-6}	1.4×10^{-6}
10^{-8}	4.1×10^{-4}	1.6×10^{-7}	1.4×10^{-8}

Case 2: Gaylor and Shapiro (1979) presented a comparison of the Mantel-Byran and one-hit methods' predicted upper confidence limits for a range of VSD's (from 10^{-2} to 10^{-6}). These calculations showed the Mantel-Bryan to be more conservative (i.e., giving a lower VSD) than the one-hit method when the experimentally determined tumor rates were high but less so when they were low.

Case 3: In 1980 the Food Safety Council presented a comparison of the results of the data from fourteen different experiments (presented in Table 22) to each of four different models (one-hit, Armitage-Doll multistage, Weibull and the gamma multi-hit). The resulting estimates of background response, information about the parameter estimates for each model, a goodness-of-fit p value for each of the models, and p values for the improvement of Weibull and gamma multihit models are presented in Table 23. Note that the lower the goodness-of-fit p value, the poorer the model handles the actual study data.

Table 23 shows that each of three models - the Armitage-Doll model, the Weibull model and the multi-hit model - has a reasonable goodness-of-fit p value (.71, .80 and .93, respectively) in the experimental range. For example, assuming the Weibull model to be correct, the probability of seeing experimental data whose fit is not as good as the data that obtained for this experiment is approximately .80, indicating a high degree of fit. However, in this case the one-hit model has a goodness-of-fit p value $< .001$, indicating that this model is a poor fit to the data. Also in Table 23 the p value for the improvement of fit for the Weibull model over the one-hit model is shown to be $< .001$. The Weibull model clearly provides a statistically significantly better fit to these data than does the one-hit model using conventional p values of .01 or .05. The goodness-of-fit p values for the one-hit, Weibull and gamma multi-hit model are based on usual chi-square tests while that for the Armitage-Doll model is based on the simulation procedure described in Crump *et al.* (1977). Likewise, the p-values for the improvement of fit for the Weibull and multihit models over the one-hit model are based on likelihood ratio procedures which are not generally available for the Armitage-Doll model.

Table 24 presents the estimates of VSD for 10^{-4} and 10^{-6} using each of the four models. These VSD's have been calculated for each model by taking $P(D_O) - P(O) = 10^{-4}$ or 10^{-6}, since $P(D_O) - P(O)$ represents the additional risk due to the added dose D_O.

Table 24 presents the VSD calculations for the four models at risk levels of 10^{-4} and 10^{-6}. Looking again at substance 11, ethylenethiourea, note that the range is from 5.5×10^{-2} to 63.0 ppm at a risk level of 10^{-4} and from 5.5×10^{-4} to 33.5 ppm at a risk level of 10^{-6}. Note that in this case the one-hit model because of the imposed low-dose linearity, yields a much smaller VSD than the other three better-fitting models which allow for low-dose non-linearity, but do not impose it. The non-linearity in the observed data for ethylenethiourea is exhibited in the VSDs in Table 24 as well as in the estimates of the α_i's for the Armitage-Doll model ($\alpha_1 = 0$) in Table 23 and the estimates of m(3.30) and k(8.23) for the Weibull and multi-hit models, respectively.

Case 4: Similar attempts have been made to evaluate the validity of the one-hit model. Carlborg (1979b) has reported that the EPA has estimated, using this model, that current exposures to DDT, dieldrin, and aflatoxin are responsible for 153,000 excess liver cancers per year in the United States. However, there are only about 7000-8000 liver cancers per year in the entire United States from all causes, including background. A similar type of assessment was made for carbon tetrachloride (Hartung, 1980), and arsenic (Downs, 1980), which led to the suggestion that the one-hit model grossly overestimated possible carcinogenic effects in humans. Carlborg's (1979a) attempt to compare the apparent occurrence of aflatoxin-induced liver cancer from several human epidemiological studies in Thailand, Kenya, Swaziland, and Mozambique, with the incidence of liver cancer predicted by animal exposure studies via several models (probit, logit, one-hit, Mantel-Bryan, Armitage-Doll multistage, Weibull and gamma hit) to be caused by environmentally relevant levels of aflatoxin yielded similar results. While the need for such attempts at validation are critical, the actual conduct of such an undertaking is difficult because of the demands made upon the epidemiological studies to precisely quantify exposure levels and estimate background cancer incidences. Extrapolation of the data from the most sensitive rat study for the four models used (99% confidence limit) revealed that the Weibull model displayed the closest fit to the human response rates derived from the epidemiological studies. The other models predicted either greater (one-hit, Armitage-Doll, and Mantel-Bryan) or lesser (probit, logit, gamma-hit) human risks than were observed (Carlborg, 1979a).

Table 25 attempts to summarize the major characteristics of the eight models presented here in terms of their operating characteristics. The performance of each model in any one particular case is dependent on the nature of the observed dose-response curve. All fit true linear data well, but respond differently to concave or convex response curves. The actual choice of model must depend on what information is available and on the professional judgment of the investigator. The authors believe that to attempt to use any purely mathematical model is wrong - that an understanding of the pharmacokinetics and mechanisms of toxicity across the dose range is an essential step in the risk assessment of carcinogens. Any mathematical model must utilize such data, and as there is now significant evidence that many of these actual response curves are multiphasic, only models which can accommodate such nonlinear response surfaces have a chance of being useful.

Risk Assessment

Having now investigated the methods that are available to extrapolate the risk of an irreversible event from a high dose range to a low dose range in the same animal species, we must now address the

TABLE 22
EXPERIMENTAL CARCINOGENICITY RESULTS FOR THIRTEEN SUBSTANCES

Dose Response Data

Dose — Number of Responses/Number of Animals

Test Number and Substance	Species	Tumor or Lesion	Dose Units							
A. Aflatoxin B₁	Rat	Liver tumor	ppb	0	1	5	15	50	100	
				0/18	2/22	1/22	4/21	20/25	28/28	
B. Bischloromethyl Ether	Rat	Respiratory tumor	# of 6 hr Exposures at 100 ppb	10	20	40	60	80	100	
				1/41	3/46	4/18	4/18	15/34	12/20	
C. Botulinum Toxin	Mouse	Death	ng	.027	.030	.034	.037	.040	.045	.050
				0/30	4/30	11/30	10/30	16/30	26/30	26/30
D. DDT	Mouse	Liver hepatoma	ppm	0	2	10	50	250		
				4/111	4/105	11/124	104	60/90		
E. Dieldrin	Mouse	Liver tumor	ppm	0	1.25	2.50	5.00			
				17/156	11/60	25/58	44/60			
F. Dimethyl-nitrosoamine	Rat	Liver tumor	ppm	0	2	5	10	20		
				0/29	0/18	4/62	2/5	15/23		
G. Ethylene-thiourea	Rat	Thyroid carcinoma	ppm	0	5	25	125	250	500	
				2/72	2/75	1/73	2/73	16/69	62/70	

TABLE 22 (cont'd)

Dose Response Data
Dose
Number of Responses/Number of Animals

Test Number and Substance	Species	Tumor or Lesion	Dose Units						
H. Hexachloro-benzene	Rat	14th rib anomoly	mg/kg	0	10	20	40	60	
				0/80	4/79	8/91	15/87	25/96	
I. NTA	Rat	Kidney tumor	% in diet	0	.02	.20	.75	1.50	2.00
				0/127	0/48	0/48	1/91	2/91	12/48
J. Sodium Saccharin	Rat	Bladder tumors	% in diet	.01	.10	1.0	5.0	7.5	
				0/25	0/27	0/27	1/25	7/29	
K. 2,3,7,8-Tetrachloro-dibenzo-p-dioxin	Rat	Intestinal anomaly	mg/kg	0	.125	.25	.50	1.0	
				0/24	0/38	1/33	3/31	3/10	
L. Rapeseed (Span) Oil	Rat	Cardio-vascular lesion	% in diet	0	5	10	15	20	
				1/10	1/10	4/10	4/10	5/10	
M. Vinyl Chloride	Rat	Liver Angiosar-coma	ppm	0	50	250	500	2500	6000
				0/58	1/59	4/59	7/59	13/59	13/60

TABLE 23

RESULTS OF FITTING FOUR DIFFERENT MODELS TO DATA ON THIRTEEN SUBSTANCES

Substance (test)	One-Hit Model Estimated VSD*	One-Hit Model Goodness-of-Fit (p-Value)	Armitage-Doll Model Estimated VSD	Armitage-Doll Model Goodness-of-Fit (p-Value)	Weibull Model Estimated VSD	Weibull Model Goodness-of-Fit (p-Value)	Weibull Model Improvement Over One Hit (p-Value)	Gamma Multi-Hit Model Estimated VSD	Gamma Multi-Hit Model Goodness-of-Fit (p-Value)	Gamma Multi-Hit Model Improvement Over One Hit
A	3.4×10^{-5}	.07	7.9×10^{-4}	.49	4.0×10^{-2}	.64	.01	.28	.54	.009
B	1.6×10^{-4}	.32	4.0×10^{-4}	.77	3.1×10^{-2}	.81	.04	3.7×10^{-2}	.89	.04
C	8.4×10^{-8}	<.001	4.2×10^{-3}	.13	4.3×10^{-3}	.22	<.001	1.3×10^{-2}	.65	<.001
D	2.8×10^{-4}	.16	6.4×10^{-4}	.47	1.7×10^{-2}	.22	.10	4.9×10^{-2}	.19	.12
E	5.7×10^{-6}	.07	2.2×10^{-5}	.36	1.2×10^{-3}	.44	.03	6.7×10^{-3}	.55	.02
F	3.2×10^{-5}	.04	1.9×10^{-2}	.57	1.9×10^{-2}	.63	.003	7.7×10^{-2}	.72	.003
G	5.5×10^{-4}	<.001	4.5	.71	6.0	.80	<.001	33.5	.93	<.001
H	2.1×10^{-4}	.99	2.2×10^{-4}	.94	2.6×10^{-4}	.96	.94	2.6×10^{-4}	.96	.95
I	2.0×10^{-5}	<.001	1.9×10^{-4}	.09	0.52	.48	<.001	0.80	.48	<.001
J	4.3×10^{-5}	.33	0.33	.72	0.53	.99	.04	1.1	7.99	.04
K	5.2×10^{-6}	.53	1.6×10^{-3}	.73	1.7×10^{-3}	.85	.12	3.8×10^{-3}	.87	.11
L	3.7×10^{-5}	.78	5.7×10^{-5}	.64	1.1×10^{-3}	.62	.67	3.8×10^{-3}	.62	.64
M	2.0×10^{-2}	.03	2.0×10^{-2}	.03	2.1×10^{-9}	.56	.002	3.9×10^{10}	.32	.002

*Virtually safe dose at 10^{-6}

TABLE 24

ESTIMATED VIRTUAL SAFE DOSE (VSD) BY FOUR MODELS FOR THIRTEEN SUBSTANCES

Test	Dose Unit	Estimated VSD at 10^{-4}				Estimated VSD at 10^{-6}			
		One Hit	Armitage-Doll	Weibull	Multi-Hit	One-Hit	Armitage-Doll	Weibull	Multi-Hit
A	ppb	3.4×10^{-3}	7.6×10^{-2}	.40	1.2	3.4×10^{-5}	7.9×10^{-4}	4.0×10^{-2}	.28
B	# of six hour exposure	1.6×10^{-2}	4.0×10^{-2}	0.47	0.48	1.6×10^{-4}	4.0×10^{-4}	3.1×10^{-2}	3.7×10^{-2}
C	ppm	8.4×10^{-6}	9.1×10^{-3}	9.2×10^{-3}	1.7×10^{-2}	8.4×10^{-8}	4.2×10^{-3}	4.3×10^{-3}	1.3×10^{-2}
D	ppm	2.8×10^{-2}	6.4×10^{-2}	0.41	0.76	2.8×10^{-4}	$6.4. \times 10^{-4}$	1.7×10^{-2}	4.9×10^{-2}
E	ppm	5.7×10^{-4}	2.2×10^{-3}	1.8×10^{-2}	5.1×10^{-2}	5.7×10^{-6}	2.2×10^{-5}	1.2×10^{-3}	6.7×10^{-3}
F	ppm	3.2×10^{-3}	0.19	.19	0.41	3.2×10^{-5}	1.9×10^{-2}	1.9×10^{-2}	7.7×10^{-2}
G	ppm	$5.5. \times 10^{-2}$	20.8	24.4	63.0	5.5×10^{-4}	4.5	6.0	33.5
H	mg/kg	2.1×10^{-2}	2.2×10^{-2}	2.4×10^{-2}	2.4×10^{-2}	2.1×10^{-4}	2.2×10^{-4}	2.6×10^{-4}	2.6×10^{-4}
I	% in diet	2.0×10^{-3}	1.9×10^{-2}	0.85	1.0	2.0×10^{-5}	1.9×10^{-4}	0.52	0.80
J	% in diet	4.3×10^{-3}	1.1	1.4	2.0	4.3×10^{-5}	0.33	0.53	1.1
K	mg/kg	5.2×10^{-4}	1.6×10^{-2}	1.7×10^{-2}	2.5×10^{-2}	5.2×10^{-6}	1.6×10^{-3}	1.7×10^{-3}	3.8×10^{-3}
L	% in diet	3.7×10^{-3}	5.7×10^{-3}	3.2×10^{-2}	6.7×10^{-2}	3.7×10^{-5}	5.7×10^{-5}	1.1×10^{-3}	3.8×10^{-3}
M	ppm	2.0	2.0	7.4×10^{-5}	3.0×10^{-5}	2.0×10^{-2}	2.0×10^{-2}	2.1×10^{-9}	3.9×10^{-10}

TABLE 25
Characteristics and Requirements for Use of Major Low Dose Extrapolation Models

	Low Dose Linearity	Extrapolates Low Dose Levels	Estimates Virtual Safe Dose	Mechanistic or Tolerance Distribution	Requires Metabolic Data	Accommodates Threshold	Takes time-to-tumor into Account	Estimate of Potential Risk of Low Doses
One-hit (Linear)	X	X	X	M				Highest
Multistage (Armitage-Doll)	X	X	X	M				High
Weibull (Chand and Hoel)			X	T		X	X	High
Multi-hit	X	X	X	M				Medium
Logit (Albert and Altshuler)	X		X	T		X	X	Medium
Probit (Mantel-Bryan)	X		X	T				Medium
Log-Probit (Gehring et. al.)		X	X	M	X	X	X	Low
Pharma-cokinetic (Cornfield)		X	X	M	X	X	X	Lowest

question of a means to extrapolate from an animal species to humans. This extrapolation has both qualitative aspects (to be discussed here) and quantitative aspects (called scaling, to be discussed later).

The qualitative aspects of species-to-species extrapolations are best addressed by a form of classification analysis (such as we reviewed in Chapter IX) tailored to the exact problem at hand. This approach identifies the physiological, metabolic, and other factors which may be involved in the risk-producing process in the model species (for example, the carcinogenesis process in test mice), establishes the similarities and differences between these factors and those in humans, and comes up with means to bridge the gaps between these two (or to identify the fact that there is no possible bridge).

Tomatis (1979) has provided an excellent evaluation of the comparability of carcinogenicity findings between rodents and man, in general finding the former to be good predictors of the end point in the latter. However, in his 1984 Stokinger lecture, Weil pointed out that the model species should respond biologically to the material as similarly as possible to man; that the routes of exposure (actual and possible) should be the same; and that there are known wide variations in response to carcinogens. Deichmann (1975), for example, has reviewed studies demonstrating that 2-naphthylamine is a human and dog carcinogen, but not active in the mouse, rat, guinea pig or rabbit.

Smith (1974) discussed interspecies variations of response to carcinogens, including N-2-fluorenyl-acetamide, which is potent for the dog, rabbit, hamster and rat (believed to be due to formation of an active metabolite by N-hydroxylation), but not in the guinea pig or steppe lemming, which do not form this metabolic derivative.

Table 26 presents an overview of the classes of factors which should be considered in the first step of a species extrapolation. Examples of such actual differences which can be classified as one of these factors are almost endless.

The absorption of compounds from the gastrointestinal tract and from the lungs is comparable among vertebrate and mammalian species. There are, however, differences between herbivorous animals and omnivorous animals due to differences in stomach structure. The problem of distribution within the body probably relates less to species than to size, and will be discussed later under scaling. Metabolism, xenobiotic metabolism of foreign compounds, metabolic activation, or toxification/detoxification mechanisms (by whatever name) is perhaps the critical factor, and this can differ widely from species to species. The increasing realization that the original compound administered is not necessarily the ultimate carcinogen makes the further study of these metabolic patterns critical.

In terms of excretory rates, the differences between the species are not very great: small animals tend to excrete compounds more

Table 26

Classes of Factors to be Considered in Species-to-Species Extrapolations in Risk Assessment

I. Sensitivity of Model Animal (Relative to Humans)
A. Pharmacologic
B. Receptor
C. Life Span
D. Size
E. Metabolic Function
F. Physiological
G. Anatomic
H. Nutritional Requirements
I. Reproductive and Developmental Processes
J. Diet
K. Critical Reflex and Behavioral Responses (as emetic reflex)
L. Behavioral
M. Rate of Cell Division
N. Other Defense Mechanisms

II. Relative Population Differences
A. Size
B. Heterogeneity
C. Selected "High Class" Nature of Test Population

III. Differences Between Test and Real World Environment
A. Physical (Temperature, Humidity, etc.)
B. Chemical
C. Nutritional

rapidly than large ones in a rather systematic way. The various cellular and intercellular barriers seem to be surprisingly constant throughout the vertebrate phylum. In addition, it is beginning to be appreciated that the receptors, such as DNA, are comparable throughout the mammalian species.

There are life-span (or temporal) differences that have not been considered adequately, either now or in the past. It takes time to develop a tumor, and at least some of that time may be taken up by the actual cell division process. Cell division rates appear to be significantly higher in smaller animals. Mouse and rat cells turn over faster than human cells - perhaps at twice the rate. On the other hand, the latent period for development of tumors is much shorter in small animals than in large ones.

Another problem is that the life-span of man is about 35 times that of the mouse or rat; thus there is a much longer time for a tumor to appear. These sorts of temporal considerations are of considerable importance.

Body size, irrespective of species, seems to be important in the rate of distribution of foreign compounds throughout the body. A simple example of this is that the cardiac output of the mouse is on the order of 1 mL/minute, and the mouse has a blood volume of about 1 mL. The mouse is turning its blood volume over every minute. In man, the cardiac output per minute is only 1/20 of its blood volume. So the mouse turns its blood over and distributes whatever is in the blood or collects excretory products over 20 times faster than man.

Another aspect of the size difference which should be considered is that the large animal has a very much greater number of susceptible cells that may interact with potential carcinogenic agents, though there is also a proportionately increased number of "dummy" cells.

Rall (1977 and 1979), Oser (1981) and Borzelleca (1984) have published articles reviewing such factors and Calabrese (1983) has published an excellent book on the subject.

Having delineated and quantified species differences (even if only having factored in comparative body weights and food consumption rates), we can now proceed to some form of quantitative extrapolation. This process is called scaling.

There are currently three major approaches to scaling in risk assessment. These are by fraction of diet, by body weight, and by body surface area (Calabrese, 1983; Schmidt-Nielsen, 1984).

The by "fraction-of-diet" method is based on converting the results in the experimental animal model to man on a mg (of test substance) / kg (diet)/day basis. When the experimental model is the mouse, this leads to an extrapolation factor which is 6-fold lower than on a body weight (mg/kg) basis (Association Food and Drug Officials, 1959). Fraction-of-diet factors are not considered accurate indices of actual dosages since the latter are influenced not only by voluntary food intake, as affected by palatability and caloric density of the diet and by single or multiple caging, but more particularly by the age of the animal. During the early stages of life, anatomic, physiologic, metabolic and immunologic capabilities are not fully developed. Moreover, the potential for toxic effect in an animal is a function of the dose ingested-ultimately, of the number of active molecules reaching the target cell. Additionally, many agents of concern do not have ingestion as the major route of intake in man. Both the Environmental Protection Agency (EPA) and the consumer Product Safety Commission (CPSC) frequently employ a fraction-of-diet scaling factor.

Human diets are generally assumed to be 600 - 700 g/day, while that in mice is 4 g/day and in rats 25 g/day (the equivalent of 50 g/kg/day).

There are several ways to perform a scaling operation on a body weight basis. The most common is to simply calculate a conversion factor (K) as

$$\frac{\text{Weight of human (70 kg)}}{\text{Weight of test animal (0.4 kg for rat)}} = K$$

More exotic methods for doing this, such as that based on a form of linear regression, are reviewed by Calabrese (1983), who believes that the body weight method is preferable.

A difficulty with this approach is that the body weights of both animals and man change throughout life. An "ideal man" or "ideal rat" weight is therefore utilized.

Finally, there are the body surface area methods, which attempt to factor in differences in metabolic rates based on the principle that these change in proportion with body surface area (since as the ratio of body surface area to body weight increases, the more energy is required to maintain constant body temperature). There are several methods for doing this, each having a ratio of dose to the animal's body weight (in mg/kg) as a starting point, resulting in a conversion factor with mg/m^2 as the units.

The EPA version is generally calculated as:

$$(M_{\text{human}}/M_{\text{animal}})^{1/3} = \text{surface factor}$$

where M = mass in kilograms. Another form is calculated based on constants that have been developed for a multitude of species of animals by actual surface area measurements (Spector, 1956). The resulting formula for this is:

$$A = KW^{2/3}$$

where A = surface area in cm^2
$\qquad$ K = constant, specific for each species
and W = weight in grams.

A scaling factor is then simply calculated as a ratio of the surface area of man over that of the model species.

The "best" scaling factor is not generally agreed upon. Though the majority opinion is that surface area is preferable where a metabolic activation or deactivation is known to be both critical to the risk producing process and present in both the model species and man, these assumptions may not always be valid. Table 27 presents a comparison of the weight and surface area extrapolation methods for eight species.

Schneiderman *et al.* (1975) and Dixon (1976) have published comparisons of these methods, but Schmidt-Nielsen (1984) should be considered the primary source on scaling in interspecies comparisons.

TABLE 27
Extrapolation of a Dose of 100 mg/kg in the Mouse to Other Species

Species	Weight (Grams)	Surface Area* (sq. cm.)	Extrapolated Dose (mg)		Ratio A/B
			Body Weight (A)	Body Surface Area (B)	
Mouse	20	46.4	2	2	1.0
Rat	400	516.7	40	22.3	1.80
Guinea Pig	400	564.5	40	24.3	1.65
Rabbit	1500	1272.0	150	54.8	2.74
Dog	12000	5766.0	1200	248.5	4.82
Cat	2000	1381.0	200	59.5	3.46
Monkey	4000	2975.0	400	128.2	3.12
Human	70000	18000.0	7000	775.8	9.8

*Surface area (except in case of man) calculated from formula:

$$\text{Surface Area (cm}^2) = K(W^{2/3})$$

where K is a constant for each species and W is body weight (values of K and surface area of man taken from Spector, 1956).

The remaining problem (or step) in performing a risk assessment is quantitating the exposure of the human population, both in terms of how many people are exposed by what routes (or means) and to what quantities of an agent they are exposed.

This process of identifying and quantitating exposure groups within the human population is beyond the scope of this text, except for some key points. Classification methods are again the key tool for identifying and properly delimiting human populations at risk. An investigator must first understand the process involved in making, shipping, using and disposing of a material. EPA recently proposed guidelines for such identification and exposure quantitation (EPA, 1984). The exposure groups can be very large or relatively small sub-populations, each with a markedly different potential for exposure. For di-(2-ethyl-hexyl) phthalate (DEHP), for example, the following at-risk populations have been identified:

IV Route: 3,000,000 receiving blood transfusions (50 mg/year)
            50,000 dialysis patients (4500 mg/year)
            10,000 hemophiliacs (760 mg/year)

Oral Route: 10,800,000 children under 3 years of age (434 mg/year)
              220,000,000 adults (dietary contamination (1.1 mg/year)

Not quantitated were possible inhalation and dermal exposure.

All such estimates of exposure in humans (and of the number of humans exposed) are subject to a large degree of uncertainity.

An alternative approach to achieving society's objective for the entire risk assessment procedure - protecting the human population from unacceptable levels of known risks - is the classical approach of using safety factors. In 1972, Weil summarized this approach as "In summary, for the evaluation of safety for man, it is necessary to: (1) design and conduct appropriate toxicologic tests, (2) statistically compare the data from treated and control animals, (3) delineate the minimum effect and maximum no ill-effect levels (Niel) for these animals, and (4) if the material is to be used, apply an appropriate safety factor, e.g., (a) 1/100 (Niel) or 1/500 (Niel) for some effects or (b) 1/500 (Niel), if the effect was a significant increase in cancer in an appropriate test." This approach has served society reasonably well over the years, once the experimental work has identified potential hazards and quantitated observable dose response relationships. Until such time as the more elegant risk assessment procedures can instill greater public confidence, the use of the safety factor approach should not be abandoned.

Both public and professional perception of the entire process leading to risk assessments of carcinogens is not good. The wide acceptance and large sales of Efron's *The Apocalyptics - Cancer and The Big Lie*, (1984), which presents a broad-based critique on the entire process surrounding our understanding of environmental carcinogenesis is an all too telling indicator of the public's increasing loss of faith. The reverses of regulatory actions on benzene and formaldehyde, in part due to the faulty nature of the risk assessments presented to support these actions, have reinforced public doubts.

Such doubts are not limited to the laiety. Gio Gori, formally a deputy director of NCI, has presented an overview and general critique (Gori, 1982) of the entire process from a regulatory perspective. Hickey (1984), addressed the specific case of low-level radiation effects (where we have the most human data) from a statisticians point of view, pointing out that existing epidemiology data does not match EPA's risk assessment. And certainly there is no consensus within toxicology, as the contents of this chapter should make clear. The consensus within the toxicology community is clearly that a more mechanistic and pharmacokinetic based modeling process is called for. Park and Snee (1983) present an excellent outline of such an approach.

The entire process of risk assessment as discussed to this point is applicable not just to carcinogens, but also to the other classes of toxic agents which result in some form of irreversible harm. The only difference is that the concept of a threshold dose level below which no ill effects are evoked is accepted for most of these other classes (the exception being mutagens).

Mutagens are not generally conceded to have thresholds, but the human health concern of those which are not established as carcinogens or teratogens is conjectural. Certainly materials identified as mutagens in an *in vivo* mammalian system (such as a dominant lethal study in mice or *in vivo* sister chromatid exchange in rabbits or rats) should be treated more conservatively than those whose mutagenicity has been established only in bacterial or biochemical test systems. EPA (1984) has proposed a regulatory process for the assessment of risks from mutagens which is not noticeably different from their approach to carcinogens, and which utilizes dose response data from many test systems (even biochemical) as a starting point.

Teratogens are now clearly established to have dose-response relationships which are subject to both time and quantity-of-dose thresholds (Jusko, 1972). The exposure of the fertilized ovum must occur within a time window when the ovum is susceptible. Likewise, the dose must be sufficient to cause an effect and yet not so great as to cause a spontaneous abortion of the embryo or fetus. Rai and Van Ruzin (1985) recently proposed a dose response model for teratogens which included two approaches to low dose extrapolation based on a one hit model. This model is also useful for mammalian dominant lethal data, which can be considered a subset of either teratogenicity or reproductive toxicity data.

Reproductive toxicants are a whole new wide world to worry about. Though Gross and Fitzhugh (1970) suggested caution in evaluating data which might be improperly suggestive of a nontoxic threshold level, there is a clear consensus that there are thresholds below which reproductive agents are inactive.

The difficulty is that such a wide variety of biochemical and physiological processes are involved in the successful operation of the reproductive process that we do not yet have adequate experimental methods to detect and quantitate all possible effects. Dixon and Nadolney (1985) have presented a brief overview of the problems involved in going from our present state of knowledge in this area to the performance of meaningful risk assessments.

Though some of the fine points may vary, one should expect that the risk assessment process for any irreversible toxicant will follow the general form and steps presented in this chapter and such assessments should be undertaken with full knowledge of the involved uncertainties, weaknesses and difficulties.

REFERENCES

Albert, R.E., and Altshuler, B. 1973: Considerations relating to the formulation of limits for unavoidable population exposures to environmental carcinogens. In *Radionuclide Carcinogenesis*, ed. J.E. Ballou et al., pp. 233–253. AEC Symposium Series, CONF-72050. NTIS Springfield.

Albert, R.E., Burns, F.J. and Altshuler, B. (1979): Reinterpretation of the Linear Non-Threshold Dose-Response Model in Terms of the Initiation - Promotion Mouse Skin Tumorigenesis, In *New Concepts In Safety Evaluation*, (M.A. Mehlman, R.E. Shapiro and H. blumenthal, Eds.) pp 88–95 Hemisphere Publishing, New York.

Anderson, M.W., Hoel, D.G., and Kaplan, N.L. (1980): A General Scheme for the Incorporation of Pharmacokinetics in Low-Dose Risk Estimation for Chemical Carcinogenesis: Example-Vinyl Chloride. *Toxicol. Appl. Pharmacol.*, 55: 154–161.

Arley, N. (1961): Theoretical Analysis of Carcinogenesis, in *Proceedings of the Fourth Berkeley Symposium on Mathematical Statistics and Probability* (J. Neyman, Ed.) pp 1–18 University of California Press, Berkeley.

Armitage, P., and Doll, R. (1961): Stochastic Models for Carcinogenesis From the Berkeley Symposium on Mathematical Statistics and Probability. pp. 19–38 University of California Press, Berkeley.

Association of Food and Drug Officials of the U.S. (1959): *Appraisal of the safety of chemicals in foods, drugs and cosmetics*. Washington, D.C.

Bennicelli, C., Camoirano, A., Petruzzelli, S., Zanacchi, P. and De Flora, S. (1983): High sensitivity of Salmonella TA102 in detecting hexavalent chromium mutagenicity and its reversal by liver and lung preparations. *Mutation Res.*, 122: 1–5.

Berkson, J. (1944): Application of the logistic function to bio-assay. *J. Am. Stat. Assoc.*; 39:357–365.

Bernstein, L.: Gold, L.S.; Ames, B.N.; Pike, M.C. and Hoel, D.G. (1985): Some Tautologous Aspects of the Comparison of Carcinogenic Potency in Rats and Mice *Fund App Toxicol.*, 5: 79–86.

Blum, H.F. (1959): *Carcinogenesis by Ultraviolet Light*. Princeton University Press. Princeton.

Borzelleca, J.F. (1984): Extrapolation of Animal Data to Man, in *Concepts in Toxicology Vol. I* (A.S. Tegeris, Ed.). pp. 294–304 Karger, New York.

Bratcher, T.L. (1977): Bayesian Analysis of a Dose-Response Experiment With Serial Sacrifices *J. Env. Path. Toxicol.*, 1: 287–292.

Bryan, W.R. and Shimkin, M.B. (1943): Quantitative Analysis of Dose-Response Data Obtained with Three Carcinogenic Hydrocarbons in Strain C3H Male Mice *J. Natl. Canc. Inst.*, 3:503–531.

Byar, D.D. (1977): Analysis of Survival Data In Heterogeneous Populations in *Recent Developments in Statistics*, (J.R. Barra, F. Brodeau, G. Romier, and B. Van Cutsem, Eds.) pp. 51–68 North-Holland Publishing Co., New York.

Cameron, T.P.; Hickman, R.L.; Korneich, M.R. and Tarone, R.E. (1985): History Survival and Growth Patterns of B6C3F1 Mice and F344 Rats in the National Cancer Institute Carcinogenesis Testing Program *Fund. App. Toxicol.*, 5:526–538.

Cairns, T. (1980): The ED_{01} Study: Introduction, Objectives, and Overview *Environ. Path. Toxicol.*, 3(3):1–7.

Calabrese, E.J. (1983): *Principles of Animal Extrapolation*, John Wiley, New York.

Carlborg, F.W. (1979a): Cancer, Mathematical Models and Aflatoxin. *Food Cosmet. Toxicol.*, 17:159–166.

Carlborg, F.W. (1979b): Comments on aspects of the EPA's water quality criteria. EPA Methodology Hearings. In: *EPA Methodology Document*. Cincinnati.

Chand, N., and Hoel, D.G. (1974): A Comparison of Models for Determining Safe Levels of Environmental Agents, in *Reliability and Biometry Statistical Analysis of Lifelength*, F. Proschan and R.J. Serfling, (Ed.), SIAM, Philadelphia.

Chu, K. (1977): *Percent Spontaneous Primary Tumors in Untreated Species Used at NCI for Carcinogen Bioassays*; NCI Clearing House.

Ciminera, J.L. (1985): Some Issues in the Design, Evaluation and Interpretation of Tumorigenicity Studies in Animals; Presented at the Symposium on Long-term Animal Carcinogenicity Studies: A Statistical Perspective, March 4-6, 1985, Bethesda, MD.

Cook, P.J., Doll, R., and Fellingham, S.A. (1969): A Mathematical Model for the Age Distribution of Cancer in Man. *Int. J. Cancer.*, 4:93–112.

Cornfield, J. (1977): Carcinogenic Risk Assessment. *Science*, 198:693–699.

Cornfield, J., Carlborg, F.W. and Van Ryzin, J. (1978). Setting Tolerance on the Basis of Mathematical Treatment of Dose-response Data Extrapolated to Low Doses. *Proc. of the First Internat. Toxicol. Congress.*, pp. 143–164 Academic Press, New York.

Cox, D.R. (1972): Regression Models and Life-Tables, *J. Royal Stat. Soc., 34B:* 187–220.

Crouch, E. and Wilson, R. (1979): Interspecies comparison of carcinogenic potency, *J. Tox. Env. Health*, 5: 1095–1118.

Crump, K.W. (1979): Dose response problems in carcinogenesis. *Biometrics*, 35: 157–167.

Crump, K.S., Hoel, D.G., Langley, C.H., and Peto, R. (1976): Fundamental carcinogenic processes and their implications for low dose risk assessment. *Cancer Res.*, 36:2973.

Day, T.D. 1967: Carcinogenic action of cigarette smoke condensate on mouse skin. *Br. J. Cancer*, 21:56–81.

De Flora, S. (1978) Metabolic deactivation of mutagens in the Salmonella/microsome test. *Nature* (London) 271:455–456.

De Flora, S., Bennicelli, C., Zanacchi, P., Camoriano, A., Petruzzelli, S. and Giuntini, C. (1984): Metabolic activiation and deactiviation of mutagens by preparations of human lung parenchyma and bronchial tree. *Mutation Res.*, 139:9–14.

De Flora, S., Morelli, A., Zanacchi, P., Bennicelli, C. and De Flora, A. (1982): Selective deactivation of ICR mutagens as related to their distinctive pulmonary carcinogenicity. *Carcinogenesis*; 3:187–194.

Dempster, A.P.; Selwyn, M.R. and Weeks, B.J. (1983): Combining historical and randomized controls for assessing trends in proportions. *J. Amer. Stat. Assoc.*, 78: 221–227.

Deichmann, W.B. (1975): Cummings Memorial Lecture - 1975. The Market Basket: Food for Thought. *Am. Ind. Hyg. Assoc. J.*, 36:411.

Dinman, B.D. (1972): "Non-concept" of "Non-threshold" chemicals in the environment. *Science*; 175:495–497.

Dinse, G.E. (1985): Estimating Tumor Prevalence, Lethality and Mortality. Presented at the Symposium on Long-term Animal Carcinogenicity Studies: A Statistical Perspective, March 4–6, 1985. Bethesda.

Dix, D. and Cohen, P. (1980): On the Role of Aging in Cancer Incidence *J. Theor. Biol.*, 83:163–173.

Dixon, R.L. (1976): Problems in Extrapolating Toxicity Data from Laboratory Animals to Man. *Envir. Hlth. Perspect.*, 13:43–50.

Dixon, R.L. and Nadolney, C.H. (1985): Assessing Risk of Reproductive Dysfunction Associated with Chemical Exposure, In *Reproductive Toxicology*; (R.L. Dixon, ED.) Raven Press, New York.

Doll, R. (1971): The Age Distribution of Cancer: Implications for Models of Carcinogenesis *J. Royal Stat Soc.*, 134:133–166.

Downs, T.D. (1980): comments on the proposed guidelines and methodology for deriving water quality criteria for the protection of human health. EPA Methodology Hearings. In: *EPA Methodology Document*. Cincinnati.

Druckrey, H. (1967): Quantitative aspects in chemical carcinogenesis. In: *Potential Carcinogenic Hazards from Drugs*, UICC Monograph Series, Vol. 7. R. Truhaut (ed.) p. 60 Springer-Verlag, Berlin.

Dumouchel, W.H. and Harris, J.E. (1983): Bayes Methods for Combining the Results of Cancer Studies in Humans and Other Species. *J. Amer Stat Assoc.*, 78: 293–315.

Efron, E. (1984): *The Apocalyptics* Simon and Schuster, New York.

Environmental Protection Agency (1976): *Federal Register*, 41: 21402, 42:10412.

EPA (1984): Proposed Guidelines For Mutagenicity Risk Assessment, *F R* 49 No. 227. (November 23) 46314–46321.

EPA (1984): Proposed Guidelines for Exposure Assessment *F R* 49 No. 227. (November 23) 46304–46312.

Epstein, S.S. (1973): The Delaney Amendment *Ecologist*; 3: 424–430.

FDA Advisory Committee on Protocols for Safety Evaluation (1971): Panel on carcinogenesis report on cancer testing in the safety evaluation of food additives and pesticides. *Toxicol. Appl. Pharmacol.*, 20:419–438.

Fears, T.R., and Tarone, R.E. (1977): Response to "Use of Statistics When Examining Life Time Studies in Rodents to Detect Carcinogenicity." *J. Tox. Environ. Health*, 3:629–632.

Fears, T.R., Tarone, R.E., and Chu, K.C. (1977): False-positive and false-negative rates for carcinogenicity screens. *Cancer Res.*, 27:1941–1945.

Feinstein, A.R. (1975): Clinical biostatistics XXII: Biologic dependency, hypothesis testing, unilateral probabilities, and other issues in scientific direction vs. statistical duplexity. *Clin. Pharmacol. Ther.*, 17:499–513.

Finney, D.J. 1952. *Statistical Methods in Biological Assay*. Hafner, New York.

Food and Drug Administration Advisory Committee on Protocols for Safety Evaluation. (1971). Panel on carcinogenesis on cancer testing in the safety evaluation of food additives and pesticides. *Toxicol. Appl. Pharmacol.*, 20:419.

Food Safety Council (1980): Quantitative Risk Assessment *Fd Cosmet Toxicol.*, 18: 711–734.

Freidman, L. (1973): Problems of evaluating the health significance of the chemicals present in foods, In: *Pharmacology and the Future of Man Vol 2*, pp. 30–41 Karger, Basel.

Gart, J.J.; Chu, K.C. and Tarone, R.E. (1979): Statistical Issues In Interpretation of Chronic Bioassay Tests for Carcinogenicity, *J. Natl. Canc. Inst.*; 62:957–974.

Gaylor, D.W. and Shapiro, R.E. (1979): Extrapolation and Risk Estimation for Carcinogenesis, In *New Concepts in Safety Evaluation* (M.A. Mehlman, R.E. Shapiro and H. Blumenthal, Eds) pp 65–87 Hemisphere Publications, New York.

Gehring, P.J. and Blau, G.E. (1977): Mechanisms of Carcinogenicity: Dose Response *J. Env Path Toxicol.*, 1:163–179.

Gehring, P.J., Watanabe, P.G. and Young, J.D. (1977): The Relevance of Dose-dependent Pharmacokinetics in the Assessment of Carcinogenic Hazards of Chemicals, in *Origins of Human Cancer, Book A*, (H. Hiatt, J.D. Watson and J.A. Winsten, Eds.) pp 187–203 Cold Spring Harbor Laboratory.

Goodman, D.G.; Ward, J.M.; Squire, R.A., Chu, K.C. and Linhart, M.S. (1979): Neoplastic and Nonneoplastic Lesions in Aging F344 Rats *Toxicol. Appl. Pharmacol.*, 48:237–248.

Gori, G.B. (1982): Regulation of Cancer-Causing Substances: Utopia or Reality *Chem. Eng. News* (September 6, 1982) 25–32.

Grasso, P and Crampton, R.F. (1972): The Value of the Mouse in Carcinogenicity Testing *Fd Cosmet Toxicol.*, 10:418–426.

Gross, M.A., Fitzhugh, O.G., and Mantel, N. (1970): Evaluation of safety for food additives: An illustration involving the influence of methyl salicylate on rat reproduction. *Biometrics*, 26:181–194.

Guess, H.A., Crump, K.S., and Peto, R. (1977): Uncertainty estimates for low-dose-rate extrapolations of animal carcinogenicity data. *Cancer Res.*, 37:3475–3483.

Guess, H.A. and Hoel, D.G. (1977): The Effect of Dose On Cancer Latency Period *J Env Path Toxicol.*, 1:279–286.

Hammond, E.C., Garfinkel, L., and Lew, E.A. (1978): Longevity, Selective Mortality, and Competitive Risks in Relation to Chemical Carcinogenesis, *Env. Res.*, 16: 153–173.

Hartley H.O. and Sielken, R.L. (1977): Estimation of "safe doses" in carcinogenic experiments. *Biometrics*; 33:1–30.

Hartung, R. (1980): Evaluation of the health effects section of the criteria document for ambient water for CCl_4. *EPA Methodology Manual*.

Haseman, J.K. (1985): False Positive Issues In Carcinogenicity Testing: An Examination of the FDA Color Studies. Presented at the Symposium on Long-term Animal Carcinogenicity Studies: A Statistical Perspective, March 4–6, 1985, Bethesda, MD.

Haseman, J.K. (1985): Issues In Carcinogencity Testing: Dose Selection *Fund App. Toxicol.*, 5:66–78.

Haseman, J.K. and Hoel, D.G. (1979): Statistical Design of Toxicity Assays: Role of Genetic Structure of Test Animal Population *J. Toxicol. Env. Health*; 5:89–101.

Hickey, R.J. (1984): Low-level radiation effects: Extrapolation as "science" *Chem. Eng. News* (January 16, 1984)

Hoel, D.G. (1972): A representation of mortality data by competing risks. *Biometrics*; 28:475–488.

Hoel, D.G., Gaylor, D.W., Kirschstein, R.L., Saffiotti, V., and Schneiderman, M.A. (1975): Estimation of risks of irreversible delayed toxicity. *J. Toxicol. Environ. Health*, 1:133.

Jusko, W.J. (1972): Pharmacodynamic Principles in Chemical Teratology: Dose-Effect Relationships, *J. Pharm. Exp. Ther.* 183:469–480.

Klaassen, C.D. and Doull, J. (1980): Evaluation of Safety: Toxicology Evaluation, In *Casarett and Doull's Toxicology* (J. Doull, C.D. Klaassen and M.O. Amdur, Eds) pp. 26 Macmillan Publishing Company, New York.

Kraybill, H.F. (1977): Newer approaches in assessment of Environmental Carcinogenesis, In. *Mycotoxins In Human and Animal Health* pp. 675–686, Pathotox Publishers, Park Forest South, Ill.

Lagakos, S. and Mosteller, F. (1981): A Case Study of Statistics in the Regulatory Process: The FD&C Red No. 40 Experiments *J. Natl. Canc. Inst.*, 66:197–212.

Lee, P.N. and O'Neill, J.A. (1971): The effect of both time and dose applied on tumor incidence rate in benzopyrene skin painting experiments. *Br. J. Cancer*; 25: 759–770.

Lijinsky, W.; Rueber, M.D. and Riggs, C.W. (1981): Dose Response Studies of Carcinogenesis in Rats by Nitrosodiethylamine, *Cancer Res*; 41:4997–5003.

Littlefield, N.A., Farmer, J.H. and Gaylor, D.W. (1980): Effects of Dose and Time in a Long-dose Carcinogenic Study, *J. Environ. Path. Toxicol.*; 3: 17–34.

Louis, T.A. and Orva, J. (1985): Adaptive Sacrifice Plans for the Carcinogen Bioassay. Presented at The Symposium on Long-term Animal Carcinogenicity Studies: A Statistical Perspective, March 4–6, 1985, Bethesda.

McKnight, B. and Crowley, J. (1984): Tests for Differences in Tumor Incidence Based on Animal Carcinogenesis Experiments *J. Amer. Stat. Assoc.*, 79:639–648.

Mantel, N. (1963): Part IV. The concept of threshold in carcinogenesis *Clin Pharmacol Therapeutics*; 4:104–109.

Mantel, N., and Bryan, W.R. (1961): Safety testing of carcinogenic agents. *J. Natl. Canc. Inst.* 27:455–470.

Mantel, N., Bohidar, N.R., Brown, C.C., Ciminera, J.L. and Tukey, J.W. (1975): An improved Mantel-Bryan procedure for "safety" testing of carcinogens. *Cancer Res.*, 35:865–872.

Mantel, N. and Schneiderman, M.A. (1975): Estimating "Safe" Levels, A Hazardous Undertaking, *Cancer Res.*, 35:1379–1386.

Meng, C. and Dempster, A.P. (1985): A Bayesian Approach to the Multiplicity Problem For Significance Testing With Binomial Data. Presented at The Symposium on Long-Term Animal Carcinogenicity Studies: A Statistical Perspective, March 4–6, 1985, Bethesda.

Miller, E.C. (1978): Some Current Perspectives on Chemical Carcinogens in Humans and Experimental Animals: Presidential Address *Cancer Res.*, 38: 1471.

Miller, E.C. and Miller, J.A. (1981): Mechanisms of Chemical Carcinogenesis *Cancer*; 47:1055–1064.

Neal, R.A. and Gibson, J.E. (1984): The Uses of Toxicology and Epidemiology in Identifying and Assessing Carcinogenic Risks in *Reducing The Carcinogenic Risks In Industry*; (P.F. Deisler, Ed.) pp. 39–65 Marcel Dekker, Inc., New York.

Nutrition Foundation (1983): *The Relevance of Mouse Liver Hepatoma To Human Carcinogenic Risk*, Nutrition Foundation, Washington.

Oser, B.L. (1981): The rat as a Model for Human Toxicology Evaluation *J. Toxicol. Envir. Health.*, 8:521–542.

Page, N.P. (1977): Concepts of a Bioassay Program In Environmental Carcinogenesis, in *Environmental Cancer* (H.F. Kraybill and M.A. Mehlman, Eds.) pp. 87–171 Hemisphere Publishing, New York.

Park, C.N. and Snee, R.D. (1983): Quantitative Risk Assessment. State-of-the-Art for Carcinogenesis *Amer. Stat.*, 37:427–441.

Peto, R. (1978): The carcinogenic effects of chronic exposure to very low levels of toxic substances. *Environ. Health Perspectives*; 22:155–159.

Peto, R. and Lee, P.N. (1973): Weibull distributions for continuous carcinogenesis experiments. *Biometrics*; 29:457–470.

Peto, R., Lee, P.N., and Paige, W.S. (1972): Statistical analysis of the bioassay of continuous carcinogens. *Roy J. Cancer*; 26:258–261.

Peto, R., Pike, M., Day, N., Gray, R., Lee, P., Parish, S., Peto, J. Richards, S., and Wahrendorf, J. (1980): "Guidelines for Simple, Sensitive Significance Tests for Carcinogenic Effects in Long-Term Animal Experiments," In *IARC Monographs on the Evaluation of the Carcinogenic Risk of Chemicals to Humans, Supplement 2, Long-Term and Short-Term Screening Assays for Carcinogens: A Critical Appraisal, Lyon*: International Agency for Research in Cancer, pp 311–346.

Petrilli, F.L. and De Flora, S. (1978a): Metabolic deactivation of hexavalent chromium mutagenicity. *Mutation Res.*, 54:139–147.

Petrilli, F.L. and De Flora, S. (1978b): Oxidation of inactive trivalent chromium to the mutagenic hexavalent form. *Mutation Res.*; 58:167–173.

Petrilli, F.L. and (1980): Mutagenicity of chromium compounds. In *Chromate Symposium 80. Focus of a Standard*. pp. 76–99 Industrial Health Foundation, Pittsburgh.

Petrilli, F.L. and De Flora, S. (1982): Interpretations on chromium mutagenicity and carcinogenicity. In *Mutagens in Our Enivornment* (Sorsa, M. and Vainio, H. Eds.) pp. 453–464 Alan R. Liss, Inc., New York.

Pike, M.C. (1966): A method of analysis of a certain class of experiments in carcinogenesis, *Biometrics*; 22:142–161.

Portier, C.J. and Hoel, D.H. (1984): Design of Animal Carcinogencity Studies for Goodness-of-Fit of Multistage Models *Fund App Tox.*, 4:949–959.

Rai, K., and Van Ryzin, J. (1979). Risk assessment of toxic environmental substances based on a generalized multihit model. *Energy and Health*, pp. 99–177. SIAM Press, Philadelphia.

Rai, K. and Van Ryzin, J. (1985): A Dose-Response Model For Teratological Experiments Involving Quantal Responses *Biomet.*, 41:1–9.

Rall, D.P. (1977) Species Differences in Carcinogenicity Testing, in *Origins of Human Cancer* (H.H. Hiatt, J.D. Watson and J.A. Winsten, Ed,) pp 1283–1290 Cold Spring Harbor Laboratories, Cold Spring Harbor, New York.

Rall, D.P. (1979): Relevance of animal experiments to humans *Environ Health Perspect.*, 32:297–300.

Robens, J.F.; Joiner, J.J. and Schueler, R.L. (1982): Methods in Testing for Carcinogenesis, in *Principles and Methods of Toxicology*; (A.W. Hayes) pp 79–105 Raven Press, New York.

Salsburg, D.S. (1977): Use of statistics when examining life time studies in rodents to detect carcinogenicity. *J. Toxicol. Environ. Health*, 3:611–628.

Salsburg, D. (1980): The Effects of Lifetime Feeding Studies on Patterns of Senile Lesions in Mice and Rats *Drug Chem Tox.*, 3:1–33.

Schmidt-Nielsen, K. (1984): *Scaling: Why Is Animal Size So Important*, Cambridge University Press, New York.

Schneiderman, M.A.; Mantel, N. and Brown, C.C. (1975): *Ann N.Y. Acad. Sci.*, 246:237–248

Smith, R.L. (1974): The Problem of Species Variations *Ann Nutr Alim.*, 28:335.

Solleveld, H.A.; Hasemen, J.K. and McConnel, E.E. (1984): Natural History of Body Weight Gain, Survival, and Neoplasia in the F344 Rat *J. Natl. Canc. Inst.* 72:929–940.

Squire, R.A. (1981): Ranking Animal Carcinogens: A Proposed Regulatory Approach *Science*; 214:877–880.

Spector, W.S. (1956): *Handbook of Biological Data* W.B. Saunders, Philadelphia.

Staffa, J.A. and Mehlman, M.A. (1980): Innovations in Cancer Risk Assessment (ED_{01} Study). *J. Env. Path. Toxicol.*, 3:1–246.

Steinhoff, D.G.; Gad, S.C. Mohr, U. and Hatfield, G.K.; Chronic Intratracheal Instillation Study of Sodium Dichromate in Rats (Submitted for publication in Experimental Pathology).

Stokinger, H.E. (1977): Toxicology and drinking water contaminants. *J. Am. Water Works Assoc.*, July, pp. 399–402.

Swenberg, J.A. (1985): The interpretation and Use of Data From Long-Term Carcinogenesis Studies in Animals *CIIT Activities* 5 No. 6.; pp. 1–6.

Tarone R.E.; Chu, K.C. and Ward, J.M. (1981): Variability in the Rates of Some Common Naturally Occurring Tumors in Fischer 344 Rats and (C57BL/6NXC3H/HEN)F[1] (B6C3F[1]) Mice *J. Natl. Canc. Inst.*, 66:1175–1181·

Tomatis, L. (1979): The Predictive Value of Rodent Carcinogenicity Tests In the Eval- of Human Risks *Ann. Rev. Pharmacol Toxicology*; 19:511–530.

Ward, J.M.; Griesemer, R.A. and Weisburger, E.K. (1979): The Mouse Liver Tumor as an Endpoint in Carcinogenesis Tests *Tox. Appl. Pharmacol.*; 51:389–397

Weil, C.S. (1972): Statistics vs Safety Factors and Scientific Judgement in the Evaluation
of Safety for Man *Tox. App. Pharmacol.*; 21:454–463.

Weil, C.S. (1984): Some Questions and Opinions: Issues In Toxicology and Risk Assessment *Am. Ind. Hyg Asoc. J.*; 45:663–670.

Wilks, S.S. (1962): *Mathematical Statistics*, pp. 290–291 John Wiley, New York.

Wilson, J.S. and Holland, L.M. (1982): The Effect of Application Frequency On Epidermal Carcinogenesis Assays, *Toxicol.*, 24:45–53.

Wittenau, M.S. and Estes, Paul (1983): The Redundancy of Mouse Carcinogenicity Bioassays, *Fund App Toxicol.*, 3:631–639.

Wolfe, B. (1977): Low-Level Radiation: Predicting the Effects *Science*, 196:1387–1389.

Yanysheva, N. Ya., and Antomonov, Yu. G. (1976): Predicting the risk of tumor-occurrence under the effect of small doses of carcinogens. *Environ. Health Perspect.*, 13:95–99.

CHAPTER 13

STRUCTURE ACTIVITY RELATIONSHIPS

Structure activity relationship (SAR) methods have become a legitimate and useful part of toxicology over the last fifteen years or so. These methods are various forms of mathematical or statistical models which seek to predict the adverse biological effects of chemicals based on their structure. The prediction may be of either a qualitative (carcinogen/noncarcinogen) or quantitative (LD_{50}) nature, with the second group usually being denoted as QSAR (quantitative structure activity relationship) models. It should be obvious at the onset that the basic techniques utilized to construct such models are those which were discussed earlier in chapters VIII (mathematical modeling) and IX (reduction of dimensionality methods).

The concept that the biological activity of a compound is a direct function of its chemical structure is now at least a century old (Crum-Brown and Fraser, 1869). During most of this century, the development and use of SAR's were the domain of pharmacology and medicinal chemistry. These two fields are responsible for the beginnings of all the basic approaches in SAR work, usually with the effort being called drug design. An introductory medicinal chemistry text (such as Foye, 1974) is strongly recommended as a starting place for SAR. Additionally, *Burger's Medicinal Chemistry* (Wolf, 1980), with its excellent overview of drug structures and activities, should enhance at least the initial stages of identifying the potential biological actions of *de novo* compounds using a pattern recognition approach.

Having already classified SAR methods into qualitative and quantitative, it should also be pointed out that both of these can be approached on two different levels. The first is on a local level, where prediction of activity (or lack of activity) is limited to other members of a congeneric series or structural near-neighbors. The accuracy of predictions via this approach is generally greater, but is of value only if one has sufficient information on some of the structures within a series of interest.

The second approach is prediction of activity over a wide range, generally based on the presence or absence of particular structural features (functional groups).

For toxicology, SAR's have a small but important number of uses at present. These can all be generalized as identifying potentially toxic effects, or restated as three main uses:

1. For the selection and design of toxicity tests to address end points of possible concern.
2. If a comprehensive or large testing program is to be conducted, SAR predictions can be used to prioritize the tests, so that outlined questions (the answers to which might preclude the need to do further testing) may be addressed first.
3. As an alternative to testing at all. Though in general it is not believed that the state-of-the-art for SAR methods allows such usage, in certain special cases (such as selecting which of several alternative candidate compounds to develop further and then test) this use may be valid and valuable.

Basic Assumptions

Starting with the initial assumption that there is a relationship between structure and biological activity, we can proceed to more readily testable assumptions.

First, that the dose of chemical is subject to a number of modifying factors (such as membrane selectivities and selective metabolic actions) which are each related in some manner to chemical structure. Indeed, absorption, metabolism, pharmacologic activity and excretion are each subject to not just structurally determined actions, but also to (in many cases) stereo-specific differential handlings.

Given these assumptions, actual elucidation of SAR's requires the following:

1. Knowledge of the biological activities of existing structures.
2. Knowledge of structural features which serve to predict activity (also called molecular parameters of interest).
3. One or more models which relate 2 to 1 with some degree of reliability.

There are now extensive sources of information as to both toxic properties of chemicals and, indeed, biological activities. These include books, journals, and manual and computerized data bases. The reader is directed to Wexler's 1982 book as a guide to accessing the different sources of toxicology information, but is cautioned to remember that there is also extensive applicable information in the realms of medicinal chemistry and pharmacology, as exemplified by Burger's (Wolff, 1980).

Molecular Parameters of Interest

Which structural and physicochemical properties of a chemical are important in predicting its toxicologic activity are both open to considerable debate (Kaufman et al., 1983; Tamura, 1983; Tute, 1983). Table 28 presents a partial list of such parameters. The reader is referred to a biologically oriented physical chemistry text (such as Chang, 1981) both for explanations of these parameters and for references to sources from which specific values may be obtained.

There are now several systems available to study the three dimensional structural aspects of molecules and their interactions. The first are the various molecular modeling sets, which can actually be very useful for some simpler problems. The second are the molecular design and analysis packages which are available for main frame computers. Lastly, molecular graphics software packages have become available recently for such microcomputers as the Apple IIe and IBM. Use of such forms of graphic structural examination as a tool or method in SAR analysis has been discussed by Cohen et al. (1974) and Gund et al. (1980). Such methods are generally called topological methods.

SAR Modeling Methods

A detailed review of even the major methodologies available for SAR/QSAR modeling in toxicology is beyond the scope of this book. Though we will briefly discuss the major approaches, the reader is directed to one of the several very readable introductory articles (Chu, 1980 or Craig, 1980) or books (Olson and Christoffersen, 1979; Topliss, 1983; or Goldberg, 1983) for somewhat detailed presentations.

To begin with, it should be made clear that all the actual techniques involved in the performance of SAR analysis have already been presented in this text. It is only their actual application to data which sets such analysis apart from the forms of modeling we have previously looked at.

All the current major SAR methods used in toxicology can be classified based on what kinds of compound-related or structural data they use and what method is used to correlate this structural data with the existing biological data.

The more classical approaches use physiocochemical data (such as molecular weight, free energies, etc.) as a starting point. The major approaches to this are by manual pattern recognition methods, cluster analysis, or by regression analysis. It is this last, in the form of Hansch or linear-free energy relationships (LFER) which actually launched all SAR work (other than that on limited congeneric cases) into the realm of being a useful approach. Indeed, still foremost among the QSAR methods is the model proposed by Hansch and his coworkers (Hansch, 1971). It was the major contribution of this group to propose the

TABLE 28
MOLECULAR PARAMETERS OF INTEREST

ELECTRONIC EFFECTS
> Ionization constants
>> Sigma substituent constant
>
> Distribution constant
> Resonance effect
> Field effect
> Molecular orbital indices*
>> Atomic/electron net charge
>> Nucleophilic superdelocalizability
>> Electrophilic superdelocalizability
>> Free radical superdelocalizability
>> Energy of the lowest empty molecular orbital
>> Energy of the highest occupied molecular orbital
>> Frontier self-atom polarizability
>> Frontier atom-atom polarizability
>> Intermolecular coulombic interaction energy
>> Electric field created at point [A] by a set of charges on a molecule

HYPROPHOBIC PARAMETERS
> Partition coefficients
> Pi substituent constants
> R_M value in liquid-liquid chromatography
> Elution time in high-pressure liquid chromatography (HPLC)
> Solubility
> Solvent partition coefficients
> pKa

STERIC EFFECTS
> Intramolecular steric effects
>> Steric substituent constant
>> Hyperconjugation correction
>
> Molar volume
> Molar refractivity, MR substituent constants
> Molecular weight
> Van der Waals radii
> Interatomic distances

SUBSTRUCTURAL EFFECTS
> Three dimensional geometry
> Fragment and molecular properties (see Chu 1980 for substituent effects)
> Chain lengths

*Calculated or theoretical parameters

incorporation of earlier observations of the importance of the relative lipophilicity to biologic activity into the formal LFER approach to provide a general QSAR model for biological effects. As a suitable measure of lipophilicity, the partition coefficient (log P) between 1-octanol and water was proposed, and it was demonstrated that this was an approximately additive and constitutive property and that it was therefore calculable, in principle, from molecular structure. Using a probabilistic model for the Hansch equation, which can be expressed as:

$$\log (1/C) = k \pi^2 = k' \pi + \rho \sigma + k''$$
$$\text{or } \log (1/C) = -k (\log P)^2 + k' (\log P) + \rho \sigma + k''$$

where C is the dose that elicits a constant biological response (e.g. ED_{50}, LD_{50}), π is the substituent lipophilicity, log P is the partition coefficient, σ is the substituent electronic effect of Hammet and k, k', ρ, and k'' are the regression coefficients derived from the statistical curve fitting. The reciprocal of the concentration reflects the fact that higher potency is associated with lower dose, and the negative sign for the π^2 or $(\log P)^2$ term reflects the expectation n of an optimum lipophilicity, designated π_0 or log P_0.

The statistical method used to determine the coefficients above is multiple linear regression. A number of statistics are derived in conjunction with such a calculation, which allow the statistical significance of the resulting correlation to be assessed. The most important of these are s, the standard deviation, r^2, the coefficient of determination or percentage of data variance accounted for by the model (r, the correlation coefficient is also commonly cited), and F, a statistic for assessing the overall significance of the derived equation, values, and confidence intervals (usually 95%) for the individual regression coefficients in the equation. Also very important in multiparameter equations are the cross-correlation coefficients between the independent variables in the equation. These must be low to assure true "independence" or orthogonality of the variables, a necessary condition for meaningful results.

In a like manner, there are a number of approaches for using structural and substructural data and correlating these to biological activities. Such approahces are generally classified as regression analysis methods, pattern recognition methods, and miscellaneous others (such as factor analysis, principal components, and probalistic analysis).

The regression analysis methods which use structural data have been, as we will see when we survey the state of the art in toxicology, the most productive and useful. "Keys" - or fragments of structure - are assigned weights as predictors of an activity, usually in some form of the Free - Wilson model (Free and Wilson, 1964) which was developed at virtually the same time as the Hansch. According to this method, the molecules of a chemical series are structurally decomposed into a common moiety (or core) that may be substituted in multiple positions. A series of linear equations of the form

$$BA_i = \sum_j a_j X_{ij} + \mu$$

are constructed where BA is the biological activity, X_j is the jth substituent with a value of 1 if present and 0 if not, a_j is the contribution of the jth substituent to BA, and μ is the overall average activity. All activity contributions at each position of substitution must sum to zero. The series of linear equations thus generated is solved by the method of least squares for the a_j and μ. There must be several more equations than unknowns and each substituent should appear more than once at a position in different combinations with substituents at other positions. The favorable aspects of this model are:

a. any set of quantitative biological data may be employed as the dependent variable,
b. no independently determined substituent constants are required,
c. the molecules comprising a sample of interest may be structurally dismembered in any desired or convenient manner,
d. multiple sites of variable substitution are readily handled by the model.

There are also several limitations: a substantial number of compounds with varying substituent combinations is required for a meaningful analysis; the derived substituent contributions give no reasonable basis for extrapolating predictions from the substituent matrix analyzed; and the model will break down if nonlinear dependence on substituent properties is important or if there are interactions between the substituents.

Pattern recognition methods comprise yet another approach to examining structural features and/or chemical properties for underlying patterns that are associated with differing biological effects. Accurate classification of untested molecules is again the primary goal. This is carried out in two stages. First, a set of compounds, designated the training set, is chosen for which the correct classification is known. A set of molecular or property descriptors (features) is generated for each compound. A suitable classification algorithm is then applied to find some combination and weight of the descriptors that allow perfect classification. Many different statistical and geometric techniques for this purpose have been used and were presented in earlier chapters. The derived classification function is then applied in the second step to compounds not included in the training set to test predictability.

In published work these have generally been other compounds of known classification also. Performance is judged by the percentage of correct predictions. Stability of the classification function is usually tested by repeating the procedure several times with slightly altered, but randomly varied, sets or samples.

The main difficulty with these methods is in "decoding" the QSAR in order to identify particular structural fragments responsible for the expression of a particular activity. And even if identified as "responsible" for activity, far harder questions for the model to answer are whether the structural fragment so identified is "sufficient" for activity, whether it is always "necessary" for activity, and to what extent its expression is modified by its molecular environment. Most pattern recognition methods use as weighting factors either the presence or absence of a particular fragment or feature (coded 1 or 0), or the frequency of occurrence of a feature. They may be made more sophisticated by coding the spatial relationship between features.

Enslein (1984) has published a good brief description of the problems involved in applying these methods in toxicology.

Applications in Toxicology

SAR methods have been developed to predict a number of toxicological end points (mutagenesis, carcinogenesis, dermal sensitization, lethality (LD_{50} values), biological oxygen demands, and

TABLE 29
Existing SAR Models for Toxicology End Points

End Point	PREDICTION Quantitative	Qualitative	Reference
Mutagenicity	X		Asher and Zervos, 1977
		X	Niculescu-Duvaz, et al., 1981
	X		Enslein et al., 1983
Carcinogenicity	X		Franke, 1973
	X		Aser and Zervos, 1977
		X	Niculescu-Duvaz, et al., 1981
	X		Enslein and Craig, 1982
Sensitization	X		Dupuis and Benezra, 1982
LD_{50}		X	Enslein et al., 1983
Teratogenicity	X		Enslein et al., 1983
Biological Oxygen Demand		X	Enslein et al., 1984

teratogenicity) with varying degrees of accuracy, and models for the prediction of other end points are under development. Some of these existing models are presented by category of use in Table 29. Additionally, both EPA and FDA have models for mutagenicity/carcinogenecity that they utilize to "flag" possible problem compounds.

It should be expected that qualitative models are more "accurate" than quantitative ones, and that the more possible mechanisms associated with an endpoint, the less accurate (or more difficult) a prediction.

REFERENCES

Asher, I.M. and Zervos, C. (1977): *Structural Correlates of Carcinogenesis and Mutagenesis,* Office of Science, FDA, Washington.

Chang, R. (1981): *Physical Chemistry with Application to Biological Systems.* MacMilliam Publishing, Inc., New York.

Chu, K.C. (1980). The Quantitative Analysis of Structure - Activity Relationships, In *Burger's Medicinal Chemistry* (M.E. Wolff, Ed). Vol. I, pp 393–418 John Wiley, New York.

Cohen, J.L.; Lee, W. and Lien, E.J. (1974): Dependence of Toxicity on Molecular Structure: Group Theory Analysis. *J Pharm Sci., 63* :1068–1072.

Crum-Brown, A. and Fraser, T. (1869): *Trans Roy Soc Edinburgh; 25*:693.

Dupuis, G. and Benezra, C. (1982): *Allergic Contact Dermatitis to Simple Chemicals - A Molecular Approach.* Marcel Dekker, Inc. New York.

Enslein, K. (1984): Estimation of Toxicological Endpoints by Structure-Activity Relationships. *Pharmacol Rev.,* 36: 131–134.

Enslein, K. and Craig, P.N. (1982) Carcinogenesis: A Predictive Structure Activity Model. *J. Toxicol. Envir. Hlth.;* 10:521–530.

Enslein, K., Lander, T.R., Tomb, M.E., Landis, W.G. (1983): Mutagenicity (Ames): A Structure-Activity Model. *J. Teratogenesis, Carcinogenesis and Mutagenesis*; 3:503–514.

Enslein, K. Tomb, M.E., Lander, T.R. (1984): Structure-Activity Models of Biological Oxygen Demand, in *QSAR in Environmental Toxicology,* (Kaiser, KLE, ed.) Reidel Publishing Co., Dordrecht.

Foye, W.O. (1974): *Principles of Medicinal Chemistry.* Lea & Febiger, Philadelphia.

Franke, R. (1973): Structure-Activity Relationships in Polycyclic Aromatic Hydrocarbons: Induction of Microsomal Aryl Hydrocarbon Hydroxylase and Its Possible Importance in Chemical Carcinogenesis *Chem-Biol Inter.,* 6:1–17.

Free, S.M., and J.W. Wilson (1964): A Mathematical Contribution to Structure-Activity Studies. *J. Med. Chem.,* 7:395–399..

Goldberg, L. (1983): *Structure-Activity Correlations as a Predictive Tool in Toxicology.* Hemisphere Publishing Corp, New York.

Gund, P.; Andosf, J.D.; Rhodes J.B., and Smith, G.M. (1980): Three-Dimensional Molecular Modeling and Drug Design. *Science;* 208:1425–1431.

Hansch, C. (1971): In *Drug Design* Vol. I Chapter 2 (E.J. Ariens, Ed.) Academic Press, New York.

Kaufman, J.J.; Lewchenko, V.; Hariharan, P.C. and Kuski, W.S. (1983): Theoretical Predictions of Toxicity, In. *Product Safety Evaluation* (A.M. Goldberg, Ed.) pp. 333–355 Mary Ann Liebert, Inc., New York.

Niculescu-Duvaz, I.; Craescu, T.; Tugulea, M.; Croisy, A. and Jacquignon, P.C. (1981): A Quantitative Structure-Activity Analysis of the Mutagenic and Carcinogenic Action of 43 Structurally Related Heterocyclic Compounds. *Carcinogenesis*; 2:269–275.

Olson, E.C. and Cristoffersen, R.E. (1979): *Computer Assisted Drug Design*. ACS, Washington.

Tamura, R.M. (1983): A Model for Toxicologic Prediction. In *Product Safety Evaluation*, (A.M. Goldberg, Ed.) pp. 317–330 Mary Ann Liebert, Inc. New York.

Topliss, J.G. (1983): *Quantitative Structure-Activity Relationships of Drugs*. Academic Press, New York.

Tute, M.S. (1983): Mathematical Modeling, In *Animals and Alternatives in Toxicity Testing* (M. Balls, R.J. Riddel and A.N. Worden, Eds.) pp. 137–166 Academic Press, New York.

Wexler, P. (1982): *Information Resources in Toxicology*, Elsevier/North Holland, New York.

Wolff, M.E. (1980): *Burger's Medicinal Chemistry*. John Wiley, New York.

CHAPTER 14

AREAS OF CONTROVERSY IN STATISTICS AS USED FOR TOXICOLOGY

It should now be clear to the reader that the use of statistics in toxicology is not a "cut and dried" matter. There are a number of areas which are (and have been) the subject of honest controversy, and it should be expected that others will arise as the two fields advance.

This volume has already presented many of the problem areas. In Chapter VII, it was seen that there is no consensus as to which *post-hoc* tests should be used after ANOVA because of some of the real-life characteristics of toxicologic data. In this same chapter, the arguments for and against the different methods of hypothesis testing for differences in organ weights were presented. In Chapter IX, the different experimental designs and computational methods for determining LD_{50} values were laid out. And in Chapter XII, the matters of risk assessment and threshold were addressed.

There remain, however, three areas to be addressed which are somewhat particular to toxicology. These are the effects of censoring on data, the direction of hypothesis testing, and the use of unbalanced designs.

Censoring

Censoring is practiced when not all the possible data arising from an experiment are available for or used in analysis. Though some would make the distinction that censored data are different from missing data in that the values for the former can be accurately estimated and those for missing data cannot, here the term is used to mean all data not included in analysis, for whatever reasons. There are four major reasons for data being censored in toxicology studies, and the degree of accuracy for which the value of such censored values can be estimated varies depending on the reason for censoring.

1. The most common reason for censoring in toxicology is death - not all the animals which start a study end it. In these cases

we have no basis to accurately estimate the observations that would have been made had the animal (or animals) lived. Censoring by death is an example of "left censoring" - unplanned, without recourse and generally during a period when the information lost would be of interest. Right censoring, on the other hand, generally is planned, there is recourse to get the information if needed and the information potentially lost is of minimal, if any, interest.

2. Data may be censored by having samples lost to measurement at intermittent periods. Such losses are the result of, for example, clotting of blood samples prior to analysis, loss of tissues during necropsy, or breakdown of instruments at critical times. Usually the values of the last observations can be estimated with some accuracy. And most such cases can be remedied by resampling (collecting more blood, for example).

3. When we judge an extreme value to be an outlier and reject it, we are censoring it. If the value is cleanly discarded, we are *de facto* saying we cannot accurately estimate its value. If, however, we use a procedure such as winsorizing and replace it with a less extreme value, we are in fact estimating the most probable, true value of the observations.

4. Finally, some observations may be censored because their values are beyond the range at which the instruments we use can accurately measure. An example is in measuring rabbit methemoglobin with an instrument designed for humans. Extreme low values are not accurately measured, and are reported as negative percentage values. In this case, we can accurately estimate a censored value as being "less than" or "greater than" a known value.

What are the consequences of censoring? The answer depends on the nature and extent of the censoring process. If only a few of a large number of values are lost and the pattern of loss is randomly distributed among all groups on study, little if any harm is done. If the extent of data loss is too severe-say because the majority of the animals in a group die-the entire experiment may have to be discarded. An intermediate case would be low, but non-random, censoring. This is not an uncommon case in toxicology, where censoring because of death tends to be concentrated in high-dose groups. In these cases, the experiment is not lost but rather truncated-some effects cannot be addressed with reference to the treatment used in highly censored groups. And, as we will discuss a little later, it may unbalance a design.

An additional common effect of censoring that should be kept in mind is its effect on the normality of the sample. If all values above a certain level (say of serum electrolytes) are censored because animals having such values die before the measurements are made, we are left with a truncated normal distribution. A special case of this was discussed by Gad and Smith (1984), in that the time-to-incapacitation values in combustion toxicology are censored because they are only measured to thirty minutes, and not beyond. Such truncated populations cannot be treated as normal for purposes of statistical analysis.

There is an entire family of methods which have been developed to address censored data sets. Bishop *et al.* (1971) present an excellent overview of some of these.

Direction of Hypothesis Testing

Which direction (or directions) we are testing a hypothesis in can be restated as asking whether we are to use a one-tailed or a two-tailed test. This is of consequence because one-tailed tests are always more sensitive (more likely to find an effect) than are two-tailed tests.

Generally, such a selection must be made prior to the start of an experiment, based on a clear statement of the question being asked (that is, the objective of the study). If we are asking if a chemical increases the incidence of cancer, then our question is one-tailed - we are not interested in the detection of any significant decrease in the incidence of cancer. Most toxicology studies, however, are of a "shot gun" nature. They are designed to detect and identify any and all effects. This is a two-tailed question - can a chemical either increase or decrease the incidence of cancer?

Feinstein (1975) provides a clear discussion of questions of direction of effect as they relate to biostatistics.

Unbalanced Designs

One of the principles of experimental design presented back in Chapter III was that of balance. This held that group sizes should be at least approximately equal. And, as we have reviewed the different methods presented in this book, we have noted that a number of them have impaired performance if the sizes of the groups are not equivalent.

Yet, it is not uncommon to lose data because of censoring in toxicology studies. And if such censoring is related to a compound or treatment effect, it is very likely that the most affected groups will not be equivalent in size to our control group at the end of an experiment.

At the same time, it should be clear that it is easier to statistically detect large effects than small effects. And, in the vast majority of cases, larger effects occur in high dose groups (not infrequently to the extent that no statistical analysis is necessary), while it is in the lower dose groups that the guidance provided by statistical analysis is most needed.

These reasons argue for the use of unbalanced designs in toxicology. That is, those treatments where it is expected that more statistical power will be needed or which are expected to suffer from an increased level of censoring due to death (where death itself is not the variable of interest) should be administered to test groups which are larger than other test groups. Farmer *et al.* (1977) have reviewed a number of options for deciding on the degree of imbalance with which to start a study.

Use of Computerized Statistical Packages

Lastly, we must recognize that for many toxicology laboratories, the approach to statistical analysis of data is to use one of the mainframe packages which automatically selects and utilizes statistical tests. It is critically important in these cases to understand the limitations and proper uses of statistical tests that are automatically employed.

REFERENCES

Bishop, Y.; Fujii, K.; Arnold, E. and Epstein, S.S. (1971): Censored Distribution Techniques in Analysis of Toxicological Data. *Experientia*, 27:1056–1059.

Farmer, J.H; Uhler, R.J. and Haley T.J. (1977): An Unbalanced Experimental Design for Dose Response Studies. *J. Environ. Path. Toxicol.*, 1:293–299.

Feinstein, A.R. (1975): Clinical Biostatistics XXXII: Biological Dependency, "Hypothesis Testing, Unilateral Probabilities, and Other Issues in Scientific Direction vs. Statistical Duplexity. *Clin. Pharmacol. Ther.*, 17: 499–513.

Gad, S.C. and Smith, A.C. (1984): Influence of Heating Rates on the Toxicity of Evolved Combustion Products: Results and a System for Research. *J. Fire Science*, 1:465–479

TABLE A: LOGARITHMS (BASE 10)

N	0	1	2	3	4	5	6	7	8	9
10	0000	0043	0086	0128	0170	0212	0253	0294	0334	0374
11	0414	0453	0492	0531	0569	0607	0645	0682	0719	0755
12	0792	0828	0864	0899	0934	0969	1004	1038	1072	1106
13	1139	1173	1206	1239	1271	1303	1335	1367	1399	1430
14	1461	1492	1523	1553	1584	1614	1644	1673	1703	1732
15	1761	1790	1818	1847	1875	1903	1931	1959	1987	2014
16	2041	2068	2095	2122	2148	2175	2201	2227	2253	2279
17	2304	2330	2355	2380	2405	2430	2455	2480	2504	2529
18	2553	2577	2601	2625	2648	2672	2695	2718	2742	2765
19	2788	2810	2833	2856	2878	2900	2923	2945	2967	2989
20	3010	3032	3054	3075	3096	3118	3139	3160	3181	3201
21	3222	3243	3263	3284	3304	3324	3345	3365	3385	3404
22	3424	3444	3464	3483	3502	3522	3541	3560	3579	3598
23	3617	3636	3655	3674	3692	3711	3729	3747	3766	3784
24	3802	3820	3838	3856	3874	3892	3909	3927	3945	3962
25	3979	3997	4014	4031	4048	4065	4082	4099	4116	4133
26	4150	4166	4183	4200	4216	4232	4249	4265	4281	4298
27	4314	4330	4346	4362	4378	4393	4409	4425	4440	4456
28	4472	4487	4502	4518	4533	4548	4564	4579	4594	4609
29	4624	4639	4654	4669	4683	4698	4713	4728	4742	4757

TABLE A: LOGARITHMS (BASE 10) (continued)

N	0	1	2	3	4	5	6	7	8	9
30	4771	4786	4800	4814	4829	4843	4857	4871	4886	4900
31	4914	4928	4942	4955	4969	4983	4997	5011	5024	5038
32	5051	5065	5079	5092	5105	5119	5132	5145	5159	5172
33	5185	5198	5211	5224	5237	5250	5263	5276	5289	5302
34	5315	5328	5340	5353	5366	5378	5391	5403	5416	5428
35	5441	5453	5465	5478	5490	5502	5514	5527	5539	5551
36	5563	5575	5587	5599	5611	5623	5635	5647	5658	5670
37	5682	5694	5705	5717	5729	5740	5752	5763	5775	5786
38	5798	5809	5821	5832	5843	5855	5866	5877	5888	5899
39	5911	5922	5933	5944	5955	5966	5977	5988	5999	6010
40	6021	6031	6042	6053	6064	6075	6085	6096	6107	6117
41	6128	6138	6149	6160	6170	6180	6191	6201	6212	6222
42	6232	6243	6253	6263	6274	6284	6294	6304	6314	6325
43	6335	6345	6355	6365	6375	6385	6395	6405	6415	6425
44	6345	6444	6454	6464	6474	6484	6493	6503	6513	6522
45	6532	6542	6551	6561	6571	6580	6590	6599	6609	6618
46	6628	6637	6646	6656	6665	6675	6684	6693	6702	6712
47	6721	6730	6739	6749	6758	6767	6776	6785	6794	6803
48	6812	6821	6830	6839	6848	6857	6866	6875	6884	6893
49	6902	6911	6920	6928	6937	6946	6955	6964	6972	6981
50	6990	6998	7007	7016	7024	7033	7042	7050	7059	7067
51	7076	7084	7093	7101	7110	7118	7126	7135	7143	7152

N	0	1	2	3	4	5	6	7	8	9
52	7160	7168	7177	7185	7193	7202	7210	7218	7226	7235
53	7243	7251	7259	7267	7275	7284	7292	7300	7308	7316
54	7324	7332	7340	7348	7356	7364	7372	7380	7388	7396
55	7404	7412	7419	7427	7435	7443	7451	7459	7466	7474
56	7482	7490	7497	7505	7513	7520	7528	7536	7543	7551
57	7559	7566	7574	7582	7589	7597	7604	7612	7619	7627
58	7634	7642	7649	7657	7664	7672	7679	7686	7694	7701
59	7709	7716	7723	7731	7738	7745	7752	7760	7767	7774
60	7782	7789	7796	7803	7810	7818	7825	7832	7839	7846
61	7853	7860	7868	7875	7882	7889	7896	7903	7910	7917
62	7924	7931	7938	7945	7952	7959	7966	7973	7980	7987
63	7993	8000	8007	8014	8021	8028	8035	8041	8048	8055
64	8062	8068	8075	8082	8089	8096	8102	8109	8116	8122
65	8129	8136	8142	8149	8156	8162	8169	8176	8182	8189
66	8195	8202	8209	8215	8222	8228	8235	8241	8248	8254
67	8261	8267	8274	8280	8287	8293	8299	8306	8312	8319
68	8325	8331	8338	8344	8351	8357	8363	8370	8376	8382
69	8388	8395	8401	8407	8414	8420	8426	8432	8439	8445
70	8451	8457	8463	8470	8476	8482	8488	8494	8500	8506
71	8513	8519	8525	8531	8537	8543	8549	8555	8561	8567
72	8573	8579	8585	8591	8597	8603	8609	8615	8621	8627
73	8633	8639	8645	8651	8657	8663	8669	8675	8681	8686
74	8692	8698	8704	8710	8716	8722	8727	8733	8739	8745

TABLE A: LOGARITHMS (BASE 10) (continued)

N	0	1	2	3	4	5	6	7	8	9
75	8751	8756	8762	8768	8774	8779	8785	8791	8797	8802
76	8808	8814	8820	8825	8831	8837	8842	8848	8854	8859
77	8865	8871	8876	8882	8887	8893	8899	8904	8910	8915
78	8921	8927	8932	8938	8943	8949	8954	8960	8965	8971
79	8976	8982	8987	8993	8998	9004	9009	9015	9020	9025
80	9031	9036	9042	9047	9053	9058	9063	9069	9074	9079
81	9085	9090	9096	9101	9106	9112	9117	9122	9128	9133
82	9138	9143	9149	9154	9159	9165	9170	9175	9180	9186
83	9191	9196	9201	9206	9212	9217	9222	9227	9232	9238
84	9243	9248	9253	9258	9263	9269	9274	9279	9284	9289
85	9294	9299	9304	9309	9315	9320	9325	9330	9335	9340
86	9345	9350	9355	9360	9365	9370	9375	9380	9385	9390
87	9395	9400	9405	9410	9415	9420	9425	9430	9435	9440
88	9445	9450	9455	9460	9465	9469	9474	9479	9484	9489
89	9494	9499	9504	9509	9513	9518	9523	9528	9533	9538
90	9542	9547	9552	9557	9562	9566	9571	9576	9581	9586
91	9590	9595	9600	9605	9609	9614	9619	9624	9628	9633
92	9638	9643	9647	9652	9657	9661	9666	9671	9575	9680
93	9685	9689	9694	9699	9703	9708	9713	9717	9722	9727
94	9731	9736	9741	9745	9750	9754	9759	9763	9768	9773
95	9777	9782	9786	9791	9795	9800	9805	9809	9814	9818
96	9823	9827	9832	9836	9841	9845	9850	9854	9859	9863
97	9868	9872	9877	9881	9886	9890	9894	9899	9903	9908
98	9912	9917	9921	9926	9930	9934	9939	9943	9948	9952
99	9956	9961	9965	9969	9974	9978	9983	9987	9991	9996

TABLE B: PROBIT TRANSFORM VALUES

%	0.0	0.1	0.2	0.3	0.4	0.5	0.6	0.7	0.8	0.9
0	...	1.9098	2.1218	2.2522	2.3479	2.4242	2.4879	2.5427	2.5911	2.6344
1	2.6737	2.7096	2.7429	2.7738	2.8027	2.8299	2.8556	2.8799	2.9031	2.9251
2	2.9463	2.9665	2.9859	3.0046	3.0226	3.0400	3.0569	3.0732	3.0890	3.1043
3	3.1192	3.1337	3.1478	3.1616	3.1750	3.1881	3.2009	3.2134	3.2256	3.2376
4	3.2493	3.2608	3.2721	3.2831	3.2940	3.3046	3.3151	3.3253	3.3354	3.3454
5	3.3551	3.3648	3.3742	3.3836	3.3928	3.4018	3.4107	3.4195	3.4282	3.4368
6	3.4452	3.4536	3.4618	3.4699	3.4780	3.4859	3.4937	3.5015	3.5091	3.5167
7	3.5242	3.5316	3.5389	3.5462	3.5534	3.5605	3.5675	3.5745	3.5813	3.5882
8	3.5949	3.6016	3.6083	3.6148	3.6213	3.6278	3.6342	3.6405	3.6468	3.6531
9	3.6592	3.6654	3.6715	3.6775	3.6835	3.6894	3.6953	3.7012	3.7070	3.7127
10	3.7184	3.7241	3.7298	3.7354	3.7409	3.7464	3.7519	3.7574	3.7628	3.7681
11	3.7735	3.7788	3.7840	3.7893	3.7945	3.7996	3.8048	3.8099	3.8150	3.8200
12	3.8250	3.8300	3.8350	3.8399	3.8448	3.8497	3.8545	3.8593	3.8641	3.8689
13	3.8736	3.8783	3.8830	3.8877	3.8923	3.8969	3.9015	3.9061	3.9107	3.9152
14	3.9197	3.9242	3.9286	3.9331	3.9375	3.9419	3.9463	3.9506	3.9550	3.9593
15	3.9636	3.9678	3.9721	3.9763	3.9806	3.9848	3.9890	3.9931	3.9973	4.0014
16	4.0055	4.0096	4.0137	4.0178	4.0218	4.0259	4.0299	4.0339	4.0379	4.0419
17	4.0458	4.0498	4.0537	4.0576	4.0615	4.0654	4.0693	4.0731	4.0770	4.0808
18	4.0846	4.0884	4.0922	4.0960	4.0998	4.1035	4.1073	4.1110	4.1147	4.1184
19	4.1221	4.1258	4.1295	4.1331	4.1367	4.1404	4.1440	4.1476	4.1512	4.1548

TABLE B: PROBIT TRANSFORM VALUES (continued)

%	0.0	0.1	0.2	0.3	0.4	0.5	0.6	0.7	0.8	0.9
20	4.1584	4.1619	4.1655	4.1690	4.1726	4.1761	4.1796	4.1831	4.1866	4.1901
21	4.1936	4.1970	4.2005	4.2039	4.2074	4.2108	4.2142	4.2176	4.2210	4.2244
22	4.2278	4.2312	4.2345	4.2379	4.2412	4.2446	4.2479	4.2512	4.2546	4.2579
23	4.2612	4.2644	4.2677	4.2710	4.2743	4.2775	4.2808	4.2840	4.2872	4.2905
24	4.2937	4.2969	4.3001	4.3033	4.3065	4.3097	4.3129	4.3160	4.3192	4.3224
25	4.3255	4.3287	4.3318	4.3349	4.3380	4.3412	4.3443	4.3474	4.3505	4.3536
26	4.3567	4.3597	4.3628	4.3659	4.3689	4.3720	4.3750	4.3781	4.3811	4.3842
27	4.3872	4.3902	4.3932	4.3962	4.3992	4.4022	4.4052	4.4082	4.4112	4.4142
28	4.4172	4.4201	4.4231	4.4260	4.4290	4.4319	4.4349	4.4378	4.4408	4.4437
29	4.4466	4.4495	4.4524	4.4554	4.4583	4.4612	4.4641	4.4670	4.4698	4.4727
30	4.4756	4.4785	4.4813	4.4842	4.4871	4.4899	4.4928	4.4956	4.4985	4.5013
31	4.5041	4.5070	4.5098	4.5126	4.5155	4.5183	4.5211	4.5239	4.5267	4.5295
32	4.5323	4.5351	4.5379	4.5407	4.5435	4.5462	4.5490	4.5518	4.5546	4.5573
33	4.5601	4.5628	4.5656	4.5684	4.5711	4.5739	4.5766	4.5793	4.5821	4.5848
34	4.5875	4.5903	4.5930	4.5957	4.5984	4.6011	4.6039	4.6066	4.6093	4.6120
35	4.6147	4.6174	4.6201	4.6228	4.6255	4.6281	4.6308	4.6335	4.6362	4.6389
36	4.6415	4.6442	4.6469	4.6495	4.6522	4.6549	4.6575	4.6602	4.6628	4.6655
37	4.6681	4.6708	4.6734	4.6761	4.6787	4.6814	4.6840	4.6866	4.6893	4.6919
38	4.6945	4.6971	4.6998	4.7024	4.7050	4.7076	4.7102	4.7129	4.7155	4.7181
39	4.7207	4.7233	4.7259	4.7285	4.7311	4.7337	4.7363	4.7389	4.7415	4.7441
40	4.7467	4.7492	4.7518	4.7544	4.7570	4.7596	4.7622	4.7647	4.7673	4.7699
41	4.7725	4.7750	4.7776	4.7802	4.7827	4.7853	4.7879	4.7904	4.7930	4.7955

%	0.0	0.1	0.2	0.3	0.4	0.5	0.6	0.7	0.8	0.9
42	4.7981	4.8007	4.8032	4.8058	4.8083	4.8109	4.8134	4.8160	4.8185	4.8211
43	4.8236	4.8262	4.8287	4.8313	4.8338	4.8363	4.8389	4.8414	4.8440	4.8465
44	4.8490	4.8516	4.8541	4.8566	4.8592	4.8617	4.8642	4.8668	4.8693	4.8718
45	4.8743	4.8769	4.8794	4.8819	4.8844	4.8870	4.8895	4.8920	4.8945	4.8970
46	4.8996	4.9021	4.9046	4.9071	4.9096	4.9122	4.9147	4.9172	4.9197	4.9222
47	4.9247	4.9272	4.9298	4.9323	4.9348	4.9373	4.9398	4.9423	4.9448	4.9473
48	4.9498	4.9524	4.9549	4.9574	4.9599	4.9624	4.9649	4.9674	4.9699	4.9724
49	4.9749	4.9774	4.9799	4.9825	4.9850	4.9875	4.9900	4.9925	4.9950	4.9975
50	5.0000	5.0025	5.0050	5.0075	5.0100	5.0125	5.0150	5.0175	5.0201	5.0226
51	5.0251	5.0276	5.0301	5.0326	5.0351	5.0376	5.0401	5.0426	5.0451	5.0476
52	5.0502	5.0527	5.0552	5.0577	5.0602	5.0627	5.0652	5.0677	5.0702	5.0728
53	5.0753	5.0778	5.0803	5.0828	5.0853	5.0878	5.0904	5.0929	5.0954	5.0979
54	5.1004	5.1030	5.1055	5.1080	5.1105	5.1130	5.1156	5.1181	5.1206	5.1231
55	5.1257	5.1282	5.1307	5.1332	5.1358	5.1383	5.1408	5.1434	5.1459	5.1484
56	5.1510	5.1535	5.1560	5.1586	5.1611	5.1637	5.1662	5.1689	5.1713	5.1738
57	5.1764	5.1789	5.1815	5.1840	5.1866	5.1891	5.1917	5.1942	5.1968	5.1993
58	5.2019	5.2045	5.2070	5.2096	5.2121	5.2147	5.2173	5.2198	5.2224	5.2250
59	5.2275	5.2301	5.2327	5.2353	5.2378	5.2404	5.2430	5.2456	5.2482	5.2508
60	5.2533	5.2559	5.2585	5.2611	5.2637	5.2666	5.2689	5.2715	5.2741	5.2767
61	5.2793	5.2819	5.2845	5.2871	5.2898	5.2924	5.2950	5.2976	5.3002	5.3029
62	5.3055	5.3081	5.3107	5.3134	5.3160	5.3186	5.3213	5.3239	5.3266	5.3292
63	5.3319	5.3345	5.3372	5.3398	5.3425	5.3451	5.3478	5.3505	5.3531	5.3558
64	5.3585	5.3611	5.3638	5.3665	5.3692	5.3719	5.3745	5.3772	5.3799	5.3826

TABLE B: PROBIT TRANSFORM VALUES (continued)

%	0.0	0.1	0.2	0.3	0.4	0.5	0.6	0.7	0.8	0.9
65	5.3853	5.3880	5.3907	5.3934	5.3961	5.3989	5.4016	5.4043	5.4070	5.4097
66	5.4125	5.4152	5.4179	5.4207	5.4234	5.4261	5.4289	5.4316	5.4344	5.4372
67	5.4399	5.4427	5.4454	5.4482	5.4510	5.4538	5.4565	5.4693	5.4621	5.4649
68	5.4677	5.4705	5.4733	5.4761	5.4789	5.4817	5.4845	5.4874	5.4902	5.4930
69	5.4959	5.4987	5.5015	5.5044	5.5072	5.5101	5.5129	5.5158	5.5187	5.5215
70	5.5244	5.5273	5.5302	5.5330	5.5359	5.5388	5.5417	5.5446	5.5476	5.5505
71	5.5534	5.5563	5.5592	5.5622	5.5651	5.5681	5.5710	5.5740	5.5769	5.5799
72	5.5828	5.5858	5.5888	5.5918	5.5948	5.5978	5.6008	5.6038	5.6068	5.6098
73	5.6128	5.6158	5.6189	5.6219	5.6250	5.6280	5.6311	5.6341	5.6372	5.6403
74	5.6433	5.6464	5.6495	5.6526	5.6557	5.6588	5.6620	5.6651	5.6682	5.6713
75	5.6745	5.6776	5.6808	5.6840	5.6871	5.6903	5.6935	5.6967	5.6999	5.7031
76	5.7063	5.7095	5.7128	5.7160	5.7192	5.7225	5.7257	5.7290	5.7323	5.7356
77	5.7388	5.7421	5.7454	5.7488	5.7521	5.7554	5.7588	5.7621	5.7655	5.7688
78	5.7722	5.7756	5.7790	5.7824	5.7858	5.7892	5.7926	5.7961	5.7995	5.8030
79	5.8064	5.8099	5.8134	5.8169	5.8204	5.8239	5.8274	5.8310	5.8345	5.8381
80	5.8416	5.8452	5.8488	5.8524	5.8560	5.8596	5.8633	5.8669	5.8705	5.8742
81	5.8779	5.8816	5.8853	5.8890	5.8927	5.8965	5.9002	5.9040	5.9078	5.9116
82	5.9154	5.9192	5.9230	5.9269	5.9307	5.9346	5.9385	5.9424	5.9463	5.9502
83	5.9542	5.9581	5.9621	5.9661	5.9701	5.9741	5.9782	5.9822	5.9863	5.9904
84	5.9945	5.9986	6.0027	6.0069	6.0110	6.0152	6.0194	6.0237	6.0279	6.0322

%	0.0	0.1	0.2	0.3	0.4	0.5	0.6	0.7	0.8	0.9
85	6.0364	6.0407	6.0450	6.0494	6.0537	6.0581	6.0625	6.0669	6.0714	6.0758
86	6.0803	6.0848	6.9893	6.0939	6.0985	6.1031	6.1077	6.1123	6.1170	6.1217
87	6.1264	6.1311	6.1359	6.1407	6.1455	6.1503	6.1552	6.1601	6.1650	6.1700
88	6.1750	6.1800	6.1850	6.1901	6.1952	6.2004	6.2055	6.2107	6.2160	6.2212
89	6.2265	6.2319	6.2372	6.2426	6.2481	6.2536	6.2591	6.2646	6.2702	6.2759
90	6.2816	6.2873	6.2930	6.2988	6.3047	6.3106	6.3165	6.3225	6.3285	6.3346
91	6.3408	6.3469	6.3532	6.3595	6.3658	6.3722	6.3787	6.3852	6.3917	6.3984
92	6.4051	6.4118	6.4187	6.4255	6.4325	6.4395	6.4466	6.4538	6.4611	6.4684
93	6.4758	6.4833	6.4909	6.4985	6.5063	6.5141	6.5220	6.5301	6.5382	6.5464
94	6.5548	6.5632	6.5718	6.5805	6.5893	6.5982	6.6072	6.6164	6.6258	6.6352
95	6.6449	6.6546	6.6646	6.6747	6.6849	6.6954	6.7060	6.7169	6.7279	6.7392
96	6.7507	6.7624	6.7744	6.7866	6.7991	6.8119	6.8250	6.8384	6.8522	6.8663
97	6.8808	6.8957	6.9110	6.9268	6.9431	6.9600	6.9774	6.9954	7.0141	7.0335
98	7.2537	7.0749	7.0969	7.1201	7.1444	7.1701	7.1973	7.2262	7.2571	7.2904
99	7.3263	7.3656	7.4087	7.4571	7.5120	7.5758	7.6520	7.7478	7.8782	8.0902

TABLE C: CHI SQUARE (X^2)*

df	.99	.98	.95	.90	.80	.70	.50	.30	.20	.10	.05	.02	.01	.001
1	.000157	.000628	.00393	.0158	.0642	.148	.455	1.074	1.642	2.706	3.841	5.412	6.635	10.827
2	.0201	.0404	.103	.211	.446	.713	1.386	2.408	3.219	4.605	5.991	7.824	9.210	13.815
3	.115	.185	.352	.584	1.005	1.424	2.366	3.665	4.642	6.251	7.815	9.837	11.345	16.268
4	.297	.429	.711	1.064	1.649	2.195	3.357	4.878	5.989	7.779	9.488	11.668	13.277	18.465
5	.554	.752	1.145	1.610	2.343	3.000	4.351	6.064	7.289	9.236	11.070	13.388	15.086	20.517
6	.872	1.134	1.635	2.204	3.070	3.828	5.348	7.231	8.558	10.645	12.592	15.033	16.812	22.457
7	1.239	1.546	2.167	2.833	3.822	4.671	6.346	8.383	9.803	12.017	14.067	16.622	18.475	24.322
8	1.646	2.032	2.733	3.490	4.594	5.527	7.344	9.524	11.030	13.362	15.507	18.168	20.090	26.125
9	2.088	2.523	3.325	4.168	5.380	6.393	8.343	10.656	12.242	14.684	16.919	19.679	21.666	27.877
10	2.558	3.059	3.940	4.865	6.179	7.267	9.342	11.781	13.422	15.987	18.307	21.161	23.209	29.588
11	3.053	3.609	4.575	5.578	6.989	8.148	10.341	12.899	14.631	17.275	19.675	22.618	24.725	31.264
12	3.571	4.178	5.226	6.304	7.807	9.034	11.310	14.011	15.812	18.549	21.026	24.054	26.217	32.909
13	4.107	4.765	5.892	7.042	8.634	9.926	12.340	15.119	16.985	19.812	22.362	25.472	27.688	34.528
14	4.660	5.368	6.571	7.790	9.467	10.821	13.338	16.222	18.151	21.064	23.685	26.873	29.141	36.123
15	5.229	5.985	7.261	8.547	10.307	11.721	14.339	17.332	19.311	22.307	24.996	28.259	30.578	37.697
16	5.812	6.614	7.962	9.312	11.152	12.624	15.338	18.418	20.465	23.542	26.296	29.633	32.000	39.252
17	6.408	7.255	8.672	10.085	12.002	13.531	16.338	19.511	21.615	24.769	27.587	30.995	33.409	40.790
18	7.015	7.906	9.390	10.865	12.857	14.440	17.338	20.601	22.760	25.989	28.869	32.346	34.805	42.312
19	7.633	8.567	10.117	11.651	13.716	15.352	18.338	21.689	23.900	27.204	30.144	33.687	36.191	43.280
20	8.260	9.237	10.851	12.443	14.578	16.266	19.337	22.775	25.038	28.412	31.410	35.020	37.566	45.315
21	8.897	9.915	11.591	13.240	15.445	17.182	20.337	23.858	26.171	29.615	32.671	36.343	38.932	46.797
22	9.542	10.600	12.338	14.041	16.314	18.101	21.337	24.939	27.301	30.813	33.924	37.659	40.289	48.268
23	10.196	11.293	13.091	14.848	17.187	19.021	22.337	26.018	28.429	32.007	35.172	38.968	41.638	49.728
24	10.856	11.992	13.848	15.659	18.062	19.943	23.337	27.096	29.553	33.196	36.415	40.270	42.980	51.179
25	11.524	12.697	14.611	16.473	18.940	20.867	24.337	28.172	30.675	34.382	37.652	41.566	44.314	52.620

df	.99	.98	.95	.90	.80	.70	.50	.30	.20	.10	.05	.02	.01	.001
26	12.198	13.409	15.379	17.292	19.820	21.792	25.336	29.246	31.795	35.563	38.885	42.856	45.642	54.052
27	12.879	14.125	16.151	18.114	20.703	22.719	26.336	30.319	32.912	36.741	40.113	44.140	46.963	55.476
28	13.565	14.847	16.928	18.939	21.588	23.647	27.336	31.391	34.027	37.916	41.337	45.419	48.278	56.893
29	14.256	15.574	17.708	19.768	22.475	24.577	28.336	32.461	35.139	39.087	42.557	46.693	49.588	58.302
30	14.953	16.306	18.493	20.599	23.364	25.508	29.336	33.530	36.250	40.256	43.773	47.962	50.892	59.703

*One tailed distribution

TABLE D: H VALUES*

SAMPLE SIZES					SAMPLE SIZES				
n_1	n_2	n_3	H (Critical value)	a	n_1	n_2	n_3	H (Critical value)	a
2	1	1	2.7000	0.500				4.7000	0.101
2	2	1	3.6000	0.200	4	4	1	6.6667	0.010
2	2	2	4.5714	0.067				6.1667	0.022
			3.7143	0.200				4.9667	0.048
3	1	1	3.2000	0.300				4.8667	0.054
3	2	1	4.2857	0.100				4.1667	0.082
			3.8571	0.133				4.0667	0.102
3	2	2	5.3572	0.029	4	4	2	7.0364	0.006
			4.7143	0.048				6.8727	0.011
			4.5000	0.067				5.4545	0.046
			4.4643	0.105				5.2364	0.052
3	3	1	5.1429	0.043				4.5545	0.098
			4.5714	0.100				4.4455	0.103
			4.0000	0.129	4	4	3	7.1439	0.010
3	3	2	6.2500	0.011				7.1364	0.011
			5.3611	0.032				5.5985	0.049
			5.1389	0.061				5.5758	0.051
			4.5556	0.100				4.5455	0.099
			4.2500	0.121				4.4773	0.102
3	3	3	7.2000	0.004	4	4	4	7.6538	0.008
			6.4889	0.011				7.5385	0.011
			5.6889	0.029				5.6923	0.049
			5.6000	0.050				5.6538	0.054
			5.0667	0.086				4.6539	0.097
			4.6222	0.100				4.5001	0.104
4	1	1	3.5714	0.200	5	1	1	3.8571	0.143
4	2	1	4.8214	0.057	5	2	1	5.2500	0.036
			4.5000	0.076				5.0000	0.048
			4.0179	0.114				4.4500	0.071
4	2	2	6.0000	0.014				4.2000	0.095
			5.3333	0.033				4.0500	0.119
			5.1250	0.052	5	2	2	6.5333	0.008
			4.4583	0.100				6.1333	0.013
			4.1667	0.105				5.1600	0.034
4	3	1	5.8333	0.021				5.0400	0.056
			5.2083	0.050				4.3733	0.090
			5.0000	0.057				4.2933	0.122
			4.0556	0.093	5	3	1	6.4000	0.012
			3.8889	0.129				4.9600	0.048

TABLE D: (Continued)

n_1	n_2	n_3	H (Critical value)	a	n_1	n_2	n_3	H (Critical value)	a
4	3	2	6.4444	0.008				4.8711	0.052
			6.3000	0.011				4.0178	0.095
			5.4444	0.046				3.8400	0.123
			5.4000	0.051	5	3	2	6.9091	0.009
			4.5111	0.098				6.8218	0.010
			4.4444	0.102				5.2509	0.049
4	3	3	6.7455	0.010				5.1055	0.052
			6.7091	0.013				4.6509	0.091
			5.7909	0.046				4.4945	0.101
			5.7273	0.050	5	3	3	7.0788	0.009
			4.7091	0.092				6.9818	0.011
5	3	3	5.6485	0.049	5	5	1	6.8364	0.011
			5.5152	0.051				5.1273	0.046
			4.5333	0.097				4.9091	0.053
			4.4121	0.109				4.1091	0.086
5	4	1	6.9545	0.008				4.0364	0.105
			6.8400	0.011	5	5	2	7.3385	0.010
			4.9855	0.044				7.2692	0.010
			4.8600	0.056				5.3385	0.047
			3.9873	0.098				5.2462	0.051
			3.9600	0.102				4.6231	0.097
5	4	2	7.2045	0.009				4.5077	0.100
			7.1182	0.010	5	5	3	7.5780	0.010
			5.2727	0.049				7.5429	0.010
			5.2682	0.050				5.7055	0.046
			4.5409	0.098				5.6264	0.051
			4.5182	0.101				4.5451	0.100
5	4	3	7.4449	0.010				4.5363	0.102
			7.3949	0.011	5	5	4	7.8229	0.010
			5.6564	0.049				7.7914	0.010
			5.6308	0.050				5.6657	0.049
			4.5487	0.099				5.6429	0.050
			4.5231	0.103				4.5229	0.099
5	4	4	7.7604	0.009				4.5200	0.101
			7.7440	0.011	5	5	5	8.0000	0.009
			5.6571	0.049				7.9800	0.010
			5.6176	0.050				5.7800	0.049
			4.6187	0.100				5.6600	0.051
			4.5527	0.102				4.5600	0.100
5	5	1	7.3091	0.009				4.5000	0.102

*Test statistics for Kruskall-Wallis nonparametric ANOVA

TABLE E: MANN-WHITNEY U VALUES

n_1	p	$n_2=2$	3	4	5	6	7	8	9	10	11	12	13	14	15	16	17	18	19	20
2	.001																			
	.005												0	0	0	0	0	0	0	0
	.01	0	0	0	0	0	0	0	0	0	0	0	1	1	1	1	1	1	2	2
	0.25	0	0	0	0	0	0	1	1	1	1	2	2	2	2	2	3	3	3	3
	.05	0	0	0	1	1	1	2	2	2	2	3	3	4	4	4	4	5	5	5
	.10	0	1	1	2	2	2	3	3	4	4	5	5	5	6	6	7	7	8	8
3	.001	0	0	0	0	0	0	0	0	0	0	0	0	0	0	0	1	1	1	1
	.005	0	0	0	0	0	0	0	1	1	1	2	2	2	3	3	3	3	4	4
	.01	0	0	0	0	0	1	1	2	2	2	3	3	3	4	4	5	5	5	6
	.025	0	0	0	1	2	2	3	3	4	4	5	5	6	6	7	7	8	8	9
	.05	0	1	1	2	3	3	4	5	5	6	6	7	8	8	9	10	10	11	12
	.10	1	2	2	3	4	5	6	6	7	8	9	10	11	11	12	13	14	15	16
4	.001	0	0	0	0	0	0	0	0	1	1	1	2	2	2	3	3	4	4	4
	.005	0	0	0	0	1	1	2	2	3	3	4	4	5	6	6	7	7	8	9
	.01	0	0	0	1	2	2	3	4	4	5	6	6	7	9	8	9	10	10	11
	.025	0	0	1	2	3	4	5	5	6	7	8	9	10	11	12	12	13	14	15
	.05	0	1	2	3	4	5	6	7	8	9	10	11	12	13	15	16	17	18	19
	.10	1	2	4	5	6	7	8	10	11	12	13	14	16	17	18	19	21	22	23
	.001	0	0	0	0	0	0	1	2	2	3	3	4	4	5	6	6	7	8	8
	.005	0	0	0	1	2	2	3	4	5	6	7	8	8	9	10	11	12	13	14

n_1	p	$n_2=2$	3	4	5	6	7	8	9	10	11	12	13	14	15	16	17	18	19	20
5	.01	0	0	1	2	3	4	5	6	7	8	9	10	11	12	13	14	15	16	17
	.025	0	1	2	3	4	6	7	8	9	10	12	13	14	15	16	18	19	20	21
	.05	1	2	3	5	6	7	9	10	12	13	14	16	17	19	20	21	23	24	26
	.10	2	3	5	6	8	9	11	13	14	16	18	19	21	23	24	26	28	29	31
6	.001	0	0	0	0	0	0	2	3	4	5	5	6	7	8	9	10	11	12	13
	.005	0	0	1	2	3	4	5	6	7	8	10	11	12	13	14	16	17	18	19
	.01	0	0	2	3	4	5	7	8	9	10	12	13	14	16	17	19	20	21	23
	.025	0	2	3	4	6	7	9	11	12	14	15	17	18	20	22	23	25	26	28
	.05	1	3	4	6	8	9	11	13	15	17	18	20	22	24	26	27	29	31	33
	.10	2	4	6	8	10	12	14	16	18	20	22	24	26	28	30	32	35	37	39
7	.001	0	0	0	0	1	2	3	4	6	7	8	9	10	11	12	14	15	16	17
	.005	0	0	1	2	4	5	7	8	10	11	13	14	16	17	19	20	22	23	25
	.01	0	1	2	4	5	7	8	10	12	13	15	17	18	20	22	24	25	27	29
	0.25	0	2	4	6	7	9	11	13	15	17	19	21	23	25	27	29	31	33	35
	.05	1	3	5	7	9	12	14	16	18	20	22	25	27	29	31	34	36	38	40
	.10	2	5	7	9	12	14	17	19	22	24	27	29	32	34	37	39	42	44	47
8	.001	0	0	0	1	2	3	5	6	7	9	10	12	13	15	16	18	19	21	22
	.005	0	0	2	3	5	7	8	10	12	14	16	18	19	21	23	25	27	29	31
	.01	0	1	3	5	7	8	10	12	14	16	18	21	23	25	27	29	31	33	35
	.025	1	3	5	7	9	11	14	16	18	20	23	25	27	30	32	35	37	39	42
	.05	2	4	6	9	11	14	16	19	21	24	27	29	32	34	37	40	42	45	48
	.10	3	6	8	11	14	17	20	23	25	28	31	34	37	40	43	46	49	52	55

TABLE E: (Continued)
U VALUES

n₁	p	$n_2=2$	3	4	5	6	7	8	9	10	11	12	13	14	15	16	17	18	19	20
9	.001	0	0	0	2	3	4	6	8	9	11	13	15	16	18	20	22	24	26	27
	.005	0	1	2	4	6	8	10	12	14	17	19	21	23	25	28	30	32	34	37
	.01	0	2	4	6	8	10	12	15	17	19	22	24	27	29	32	34	37	39	41
	.025	1	3	5	8	11	13	16	18	21	24	27	29	32	35	38	40	43	46	49
	.05	2	5	7	10	13	16	19	22	25	28	31	34	37	40	43	46	49	52	55
	.10	3	6	10	13	16	19	23	26	29	32	36	39	42	46	49	53	56	59	63
17	.001	0	1	3	6	10	14	18	22	26	30	35	39	44	48	53	58	62	67	71
	.005	0	3	7	11	16	20	25	30	35	40	45	50	55	61	66	71	76	82	87
	.01	1	5	9	14	19	24	29	34	39	45	50	56	61	67	72	78	83	89	94
	0.25	3	7	12	18	23	29	35	40	46	52	58	64	70	76	82	88	94	100	106
	.05	4	10	16	21	27	34	40	46	52	58	65	71	78	84	90	97	103	110	116
	.10	7	13	19	26	32	39	46	53	59	66	73	80	86	93	100	114	121	128	128
18	.001	0	1	4	7	11	15	19	24	28	33	38	43	47	52	57	62	67	72	77
	.005	0	3	7	12	17	22	27	32	38	43	48	54	59	65	71	76	82	88	93
	.01	1	5	10	15	20	25	31	37	42	48	54	60	66	71	77	83	89	95	101
	.025	3	8	13	19	25	31	37	43	49	56	62	68	75	81	87	94	100	107	113
	.05	5	10	17	23	29	36	42	49	56	62	69	76	83	89	96	103	110	117	124
	.10	7	14	21	28	35	42	49	56	63	70	78	85	92	99	107	114	121	129	136

n_1	p	$n_2=2$	3	4	5	6	7	8	9	10	11	12	13	14	15	16	17	18	19	20
19	.001	0	1	4	8	12	16	21	26	30	35	41	46	51	56	61	67	72	78	83
	.005	1	4	8	13	18	23	29	34	40	46	52	58	64	70	75	82	88	94	100
	.01	2	5	10	16	21	27	33	39	45	51	57	64	70	76	83	89	95	102	108
	.025	3	8	14	20	26	33	39	46	53	59	66	73	79	86	93	100	107	114	120
	.05	5	11	18	24	31	38	45	52	59	66	73	81	88	95	102	110	117	124	131
	.10	8	15	22	29	37	44	52	59	67	74	82	90	98	105	113	121	129	136	144
20	.001	0	1	4	8	13	17	22	27	33	38	43	49	55	60	66	71	77	83	89
	.005	1	4	9	14	19	25	31	37	43	49	55	61	68	74	80	87	93	100	106
	.01	2	6	11	17	23	29	35	41	48	54	61	68	74	81	88	94	101	108	115
	.025	3	9	15	21	28	35	42	49	56	63	70	77	84	91	99	106	113	120	128
	.05	5	12	19	26	33	40	48	55	63	70	78	85	93	101	108	116	124	131	139
	.10	8	16	23	31	39	47	55	63	71	79	87	95	103	111	120	128	136	144	152

TABLE F: t Test Critical Values*

df	.1	p≤ .05	.01	.001
1	6.314	12.706	63.657	636.619
2	2.920	4.303	9.925	31.598
3	2.353	3.182	5.841	21.941
4	2.132	2.776	4.604	8.610
5	2.015	2.571	4.032	6.859
6	1.943	2.447	3.707	5.959
7	1.895	2.365	3.499	5.405
8	1.860	2.306	3.355	5.041
9	1.833	2.262	3.250	4.781
10	1.812	2.228	3.169	4.587
11	1.796	2.201	3.106	4.437
12	1.782	2.179	3.055	4.318
13	1.771	2.160	3.012	4.221
14	1.761	2.145	2.977	4.140
15	1.753	2.131	2.947	4.073
16	1.746	2.120	2.921	4.015
17	1.740	2.110	2.898	3.965
18	1.734	2.101	2.878	3.922
19	1.729	2.093	2.861	3.883
20	1.725	2.086	2.845	3.850
21	1.721	2.080	2.831	3.819
22	1.717	2.074	2.819	3.792
23	1.714	2.069	2.807	3.767
24	1.711	2.064	2.797	3.745
25	1.708	2.060	2.787	3.725
26	1.706	2.056	2.779	3.707
27	1.703	2.052	2.771	3.690
28	1.701	2.048	2.763	3.674
29	1.699	2.045	2.756	3.659
30	1.697	2.042	2.750	3.646
40	1.684	2.021	2.704	3.551
60	1.671	2.000	2.660	3.460
120	1.658	1.980	2.617	3.373
	1.645	1.960	2.576	3.294

*Two tailed t - distribution values

TABLE G: F Distribution Values*
(1) p < 0.05
Sample size (N) for greater mean square (MS_{bg})

Sample Size (N) for MS_{wg}	1	2	3	4	5	6	7	8	9	10	12	15	20	24	30	40	60	120	∞
1	161.4	199.5	215.7	224.6	230.2	234.0	236.8	238.9	240.5	241.9	243.9	245.9	248.0	249.1	250.1	251.1	252.2	253.3	254.3
2	18.51	19.00	19.16	19.25	19.30	19.33	19.35	19.37	19.38	19.40	19.41	19.43	19.45	19.45	19.46	19.47	19.48	19.49	19.50
3	10.13	9.55	9.28	9.12	9.01	8.94	8.89	8.85	8.81	8.74	8.74	8.70	8.66	8.64	8.62	8.62	8.57	8.55	8.53
4	7.71	6.94	6.59	6.39	6.26	6.16	6.09	6.04	6.00	5.96	5.91	5.86	5.80	5.77	5.75	5.72	5.69	5.66	5.63
5	6.61	5.79	5.41	5.19	5.05	4.95	4.88	4.82	4.77	4.74	4.68	4.62	4.56	4.53	4.50	4.46	4.43	4.40	4.36
6	5.99	5.14	4.76	4.53	4.39	4.28	4.21	4.15	4.10	4.06	4.00	3.94	3.87	3.84	3.81	3.77	3.74	3.70	3.67
7	5.59	4.74	4.35	4.12	3.97	3.87	3.79	3.73	3.68	3.64	3.57	3.51	3.44	3.41	3.38	3.34	3.30	3.27	3.23
8	5.32	4.46	4.07	3.84	3.69	3.58	3.50	3.44	3.39	3.35	3.28	3.22	3.15	3.12	3.08	3.04	3.01	2.97	2.93
9	5.12	4.26	3.86	3.63	3.48	3.37	3.29	3.23	3.18	3.14	3.07	3.01	2.94	2.90	2.86	2.83	2.79	2.75	1.71
10	4.96	4.10	3.71	3.48	3.33	3.22	3.14	3.07	3.02	2.98	2.91	2.85	2.77	2.74	2.70	2.66	2.62	2.58	2.54
11	4.84	3.98	3.59	3.36	3.20	3.09	3.01	2.95	2.90	2.85	2.79	2.72	2.65	2.61	2.57	2.53	2.49	2.45	2.40
12	4.75	3.89	3.49	3.26	3.11	3.00	2.91	2.85	2.80	2.75	2.69	2.62	2.54	2.51	2.47	2.43	2.38	2.34	2.30
13	4.67	3.81	3.41	3.18	3.03	2.92	2.83	2.77	2.71	2.67	2.60	2.53	2.46	2.42	2.38	2.34	2.30	2.25	2.21
14	4.60	3.74	3.34	3.11	2.96	2.85	2.76	2.70	2.65	2.60	2.53	2.46	2.39	2.35	2.31	2.27	2.22	2.18	2.13
15	4.54	3.68	3.29	3.06	2.90	2.79	2.71	2.64	2.59	2.54	2.48	2.40	2.33	2.29	2.25	2.20	2.16	2.11	2.07
16	4.49	3.63	3.24	3.01	2.85	2.74	2.66	2.59	2.54	2.49	2.42	2.35	2.28	2.24	2.19	2.15	2.11	2.06	2.01
17	4.45	3.59	3.20	2.96	2.81	2.70	2.61	2.55	2.49	2.45	2.38	2.31	2.23	2.19	2.13	2.10	2.06	2.01	1.96
18	4.41	3.55	3.16	2.93	2.77	2.66	2.58	2.51	2.46	2.41	2.34	2.27	2.19	2.15	2.11	2.06	2.02	1.97	1.92
19	4.38	3.52	3.13	2.90	2.74	2.63	2.54	2.48	2.42	2.38	2.31	2.23	2.16	2.11	2.07	2.03	1.98	1.93	1.88

For F test, ANOVA, ANCOVA

TABLE G: F Distribution Values*
(1) $p < 0.05$

Sample size $^{(N)}$ for greater mean square (MS_{bg})

Sample Size (N) for MS_{wg}	1	2	3	4	5	6	7	8	9	10	12	15	20	24	30	40	60	120	∞
20	4.35	3.49	3.10	2.87	2.71	2.60	2.51	2.45	2.39	2.35	2.28	2.20	2.12	2.08	2.04	1.99	1.95	1.90	1.84
21	4.32	3.47	3.07	2.84	2.68	2.57	2.49	2.42	2.37	2.32	2.25	2.18	2.10	2.05	2.01	1.96	1.92	1.87	1.81
22	4.30	3.44	3.05	2.82	2.66	2.55	2.46	2.40	2.34	2.30	2.23	2.15	2.07	2.03	1.98	1.94	1.89	1.84	1.78
23	4.28	3.42	3.03	2.80	2.64	2.53	2.44	2.37	2.32	2.27	2.20	2.13	2.05	2.01	1.96	1.91	1.86	1.81	1.76
24	4.26	3.40	3.01	2.78	2.62	2.51	2.42	2.36	2.30	2.25	2.18	2.11	2.03	1.98	1.94	1.89	1.84	1.79	1.73
25	4.24	3.39	2.99	2.76	2.60	2.49	2.40	2.34	2.28	2.24	2.16	2.09	2.01	1.96	1.92	1.87	1.82	1.77	1.71
26	4.23	3.37	2.98	2.74	2.59	2.47	2.39	2.32	2.27	2.22	2.15	2.07	1.99	1.95	1.90	1.85	1.80	1.75	1.69
27	4.21	3.35	2.96	2.73	2.57	2.46	2.37	2.31	2.25	2.20	2.13	2.06	1.97	1.93	1.88	1.84	1.79	1.73	1.67
28	4.20	3.34	2.95	2.71	2.56	2.45	2.36	2.29	2.24	2.19	2.12	2.04	1.96	1.91	1.87	1.82	1.77	1.71	1.65
29	4.18	3.33	2.93	2.70	2.55	2.43	2.35	2.28	2.22	2.18	2.10	2.03	1.94	1.90	1.85	1.81	1.75	1.70	1.64
30	4.17	3.32	2.92	2.69	2.53	2.42	2.33	2.27	2.21	2.16	2.09	2.01	1.93	1.89	1.84	1.79	1.74	1.68	1.62
40	4.08	3.23	2.84	2.61	2.45	2.34	2.25	2.18	2.12	2.08	2.00	1.92	1.84	1.79	1.74	1.69	1.64	1.58	1.51
60	4.00	3.15	2.76	2.53	2.37	2.25	2.17	2.10	2.04	1.99	1.92	1.84	1.75	1.70	1.65	1.59	1.53	1.47	1.39
120	3.92	3.07	2.68	2.45	2.29	2.17	2.09	2.02	1.96	1.91	1.83	1.75	1.66	1.61	1.55	1.50	1.43	1.35	1.25
∞	3.83	3.00	2.60	2.37	2.21	2.10	2.01	1.94	1.88	1.83	1.75	1.67	1.57	1.52	1.46	1.39	1.32	1.22	1.00

For F test, ANOVA, ANCOVA

TABLE G: F Distribution Values
(2) p < 0.001
Sample size (N) for greater mean square (MS$_{bg}$)

Sample Size (N) for MS$_{wg}$	1	2	3	4	5	6	7	8	9	10	12	15	20	24	30	40	60	120	∞
1	4052	4999.50	5403	5625	5764	5859	5928	5982	6022	6056	6106	6157	6209	6235	6261	6287	6313	6339	6366
2	98.50	99.00	99.17	99.25	99.30	99.33	99.36	99.37	99.39	99.40	99.42	99.43	99.45	99.46	99.47	99.47	99.48	99.49	99.50
3	34.12	30.82	29.46	28.71	28.24	27.91	27.67	27.49	27.35	27.23	27.05	26.87	26.69	26.60	26.50	26.41	26.32	26.22	26.13
4	21.20	18.00	16.69	15.98	15.52	15.21	14.98	14.80	14.66	14.55	14.37	14.20	14.02	13.93	13.84	13.75	13.65	13.56	13.46
5	16.26	13.27	12.06	11.39	10.97	10.67	10.46	10.29	10.16	10.05	9.89	9.72	9.55	9.47	9.38	9.29	9.20	9.11	9.02
6	13.75	10.92	9.78	9.15	8.75	8.47	8.26	8.10	7.98	7.87	7.72	7.56	7.40	7.31	7.23	7.14	7.06	6.97	6.88
7	12.25	9.55	8.45	7.85	7.46	7.19	6.99	6.84	6.72	6.62	6.47	6.31	6.16	6.07	5.99	5.91	5.82	5.74	5.65
8	11.26	8.65	7.59	7.01	6.63	6.37	6.18	6.03	5.91	5.81	5.67	5.52	5.36	5.28	5.20	5.12	5.03	4.95	4.86
9	10.56	8.02	6.99	6.42	6.06	5.80	5.61	5.47	5.35	5.26	5.11	4.96	4.81	4.73	4.65	4.57	4.48	4.40	4.31
10	10.04	7.56	6.55	5.99	5.64	5.39	5.20	5.06	4.94	4.85	4.71	4.56	4.41	4.33	4.25	4.17	4.08	4.00	3.91
11	9.65	7.21	6.22	5.67	5.32	5.07	4.89	4.74	4.63	4.54	4.40	4.25	4.10	4.02	3.94	3.86	3.78	3.69	3.60
12	9.33	6.93	5.95	5.41	5.06	4.82	4.64	4.50	4.39	4.30	4.16	4.01	3.86	3.78	3.70	3.62	3.54	3.45	3.36
13	9.07	6.70	5.74	5.21	4.86	4.62	4.44	4.30	4.19	4.10	3.96	3.82	3.66	3.59	3.51	3.43	3.34	3.25	3.17
14	8.86	6.51	5.56	5.04	4.69	4.46	4.28	4.14	4.03	3.94	3.80	3.66	3.51	3.43	3.35	3.27	3.18	3.09	3.00
15	8.68	6.36	5.42	4.89	4.56	4.32	4.14	4.00	3.89	3.80	3.67	3.52	3.37	3.29	3.21	3.13	3.05	2.96	2.87
16	8.53	6.23	5.29	4.77	4.44	4.20	4.03	3.89	3.78	3.69	3.55	3.41	3.26	3.18	3.10	3.02	2.93	2.84	2.75
17	8.40	6.11	5.18	4.67	4.34	4.10	3.93	3.79	3.68	3.59	3.46	3.31	3.16	3.08	3.00	2.92	2.83	2.75	2.65
18	8.29	6.01	5.09	4.58	4.25	4.01	3.84	3.71	3.60	3.51	3.37	3.23	3.08	3.00	2.92	2.84	2.75	2.66	2.57
19	8.18	5.93	5.01	4.50	4.17	3.94	3.77	3.63	3.52	3.43	3.30	3.15	3.00	2.92	2.84	2.76	2.67	2.58	2.49
20	8.10	5.85	4.94	4.43	4.10	3.87	3.70	3.56	3.46	3.37	3.23	3.09	2.94	2.86	2.78	2.69	2.61	2.52	2.42
21	8.02	5.78	4.87	4.37	4.04	3.81	3.64	3.51	3.40	3.31	3.17	3.03	2.88	2.80	2.72	2.64	2.55	2.46	2.36
22	7.95	5.72	4.82	4.31	3.99	3.76	3.59	3.45	3.35	3.26	3.12	2.98	2.83	2.75	2.67	2.58	2.50	2.40	2.31
23	7.88	5.66	4.76	4.26	3.94	3.71	3.54	3.41	3.30	3.21	3.07	2.93	2.78	2.70	2.62	2.54	2.45	2.35	2.26
24	7.82	5.61	4.72	4.22	3.90	3.67	3.50	3.36	3.26	3.17	3.03	2.89	2.74	2.66	2.58	2.49	2.40	2.31	2.21

TABLE G: F Distribution Values*
(2) $p < 0.01$ (continued)

Sample size (N) for greater mean square (MS_{bg})

Sample Size (N) for MS_{wg}	1	2	3	4	5	6	7	8	9	10	12	15	20	24	30	40	60	120	∞
25	7.77	5.57	4.68	4.18	3.85	3.63	3.46	3.32	3.22	3.13	2.99	2.85	2.70	2.62	2.54	2.45	2.36	2.27	2.17
26	7.72	5.53	4.64	4.14	3.82	3.59	3.42	3.29	3.18	3.09	2.96	2.81	2.66	2.58	2.50	2.42	2.33	2.23	2.13
27	7.68	5.49	4.60	4.11	3.78	3.56	3.39	3.26	3.15	3.06	2.93	2.78	2.63	2.55	2.47	2.38	2.29	2.20	2.10
28	7.64	5.45	4.57	4.07	3.75	3.53	3.36	3.23	3.12	3.03	2.90	2.75	2.60	2.52	2.44	2.35	2.26	2.17	2.06
29	7.60	5.42	4.54	4.04	3.73	3.50	3.33	3.20	3.09	3.00	2.87	2.73	2.57	2.49	2.41	2.33	2.23	2.14	2.03
30	7.56	5.39	4.51	4.02	3.70	3.47	3.30	3.17	3.07	2.98	2.84	2.70	2.55	2.47	2.39	2.30	2.21	2.11	2.01
40	7.31	5.18	4.31	3.83	3.51	3.29	3.12	2.99	2.89	2.80	2.66	2.52	2.37	2.29	2.20	2.11	2.02	1.92	1.80
60	7.08	4.98	4.13	3.65	3.34	3.12	2.95	2.82	2.72	2.63	2.50	2.35	2.20	2.12	2.03	1.94	1.84	1.73	1.60
120	6.85	4.79	3.95	3.48	3.17	2.96	2.79	2.66	2.56	2.47	2.34	2.19	2.03	1.95	1.86	1.76	1.66	1.53	1.38
∞	6.63	4.61	3.78	3.32	3.02	2.80	2.64	2.51	2.41	2.32	2.18	2.04	1.88	1.79	1.70	1.59	1.47	1.32	1.00

TABLE G: F Distribution Values
(3) $p < 0.001$

Sample size $^{(N)}$ for greater mean square (MS_{bg})

	1	2	3	4	5	6	7	8	9	10	12	15	20	24	30	40	60	120	∞
1	4053*	5000*	5404*	5625*	5764*	5859*	5929*	5981*	6023*	6056*	6107*	6158*	6209*	6235*	6261*	6287*	6313*	6340*	6366*
2	998.5	999.0	999.2	999.2	999.3	999.3	999.4	999.4	999.4	999.4	999.4	999.4	999.4	999.5	999.5	999.5	999.5	999.5	999.5
3	167.0	148.5	141.1	137.1	134.6	132.8	131.6	130.6	129.9	129.2	128.3	127.4	126.4	125.9	125.4	125.0	124.5	124.0	123.5
4	74.14	61.25	56.18	53.44	51.71	50.53	49.66	49.00	48.47	48.05	47.41	46.76	46.10	45.77	45.43	45.09	44.75	44.40	44.05
5	47.18	37.12	33.20	31.09	29.75	28.84	28.16	27.64	27.24	26.92	26.42	25.91	25.39	25.14	24.87	24.60	24.33	24.06	23.79
6	35.51	27.00	23.70	21.92	20.81	20.03	19.46	19.03	18.69	18.41	17.99	17.56	17.12	16.89	16.67	16.44	16.21	15.99	15.75
7	29.25	21.69	18.77	17.19	16.21	15.52	15.02	14.63	14.33	14.08	13.71	13.32	12.93	12.73	12.53	12.33	12.12	11.91	11.70
8	25.42	18.49	15.83	14.39	13.49	12.86	12.40	12.04	11.77	11.54	11.19	10.84	10.48	10.30	10.11	9.92	9.73	9.53	9.33
9	22.86	16.39	13.90	12.56	11.71	11.13	10.70	10.37	10.11	9.89	9.57	9.24	8.90	8.72	8.55	8.37	8.19	8.00	7.81
10	21.04	14.91	12.55	11.28	10.48	9.92	9.52	9.20	8.96	8.75	8.45	8.13	7.80	7.64	7.47	7.30	7.12	6.94	6.76
11	19.69	13.81	11.56	10.35	9.58	9.05	8.66	8.35	8.12	7.92	7.63	7.32	7.01	6.85	6.68	6.52	6.35	6.17	6.00
12	18.64	12.97	10.80	9.63	8.89	8.38	8.00	7.71	7.48	7.29	7.00	6.71	6.40	6.25	6.09	5.93	5.76	5.59	5.42
13	17.81	12.31	10.21	9.07	8.35	7.86	7.49	7.21	6.98	6.80	6.52	6.23	5.93	5.78	5.63	5.47	5.30	5.14	4.97
14	17.14	11.78	9.73	8.62	7.92	7.43	7.08	6.80	6.58	6.40	6.13	5.85	5.56	5.41	5.25	5.10	4.94	4.77	4.60
15	16.59	11.34	9.34	8.25	7.57	7.09	6.74	6.47	6.26	6.08	5.81	5.54	5.25	5.10	4.95	4.80	4.64	4.47	4.31
16	16.12	10.97	9.00	7.94	7.27	6.81	6.46	6.19	5.98	5.81	5.55	5.27	4.99	4.85	4.70	4.54	4.39	4.23	4.06
17	15.72	10.66	8.73	7.68	7.02	6.56	6.22	5.96	5.75	5.58	5.32	5.05	4.78	4.63	4.48	4.33	4.18	4.02	3.85
18	15.38	10.39	8.49	7.46	6.81	6.35	6.02	5.76	5.56	5.39	5.13	4.87	4.59	4.45	4.30	4.15	4.00	3.84	3.67
19	15.08	10.16	8.28	7.26	6.62	6.18	5.85	5.59	5.39	5.22	4.97	4.70	4.43	4.29	4.14	3.99	3.84	3.68	3.51
20	14.82	9.95	8.10	7.10	6.46	6.02	5.69	5.44	5.24	5.08	4.82	4.56	4.29	4.15	4.00	3.86	3.70	3.54	3.38
21	14.59	9.77	7.94	6.95	6.32	5.88	5.56	5.31	5.11	4.95	4.70	4.44	4.17	4.03	3.88	3.74	3.58	3.42	3.26
22	14.38	9.61	7.80	6.81	6.19	5.76	5.44	5.19	4.99	4.83	4.58	4.33	4.06	3.92	3.78	3.63	3.48	3.32	3.05
23	14.19	9.47	7.67	6.69	6.08	5.65	5.35	5.09	4.89	4.73	4.48	4.23	3.96	3.82	3.68	3.53	3.38	3.22	3.05
24	14.03	9.34	7.55	6.59	5.98	5.55	5.23	4.99	4.80	4.64	4.39	4.14	3.87	3.74	3.59	3.45	3.29	3.14	2.97

TABLE G: F Distribution Values*
(3) p < 0.001 (continued)

Sample size (N) for greater mean square (MS_{bg})

Sample Size (N) for MS_{wg}

	1	2	3	4	5	6	7	8	9	10	12	15	20	24	30	40	60	120	∞
25	13.88	9.22	7.45	6.49	5.88	5.46	5.15	4.91	4.71	4.56	4.31	4.06	3.79	3.66	3.52	3.37	3.22	3.06	2.89
26	13.74	9.12	7.36	6.41	5.80	5.38	5.07	4.83	4.64	4.48	4.24	3.99	3.72	3.59	3.44	3.30	3.15	2.99	2.82
27	13.61	9.02	7.27	6.33	5.73	5.31	5.00	4.76	4.57	4.41	4.17	3.92	3.66	3.52	3.38	3.23	3.08	2.92	2.75
28	13.50	8.93	7.19	6.25	5.66	5.24	4.93	4.69	4.50	4.35	4.11	3.86	3.60	3.46	3.32	3.18	3.02	2.86	2.69
29	13.39	8.85	7.12	619	5.59	5.18	4.87	4.64	4.45	4.29	4.05	3.80	3.54	3.41	3.27	3.12	2.97	2.81	2.64
30	13.29	8.77	7.05	6.12	5.53	5.12	4.82	4.58	4.39	4.24	4.00	3.75	3.49	3.36	3.22	3.07	2.92	2.76	2.59
40	12.61	8.25	6.60	5.70	5.13	4.73	4.44	4.21	4.02	3.87	3.64	3.40	3.15	3.01	2.87	2.73	2.57	2.41	2.23
60	11.97	7.76	6.17	5.31	4.76	4.37	4.09	3.87	3.69	3.54	3.31	3.08	2.83	2.69	2.55	2.41	2.25	2.08	1.89
120	11.38	7.32	5.79	4.95	4.42	4.04	3.77	3.55	3.38	3.24	3.02	2.78	2.53	2.40	2.26	2.11	1.95	1.76	1.54
∞	10.83	6.91	5.42	4.62	4.10	3.74	3.47	3.27	3.10	2.96	2.74	2.51	2.27	2.13	1.99	1.84	1.66	1.45	1.00

TABLE H: Z SCORES FOR NORMAL DISTRIBUTION

z	PROPORTIONAL PARTS									
	0.00	0.01	0.02	0.03	0.04	0.05	0.06	0.07	0.08	0.09
0.0	0.5000	0.4960	0.4920	0.4880	0.4840	0.4801	0.4761	0.4721	0.4681	0.4641
0.1	0.4602	0.4562	0.4522	0.4483	0.4443	0.4404	0.4364	0.4325	0.4286	0.4247
0.2	0.4207	0.4168	0.4129	0.4090	0.4052	0.4013	0.3974	0.3936	0.3897	0.3859
0.3	0.3821	0.3783	0.3745	0.3707	0.3669	0.3632	0.3594	0.3557	0.3520	0.3483
0.4	0.3446	0.3409	0.3372	0.3336	0.3300	0.3264	0.3228	0.3192	0.3156	0.3121
0.5	0.3085	0.3050	0.3015	0.2981	0.2946	0.2912	0.2877	0.2843	0.2810	0.2776
0.6	0.2743	0.2709	0.2676	0.2643	0.2611	0.2578	0.2546	0.2514	0.2483	0.2451
0.7	0.2420	0.2389	0.2358	0.2327	0.2296	0.2266	0.2236	0.2206	0.2177	0.2148
0.8	0.2119	0.2090	0.2061	0.2033	0.2005	0.1977	0.1949	0.1922	0.1894	0.1867
0.9	0.1841	0.1814	0.1788	0.1762	0.1736	0.1711	0.1685	0.1660	0.1635	0.1611
1.0	0.1587	0.1562	0.1539	0.1515	0.1492	0.1469	0.1446	0.1423	0.1401	0.1379
1.1	0.1357	0.1335	0.1314	0.1292	0.1271	0.1251	0.1230	0.1210	0.1190	0.1170
1.2	0.1151	0.1131	0.1112	0.1093	0.1075	0.1056	0.1038	0.1020	0.1003	0.0985
1.3	0.0968	0.0951	0.0934	0.0918	0.0901	0.0885	0.0869	0.0853	0.0838	0.0823
1.4	0.0808	0.0793	0.0778	0.0764	0.0749	0.0735	0.0721	0.0708	0.0694	0.0681
1.5	0.0668	0.0655	0.0643	0.0630	0.0618	0.0606	0.0594	0.0582	0.0571	0.0559
1.6	0.0548	0.0537	0.0526	0.0516	0.0505	0.0495	0.0485	0.0475	0.0465	0.0455
1.7	0.0446	0.0436	0.0427	0.418	0.409	0.0401	0.0392	0.0384	0.0375	0.0367
1.8	0.0359	0.0351	0.0344	0.0336	0.0329	0.0322	0.0314	0.0307	0.0301	0.0294
1.9	0.0287	0.0281	0.0274	0.0268	0.0262	0.0256	0.0250	0.0244	0.0239	0.0233

TABLE H: Z SCORES FOR NORMAL DISTRIBUTION (continued)

z	0.00	0.01	0.02	0.03	0.04	0.05	0.06	0.07	0.08	0.09
2.0	0.0228	0.0222	0.0217	0.0212	0.0207	0.0202	0.0197	0.0192	0.0188	0.0183
2.1	0.0179	0.0174	0.0170	0.0166	0.0162	0.0158	0.0154	0.0150	0.0146	0.0143
2.2	0.0139	0.0136	0.0132	0.0129	0.0125	0.0122	0.0119	0.0116	0.0113	0.0110
2.3	0.0107	0.0104	0.0102	0.0099	0.0096	0.0094	0.0091	0.0089	0.0087	0.0084
2.4	0.0082	0.0080	0.0078	0.0075	0.0073	0.0071	0.0069	0.0068	0.0066	0.0064
2.5	0.0062	0.0060	0.0059	0.0057	0.0055	0.0054	0.0052	0.0051	0.0049	0.0048
2.6	0.0047	0.0045	0.0044	0.0043	0.0041	0.0040	0.0039	0.0038	0.0037	0.0036
2.7	0.0035	0.0034	0.0033	0.0032	0.0031	0.0030	0.0029	0.0028	0.0027	0.0026
2.8	0.0026	0.0025	0.0024	0.0023	0.0023	0.0022	0.0021	0.0021	0.0020	0.0019
2.9	0.0019	0.0018	0.0018	0.0017	0.0016	0.0016	0.0015	0.0015	0.0014	0.0014
3.0	0.0013	0.0013	0.0013	0.0012	0.0012	0.0011	0.0011	0.0011	0.0010	0.0010
3.1	0.0010	0.0009	0.0009	0.0009	0.0008	0.0008	0.0008	0.0008	0.0007	0.0007
3.2	0.0007	0.0007	0.0006	0.0006	0.0006	0.0006	0.0006	0.0005	0.0005	0.0005
3.3	0.0005	0.0005	0.0005	0.0004	0.0004	0.0004	0.0004	0.0004	0.0004	0.0004
3.4	0.0003	0.0003	0.0003	0.0003	0.0003	0.0003	0.0003	0.0003	0.0003	0.0002
3.5	0.0002	0.0002	0.0002	0.0002	0.0002	0.0002	0.0002	0.0002	0.0002	0.0002
3.6	0.0002	0.0002	0.0001	0.0001	0.0001	0.0001	0.0001	0.0001	0.0001	0.0001
3.7	0.0001	0.0001	0.0001	0.0001	0.0001	0.0001	0.0001	0.0001	0.0001	0.0001
3.8	0.0001	0.0001	0.0001	0.0001	0.0001	0.0001	0.0001	0.0001	0.0001	0.0001
3.9	0.0000	0.0000	0.0000	0.0000	0.0000	0.0000	0.0000	0.0000	0.0000	0.0000

PROPORTIONAL PARTS

TABLE I
TABLE FOR CALCULATION OF MEDIAN-EFFECTIVE DOSE BY MOVING AVERAGE

	n = 2, K = 3			n = 4, K = 3			n = 5, K = 3	
r-values	f	σf	r-values	f	σf	r-values	f	σf
0,0,1,2	1.00000	0.50000	2,0,3,4	0.50000	0.57735	0,1,2,5	0.90000	0.31623
0,0,2,2	0.50000	0.00000	2,0,4,4	0.00000	0.57735	0,1,3,5	0.7000	0.31623
0,1,1,2	0.50000	0.70711	2,1,1,4	1.00000	0.70711	0,1,4,5	0.50000	0.28284
0,1,2,2	0.00000	0.50000	2,1,2,4	0.50000	0.81650	0,1,5,5	0.30000	0.20000
1,0,1,2	1.00000	1.00000	2,1,3,4	0.00000	0.91287	0,2,2,5	0.70000	0.34641
1,0,2,2	0.00000	1.00000	2,2,2,4	0.00000	1.00000	0,2,3,5	0.50000	0.34641
1,1,1,2	0.00000	1.73205	3,0,2,4	1.00000	1.15470	0,2,4,5	0.30000	0.31623
0,0,2,1	1.00000	1.00000	3,0,3,4	0.00000	1.41421	0,2,5,5	0.10000	0.24495
0,1,1	1.00000	1.73205	3,1,1,4	1.00000	1.41421	0,3,3,5	0.30000	0.34641
0,1,2,1	0.00000	1.00000	3,1,2,4	0.00000	1.82574	0,3,4,5	0.10000	0.31623
			0,0,3,3	1.00000	0.47140	1,0,3,5	0.87500	0.30778
	n = 3, K = 3		0,0,4,3	0.66667	0.22222	1,0,4,5	0.62500	0.26700
			0,1,2,3	1.00000	0.60858	1,0,5,5	0.37500	0.15625
0,0,2,3	0.83333	0.33333	0,1,3,3	0.66667	0.52116	1,1,2,5	0.87500	0.39652
0,0,3,3	0.50000	0.00000	0,1,4,3	0.33333	0.35136	1,1,3,5	0.62500	0.40625
0,1,1,3	0.83333	0.47140	0,2,2,3	0.66667	0.58794	1,1,4,5	0.37500	0.38654
0,1,2,3	0.50000	0.47140	0,2,3,3	0.33333	0.52116	1,1,5,5	0.12500	0.33219

TABLE I (continued)
TABLE FOR CALCULATION OF MEDIAN-EFFECTIVE DOSE BY MOVING AVERAGE

n = 2, K = 3

r-values	f
0,1,3,3	0.33333
0,2,2,3	0.47140
1,0,2,3	0.51539
1,0,3,3	0.37500
1,1,1,3	0.71807
1,1,2,3	0.25000
1,1,3,3	0.80039
2,0,2,3	1.11803
0,0,3,2	0.37500
0,1,2,2	0.80039
0,1,3,2	0.51539
0,2,2,2	0.71807
0,1,3,1	1.11803

n = 4, K = 3

r-values	f	f
0,2,4,3	0.00000	0.38490
0,3,3,3	0.00000	0.47140
1,0,3,3	1.00000	0.70711
1,0,4,3	0.50000	0.35355
1,1,2,3	1.00000	0.91287
1,1,3,3	0.50000	0.79057
1,1,4,3	0.00000	0.70711
1,2,2,3	0.50000	0.88976
1,2,3,3	0.00000	0.91287
2,0,3,3	1.00000	1.41421
2,0,4,3	0.00000	1.15470
2,1,2,3	1.00000	1.82574
2,1,3,3	0.00000	1.82574
2,2,2,3	0.00000	2.00000
0,0,4,2	1.00000	0.57735
0,1,3,2	1.00000	0.91287
0,1,4,2	0.50000	0.57735
0,2,2,2	1.00000	1.00000
0,0,2,4	1.00000	0.28868
0,0,3,4	0.75000	0.25000
0,0,4,4	0.50000	0.00000

n = 5, K = 3

r-values	f	f
1,2,2,5	0.62500	0.44304
1,2,3,5	0.37500	0.46034
1,2,4,5	0.12500	0.45178
1,3,3,5	0.12500	0.48513
2,0,3,5	0.83333	0.41388
2,0,4,5	0.50000	0.39087
2,0,5,5	0.16667	0.34021
2,1,2,5	0.83333	0.53142
2,1,3,5	0.50000	0.56519
2,1,4,5	0.16667	0.58134
2,2,2,5	0.50000	0.61237
2,2,3,5	0.16667	0.67013
0,0,4,4	0.87500	0.33219
0,0,5,4	0.62500	0.15625
0,1,3,4	0.87500	0.45178
0,1,4,4	0.62500	0.38654
0,1,5,4	0.37500	0.26700
0,2,2,4	0.87500	0.48513

n = 2, K = 3

r-values	f	σf
0,1,1,4	1.00000	0.35355
0,1,2,4	0.75000	0.38188
0,1,3,4	0.50000	0.35355
0,1,4,4	0.25000	0.25000
0,2,2,4	0.50000	0.40825
0,2,3,4	0.25000	0.38188
0,2,4,4	0.00000	0.28868
0,3,3,4	0.00000	0.35355
1,0,2,4	1.00000	0.38490
1,0,3,4	0.66667	0.35136
1,0,4,4	0.33333	0.22222
1,1,1,4	1.00000	0.47140
1,1,2,4	0.66667	0.52116
1,1,3,4	0.33333	0.52116
1,1,4,4	0.00000	0.47140
1,2,2,4	0.33333	0.58794
1,2,3,4	0.00000	0.60858
2,0,2,4	1.00000	0.57735

n = 4, K = 3

r-values	f	σf
0,2,3,2	0.50000	0.81650
0,2,4,2	0.00000	0.57735
0,3,3,2	0.00000	0.70711
1,0,4,2	1.00000	1.15470
1,1,3,2	1.00000	1.82574
1,1,4,2	0.00000	1.41421
1,2,2,2	1.00000	2.00000
1,2,3,2	0.00000	1.82574
0,2,3,1	1.00000	1.82574
0,2,4,1	0.00000	1.15470
0,3,3,1	0.00000	1.41421
0,1,4,1	1.00000	1.41421

n = 5, K = 3

r-values	f	σf
0,0,3,5	0.90000	0.24495
0,0,4,5	0.70000	0.20000
0,0,5,5	0.50000	0.00000

n = 5, K = 3

r-values	f	σf
0,2,3,4	0.62500	0.46034
0,2,4,4	0.37500	0.40625
0,2,5,4	0.12500	0.30778
0,3,3,4	0.37500	0.44304
0,3,4,4	0.12500	0.39652
1,0,4,4	0.83333	0.43744
1,0,5,4	0.50000	0.23570
1,1,3,4	0.83333	0.59835
1,1,4,4	0.50000	0.52705
1,1,5,4	0.16667	0.43744
1,2,2,4	0.83333	0.64310
1,2,3,4	0.50000	0.62361
1,2,4,4	0.16667	0.59835
1,3,3,4	0.16667	0.64310
2,0,4,4	0.75000	0.64348
2,0,5,4	0.25000	0.47598
2,1,3,4	0.75000	0.88829
2,1,4,4	0.25000	0.85239

*Portion reprinted from *Biometrics* with permission of Trustees

TABLE I (Continued)
TABLE FOR CALCULATION OF MEDIAN-EFFECTIVE DOSE BY MOVING AVERAGE

n = 5, K = 3

r-values	f
2,2,2,4	0.75000
2,2,3,4	0.25000
0,0,5,3	0.83333
0,1,4,3	0.83333
0,1,5,3	0.50000
0,2,3,3	0.83333
0,2,4,3	0.50000
0,2,5,3	0.16667
0,3,3,3	0.50000
0,3,4,3	0.16667
1,0,5,3	0.75000
1,1,4,3	0.75000
1,1,5,3	0.25000
1,2,3,3	0.75000
1,2,4,3	0.25000
1,3,3,3	0.25000

n = 6, K = 3

r-values	f	f
0,0,3,6	1.00000	0.22361

n = 6, K = 3

r-values	f	f
1,4,4,6	0.00000	0.36878
2,0,3,6	1.00000	0.33541
2,0,4,6	0.75000	0.32596
2,0,5,6	0.50000	0.29580
2,0,6,6	0.25000	0.23717
2,1,2,6	1.00000	0.40311
2,1,3,6	0.75000	0.42573
2,1,4,6	0.50000	0.43301
2,1,5,6	0.25000	0.42573
2,1,6,6	0.00000	0.29580
2,2,2,6	0.75000	0.45415
2,2,3,6	0.50000	0.48734
2,2,4,6	0.25000	0.50621
2,2,5,6	0.00000	0.43301
2,3,3,6	0.25000	0.53033
2,3,4,6	0.00000	0.48734
3,0,3,6	1.00000	0.44721
3,0,4,6	0.66667	0.43885
3,0,5,6	0.33333	0.44721
3,0,6,6	0.00000	0.44721

n = 6, K = 3

r-values	f	f
0,3,6,5	0.00000	0.26833
0,4,4,5	0.20000	0.36000
0,4,5,5	0.00000	0.32249
1,0,4,5	1.00000	0.40311
1,0,5,5	0.75000	0.31869
1,0,6,5	0.50000	0.17678
1,1,3,5	1.00000	0.48734
1,1,4,5	0.75000	0.44896
1,1,5,5	0.50000	0.39528
1,1,6,5	0.25000	0.31869
1,2,2,5	1.00000	0.51235
1,2,3,5	0.75000	0.50156
1,2,4,5	0.50000	0.48088
1,2,5,5	0.25000	0.44896
1,2,6,5	0.00000	0.40311
1,3,3,5	0.50000	0.50621
1,3,4,5	0.25000	0.50156
1,3,5,5	0.00000	0.48734
1,4,4,5	0.00000	0.51235
2,0,4,5	1.00000	0.53748

r-values	n = 6, K = 3 f	σf	r-values	f	σf	r-values	n = 6, K = 3 f	σf
0,0,4,6	0.83333	0.21082	3,1,2,6	1.00000	0.53748	2,0,5,5	0.66667	0.42455
0,0,5,6	0.66667	0.16667	3,1,3,6	0.66667	0.57090	2,0,6,5	0.33333	0.30225
0,0,6,6	0.50000	0.00000	3,1,4,6	0.33333	0.61464	2,1,3,5	1.00000	0.64979
0,1,2,6	1.00000	0.26874	3,1,5,6	0.00000	0.64979	2,1,4,5	0.66667	0.59835
0,1,3,6	0.83333	0.27889	3,2,2,6	0.66667	0.60858	2,1,5,5	0.33333	0.55998
0,1,4,6	0.66667	0.26874	3,2,3,6	0.33333	0.68313	2,1,6,5	0.00000	0.53748
0,1,5,6	0.50000	0.23570	3,2,4,6	0.00000	0.74536	2,2,2,5	1.00000	0.68313
0,1,6,6	0.33333	0.16667	3,3,3,6	0.00000	0.77460	2,2,3,5	0.66667	0.66852
0,2,2,6	0.83333	0.29814	4,0,3,6	1.00000	0.67082	2,2,4,5	0.33333	0.66852
0,2,3,6	0.66667	0.30732	4,0,4,6	0.50000	0.70711	2,2,5,5	0.00000	0.68313
0,2,4,6	0.50000	0.29814	4,0,5,6	0.00000	0.80622	2,3,3,5	0.33333	0.70097
0,2,5,6	0.33333	0.26874	4,1,2,6	1.00000	0.80622	2,3,4,5	0.00000	0.74536
0,2,6,6	0.16667	0.21082	4,1,3,6	0.50000	0.89443	3,0,4,5	1.00000	0.80622
0,3,3,6	0.50000	0.31623	4,1,4,6	0.00000	1.02470	3,0,5,5	0.50000	0.65192
0,3,4,6	0.33333	0.30732	4,2,2,6	0.50000	0.94888	3,0,6,5	0.00000	0.67082
0,3,5,6	0.16667	0.27889	4,2,3,6	0.00000	1.11803	3,1,3,5	1.00000	0.92195
0,3,6,6	0.00000	0.22361	5,0,3,6	1.00000	1.34164	3,1,4,5	0.50000	0.90830
0,4,4,6	0.16667	0.29814	5,0,4,6	0.00000	1.61245	3,1,5,5	0.00000	0.92195
0,4,5,6	0.00000	0.26874	5,1,2,6	1.00000	1.61245	3,2,2,5	1.00000	1.02470
1,0,3,6	1.00000	0.26833	5,1,3,6	0.00000	1.94936	3,2,3,5	0.50000	1.01242
1,0,4,6	0.80000	0.25612	5,2,2,6	0.00000	2.04939	3,2,4,5	0.00000	1.11803
1,0,5,6	0.60000	0.21541	0,0,4,5	1.00000	0.26833	3,3,3,5	0.00000	1.16190
1,0,6,6	0.40000	0.12000	0,0,5,5	0.80000	0.25612	4,0,4,5	1.00000	1.61245
1,1,2,6	1.00000	0.32249	0,0,6,5	0.60000	0.12000	4,0,5,5	0.00000	1.61245

TABLE I (Continued)

TABLE FOR CALCULATION OF MEDIAN-EFFECTIVE DOSE BY MOVING AVERAGE

r-values	n = 6, K = 3 f	σf	r-values	n = 6, K = 3 f	σf	r-values	n = 6, K = 3 f	σf
1,1,3,6	0.80000	0.33704	0,1,3,5	1.00000	0.34641	4,1,3,5	1.00000	1.94936
1,1,4,6	0.60000	0.33226	0,1,4,5	0.80000	0.36000	4,1,4,5	0.00000	2.04939
1,1,5,6	0.40000	0.30724	0,1,5,5	0.60000	0.30724	4,2,2,5	1.00000	2.04939
1,1,6,6	0.20000	0.25612	0,1,6,5	0.40000	0.21541	4,2,3,5	0.00000	2.23607
1,2,2,6	0.80000	0.36000	0,2,2,5	1.00000	0.36878	0,0,5,4	1.00000	0.29580
1,2,3,6	0.60000	0.37736	0,2,3,5	0.80000	0.40200	0,0,6,4	0.75000	0.23717
1,2,4,6	0.40000	0.37736	0,2,4,5	0.60000	0.37736	0,1,4,4	1.00000	0.43301
1,2,5,6	0.20000	0.36000	0,2,5,5	0.40000	0.33226	0,1,5,4	0.75000	0.42573
1,2,6,6	0.00000	0.26833	0,2,6,5	0.20000	0.25612	0,1,6,4	0.50000	0.29580
1,3,3,6	0.40000	0.39799	0,3,3,5	0.60000	0.39799	0,2,3,4	1.00000	0.48734
1,3,4,6	0.20000	0.40200	0,3,4,5	0.40000	0.37736	0,2,4,4	0.75000	0.50621
1,3,5,6	0.00000	0.34641	0,3,5,5	0.20000	0.33704	0,2,5,4	0.50000	0.43301
0,2,6,4	0.25000	0.32596	2,3,4,4	0.00000	1.11803	1,3,5,3	0.00000	0.92195
0,3,3,4	0.75000	0.53033	3,0,5,4	1.00000	1.67332	1,4,4,3	0.00000	1.02470
0,3,4,4	0.50000	0.48734	3,0,6,4	0.00000	1.34164	2,0,6,3	1.00000	1.34164
0,3,5,4	0.25000	0.42573	3,1,4,4	1.00000	2.09762	2,1,5,3	1.00000	1.94936
0,3,6,4	0.00000	0.33541	3,1,5,4	0.00000	1.94936	2,1,6,3	0.00000	1.67332
0,4,4,4	0.25000	0.45415	3,2,3,4	1.00000	2.28035	2,2,4,3	1.00000	2.23607
0,4,5,4	0.00000	0.40311	3,2,4,4	0.00000	2.23607	2,2,5,3	0.00000	2.09762

n = 6, K = 3

r-values	f	σf
1,0,5,4	1.00000	0.53748
1,0,6,4	0.66667	0.30225
1,1,4,4	1.00000	0.68313
1,1,5,4	0.66667	0.55998
1,1,6,4	0.33333	0.42455
1,2,3,4	1.00000	0.74536
1,2,4,4	0.66667	0.66852
1,2,5,4	0.33333	0.59835
1,2,6,4	0.00000	0.53748
1,3,3,4	0.66667	0.70097
1,3,4,4	0.33333	0.66852
1,3,5,4	0.00000	0.64979
1,4,4,4	0.00000	0.68313
2,1,6,4	0.00000	0.80622
2,2,3,4	1.00000	1.11803
2,2,4,4	0.50000	1.00000
2,2,5,4	0.00000	1.02470
2,3,3,4	0.50000	1.04881

n = 10, K = 3

r-values	f	σf
0,0,5,10	1.0	0.16667
0,0,6,10	0.9	0.16330

n = 6, K = 3

r-values	f	σf
3,3,3,4	0.00000	2.32379
0,0,6,3	1.00000	0.44721
0,1,5,3	1.00000	0.64979
0,1,6,3	0.66667	0.44721
0,2,4,3	1.00000	0.74536
0,2,5,3	0.66667	0.61464
0,2,6,3	0.33333	0.43885
0,3,3,3	1.00000	0.77460
0,3,4,3	0.66667	0.68313
0,3,5,3	0.33333	0.57090
0,3,6,3	0.00000	0.44721
0,4,4,3	0.33333	0.60858
0,4,5,3	0.00000	0.53748
1,2,5,3	0.50000	0.90830
1,2,6,3	0.00000	0.80622
1,3,3,3	1.00000	1.16190
1,3,4,3	0.50000	1.01242

n = 10, K = 3

r-values	f	σf
1,1,5,10	0.88889	0.21631
1,1,6,10	0.77778	0.21419

n = 6, K = 3

r-values	f	σf
2,3,3,3	1.00000	2.32379
2,3,4,3	0.00000	2.28035
0,1,6,2	1.00000	0.80622
0,2,5,2	1.00000	1.02470
0,2,6,2	0.50000	0.70711
0,3,4,2	1.00000	1.11803
0,3,5,2	0.50000	0.89443
0,3,6,2	0.00000	0.67082
0,4,4,2	0.50000	0.94868
0,4,5,2	0.00000	0.80622
1,1,6,2	1.00000	1.61245
1,2,5,2	1.00000	2.04939
1,2,6,2	0.00000	1.61245
0,3,5,1	1.00000	1.94936
0,3,6,1	0.00000	1.34164
0,4,4,1	1.00000	2.04939
0,4,5,1	0.00000	1.61245

n = 10, K = 3

r-values	f	σf
2,2,7,10	0.50000	0.26021
2,2,8,10	0.37500	0.24694

TABLE I (Continued)
TABLE FOR CALCULATION OF MEDIAN-EFFECTIVE DOSE BY MOVING AVERAGE

r-values	n = 10, K = 3 f	σf	r-values	n = 10, K = 3 f	σf	r-values	n = 10, K = 3 f	σf
0,0,7,10	0.8	0.15275	1,1,7,10	0.66667	0.20621	2,2,9,10	0.25000	0.24296
0,0,8,10	0.7	0.13333	1,1,8,10	0.55556	0.19166	2,2,10,10	0.12500	0.22140
0,0,9,10	0.6	0.10000	1,1,9,10	0.44444	0.16882	2,3,3,10	0.87500	0.27043
0,0,10,10	0.5	0.00000	1,1,10,10	0.33333	0.13354	2,3,4,10	0.75000	0.28106
0,1,4,10	1.0	0.19149	1,2,3,10	1.00000	0.22529	2,3,5,10	0.62500	0.28603
0,1,5,10	0.9	0.19436	1,2,4,10	0.88889	0.23457	2,3,6,10	0.50000	0.28565
0,1,6,10	0.8	0.19149	1,2,5,10	0.77778	0.23843	2,3,7,10	0.37500	0.27990
0,1,7,10	0.7	0.18257	1,2,6,10	0.66667	0.23715	2,3,8,10	0.25000	0.28260
0,1,8,10	0.6	0.16667	1,2,7,10	0.55556	0.23064	2,3,9,10	0.12500	0.27081
0,1,9,10	0.5	0.14142	1,2,8,10	0.44444	0.21842	2,3,10,10	0.00000	0.25345
0,1,10,10	0.4	0.10000	1,2,9,10	0.33333	0.19945	2,4,4,10	0.62500	0.29204
0,2,3,10	1.0	0.20276	1,2,10,10	0.22222	0.17151	2,4,5,10	0.500000	0.29756
0,2,4,10	0.9	0.21082	1,3,3,10	0.88889	0.24034	2,4,6,10	0.37500	0.29789
0,2,5,10	0.8	0.21344	1,3,4,10	0.77778	0.24968	2,4,7,10	0.25000	0.30619
0,2,6,10	0.7	0.21082	1,3,5,10	0.66667	0.25391	2,4,8,10	0.12500	0.30117
0,2,7,10	0.6	0.20276	1,3,6,10	0.55556	0.25331	2,4,9,10	0.00000	0.29166
0,2,8,10	0.5	0.18856	1,3,7,10	0.44444	0.24784	2,5,5,10	0.37500	0.30369
0,2,9,10	0.4	0.16667	1,3,8,10	0.33333	0.23715	2,5,6,10	0.25000	0.31732
0,2,10,10	0.3	0.13333	1,3,9,10	0.22222	0.22050	2,5,7,10	0.12500	0.31799
0,3,3,10	0.9	0.21602	1,3,10,10	0.11111	0.19637	2,5,8,10	0.00000	0.31458

n = 10, K = 3		
r-values	f	f
0,3,4,10	0.8	0.22361
0,3,5,10	0.7	0.22608
0,3,6,10	0.6	0.22361
0,3,7,10	0.5	0.21602
0,3,8,10	0.4	0.20276
0,3,9,10	0.3	0.18257
0,3,10,10	0.2	0.15275
0,4,4,10	0.7	0.23094
0,4,5,10	0.6	0.23336
0,4,6,10	0.5	0.23094
0,4,7,10	0.4	0.22361
0,4,8,10	0.3	0.21082
0,4,9,10	0.2	0.19149
0,4,10,10	0.1	0.16330
0,5,5,10	0.5	0.23570
0,5,6,10	0.4	0.23336
0,5,7,10	0.3	0.22608
0,5,8,10	0.2	0.21344
0,5,9,10	0.1	0.19436
0,5,10,10	0.0	0.16667
0,6,6,10	0.3	0.23094
0,6,7,10	0.2	0.22361
0,6,8,10	0.1	0.21082

n = 10, K = 3		
r-values	f	f
1,4,4,10	0.66667	0.25926
1,4,5,10	0.55556	0.26392
1,4,6,10	0.44444	0.26392
1,4,7,10	0.33333	0.25926
1,4,8,10	0.22222	0.24968
1,4,9,10	0.11111	0.23457
1,4,10,10	0.00000	0.21276
1,5,5,10	0.44444	0.26907
1,5,6,10	0.33333	0.26963
1,5,7,10	0.22222	0.26565
1,5,8,10	0.11111	0.25690
1,5,9,10	0.00000	0.24287
1,6,6,10	0.22222	0.27076
1,6,7,10	0.11111	0.26736
1,6,8,10	0.00000	0.25926
1,7,7,10	0.00000	0.26450
2,0,5,10	1.00000	0.20833
2,0,6,10	0.87500	0.20465
2,0,7,10	0.75000	0.19320
2,0,8,10	0.62500	0.17237
2,0,9,10	0.50000	0.10534
2,0,10,10	0.37500	0.07365
2,1,4,10	1.00000	0.23936

n = 10, K = 3		
r-values	f	f
2,6,6,10	0.12500	0.32340
2,6,7,10	0.00000	0.32543
3,0,5,10	1.00000	0.23809
3,0,6,10	0.85714	0.23536
3,0,7,10	0.71429	0.22695
3,0,8,10	0.57143	0.21695
3,0,9,10	0.42857	0.18962
3,0,10,10	0.28571	0.15587
3,1,4,10	1.00000	0.27355
3,1,5,10	0.85714	0.27941
3,1,6,10	0.71429	0.28057
3,1,7,10	0.57143	0.28074
3,1,8,10	0.42857	0.26877
3,1,9,10	0.28571	0.25517
3,1,10,10	0.14286	0.23536
3,2,3,10	1.00000	0.28965
3,2,4,10	0.85714	0.30278
3,2,5,10	0.71429	0.31122
3,2,6,10	0.57143	0.31857
3,2,7,10	0.42857	0.31536
3,2,8,10	0.28571	0.31122
3,2,9,10	0.14286	0.30278
3,2,10,10	0.00000	0.28965

TABLE I (Continued)
TABLE FOR CALCULATION OF MEDIAN-EFFECTIVE DOSE BY MOVING AVERAGE

	n = 10, K = 3			n = 10, K = 3			n = 10, K = 3	
r-values	f	σf	r-values	f	σf	r-values	f	σf
0,6,9,10	0.0	0.19149	2,1,5,10	0.87500	0.22902	3,3,3,10	0.85714	0.31018
0,7,7,10	0.1	0.21602	2,1,6,10	0.75000	0.24116	3,3,4,10	0.71429	0.32546
0,7,8,10	0.0	0.20276	2,1,7,10	0.62500	0.23246	3,3,5,10	0.57143	0.33926
1,0,5,10	1.0	0.18518	2,1,8,10	0.50000	0.21651	3,3,6,10	0.42857	0.34291
1,0,6,10	0.88889	0.18186	2,1,9,10	0.37500	0.19151	3,3,7,10	0.28571	0.34574
1,0,7,10	0.77778	0.17151	2,1,10,10	0.25000	0.17678	3,3,8,10	0.14286	0.34480
1,0,8,10	0.66667	0.15270	2,2,3,10	1.00000	0.25345	3,3,9,10	0.00000	0.34007
1,0,9,10	0.55556	0.12159	2,2,4,10	0.87500	0.26393	3,4,4,10	0.57143	0.34588
1,0,10,10	0.44444	0.06172	2,2,5,10	0.75000	0.26842	3,4,5,10	0.42857	0.35589
1,1,4,10	1.00000	0.21276	2,2,6,10	0.62500	0.26717	3,4,6,10	0.28571	0.36488
3,4,7,10	0.14286	0.37017	5,3,4,10	0.60000	0.46667	9,0,6,10	0.00000	1.77951
3,4,8,10	0.00000	0.37192	5,3,5,10	0.40000	0.48990	9,1,4,10	1.00000	1.77951
3,5,5,10	0.28571	0.37104	5,3,6,10	0.20000	0.52068	9,1,5,10	0.00000	2.18581
3,5,6,10	0.14286	0.38223	5,3,7,10	0.00000	0.54569	9,2,3,10	1.00000	2.02759
3,5,7,10	0.00000	0.38978	5,4,4,10	0.40000	0.49889	9,2,4,10	0.00000	2.33333
3,6,6,10	0.00000	0.39555	5,4,5,10	0.20000	0.53748	9,3,3,10	0.00000	2.38048
4,0,5,10	1.00000	0.27778	5,4,6,10	0.00000	0.56960	0,0,6,9	1.00000	0.21276
4,0,6,10	0.83333	0.27592	5,5,5,10	0.00000	0.57735	0,0,7,9	0.88889	0.19637
4,0,7,10	0.66667	0.27027	6,0,5,10	1.00000	0.41667	0,0,8,9	0.77778	0.17151
4,0,8,10	0.50000	0.26058	6,0,6,10	0.75000	0.45644	0,0,9,9	0.66667	0.13354

n = 10, K = 3				n = 10, K = 3				n = 10, K = 3		
r-values	f	σf		r-values	f	σf		r-values	f	σf
4,0,9,10	0.33333	0.24637		6,0,7,10	0.50000	0.43301		0,0,10,9	0.55556	0.06172
4,0,10,10	0.16667	0.22680		6,0,8,10	0.25000	0.45262		0,1,5,9	1.00000	0.24287
4,1,4,10	1.00000	0.31914		6,0,9,10	0.00000	0.47871		0,1,6,9	0.88889	0.23457
4,1,5,10	0.83333	0.32710		6,1,4,10	1.00000	0.47871		0,1,7,9	0.77778	0.22050
4,1,6,10	0.66667	0.33178		6,1,5,10	0.75000	0.52705		0,1,8,9	0.66667	0.19945
4,1,7,10	0.50000	0.33333		6,1,6,10	0.50000	0.52042		0,1,9,9	0.55555	0.16882
4,1,8,10	0.33333	0.33178		6,1,7,10	0.25000	0.54962		0,1,10,9	0.44444	0.12159
4,1,9,10	0.16667	0.32710		6,1,8,10	0.00000	0.58333		0,2,4,9	1.00000	0.25926
4,1,10,10	0.00000	0.31914		6,2,3,10	1.00000	0.50690		0,2,5,9	0.88889	0.25690
4,2,3,10	1.00000	0.33793		6,2,4,10	0.75000	0.56519		0,2,6,9	0.77778	0.24968
4,2,4,10	0.83333	0.35428		6,2,5,10	0.50000	0.57130		0,2,7,9	0.66667	0.23715
4,2,5,10	0.66667	0.36711		6,2,6,10	0.25000	0.60953		0,2,8,9	0.55556	0.21842
4,2,6,10	0.50000	0.37679		6,2,7,10	0.00000	0.65085		0,2,9,9	0.44444	0.19166
4,2,7,10	0.33333	0.38356		6,3,3,10	0.75000	0.57735		0,2,10,9	0.33333	0.15270
4,2,8,10	0.16667	0.38756		6,3,4,10	0.50000	0.59512		0,3,3,9	1.00000	0.26450
4,2,9,10	0.00000	0.38889		6,3,5,10	0.25000	0.64280		0,3,4,9	0.88889	0.26736
4,3,3,10	0.83333	0.36289		6,3,6,10	0.00000	0.69222		0,3,5,9	0.77778	0.26565
4,3,4,10	0.66667	0.38356		6,4,4,10	0.25000	0.65352		0,3,6,9	0.66667	0.25926
4,3,5,10	0.50000	0.40062		6,4,5,10	0.00000	0.71200		0,3,7,9	0.55556	0.24784
4,3,6,10	0.33333	0.41450		7,0,5,10	1.00000	0.55556		0,3,8,9	0.44444	0.23064
4,3,7,10	0.16667	0.42552		7,0,6,10	0.66667	0.57013		0,3,9,9	0.33333	0.20621
4,3,8,10	0.00000	0.43390		7,0,7,10	0.33333	0.61195		0,3,10,9	0.22222	0.17151
4,4,4,10	0.50000	0.48025		7,0,8,10	0.00000	0.67586		0,4,4,9	0.77778	0.27076

TABLE I (Continued)
TABLE FOR CALCULATION OF MEDIAN-EFFECTIVE DOSE BY MOVING AVERAGE

r-values	n = 10, K = 3 f	σf	r-values	n = 10, K = 3 f	σf	r-values	n = 10, K = 3 f	σf
4,4,5,10	0.33333	0.42913	7,1,4,10	1.00000	0.63828	0,4,5,9	0.66667	0.26963
4,4,6,10	0.16667	0.44675	7,1,5,10	0.66667	0.66975	0,4,6,9	0.55556	0.26392
4,4,7,10	0.00000	0.46148	7,1,6,10	0.33333	0.72293	0,4,7,9	0.44444	0.25331
4,5,5,10	0.16667	0.45361	7,1,7,10	0.00000	0.79349	0,4,8,9	0.33333	0.23715
4,5,6,10	0.00000	0.47466	7,2,3,10	1.00000	0.67586	0,4,9,9	0.22222	0.21419
5,0,5,10	1.00000	0.33333	7,2,4,10	0.66667	0.72293	0,4,10,9	0.11111	0.18186
5,0,6,10	0.80000	0.33333	7,2,5,10	0.33333	0.78829	0,5,5,9	0.55556	0.26907
5,0,7,10	0.60000	0.33333	7,2,6,10	0.00000	0.86780	0,5,6,9	0.44444	0.26392
5,0,8,10	0.40000	0.33333	7,3,3,10	0.66667	0.73981	0,5,7,9	0.33333	0.25391
5,0,9,10	0.20000	0.33333	7,3,4,10	0.33333	0.81901	0,5,8,9	0.22222	0.23843
5,0,10,10	0.00000	0.33333	7,3,5,10	0.00000	0.90948	0,5,9,9	0.11111	0.21631
5,1,4,10	1.00000	0.38297	7,4,4,10	0.00000	0.92296	0,5,10,9	0.00000	0.18518
5,1,5,10	0.80000	0.39440	8,0,5,10	1.00000	0.83333	0,6,6,9	0.33333	0.25926
5,1,6,10	0.60000	0.40552	8,0,6,10	0.50000	0.88192	0,6,7,9	0.22222	0.24968
5,1,7,10	0.40000	0.41633	8,0,7,10	0.00000	1.01379	0,6,8,9	0.11111	0.23457
5,1,8,10	0.20000	0.42687	8,1,4,10	1.00000	0.95743	0,6,9,9	0.00000	0.21276
5,1,9,10	0.00000	0.43716	8,1,5,10	0.50000	1.02740	0,7,7,9	0.11111	0.24034
5,2,3,10	1.00000	0.40552	8,1,6,10	0.00000	1.16667	0,7,8,9	0.00000	0.22529
5,2,4,10	0.80000	0.42688	8,2,3,10	1.00000	1.01379	1,0,6,9	1.00000	0.23936

r-values	n = 10, K = 3 f	σf	r-values	n = 10, K = 3 f	σf	r-values	n = 10, K = 3 f	σf
5,2,5,10	0.60000	0.44721	8,2,4,10	0.50000	1.10554	1,0,7,9	0.87500	0.22060
5,2,6,10	0.40000	0.46667	8,2,5,10	0.00000	1.25830	1,0,8,9	0.75000	0.19376
5,2,7,10	0.20000	0,48534	8,3,3,10	0.50000	1.13039	1,0,9,9	0.62500	0.15468
5,2,8,10	0.00000	0.50332	8,3,4,10	0.00000	1.30171	1,0,10,9	0.50000	0.08838
5,3,3,10	0.80000	0.43716	9,0,5,10	1.00000	1.66667	1,1,5,9	1.00000	0.27323
11,6,9	0.87500	0.26363	2,3,6,9	0.57143	0.34194	4,1,6,9	0.80	0.42016
11,7,9	0.75000	0.24869	2,3,7,9	0.42857	0.33423	4,1,7,9	0.60	0.40596
11,8,9	0.62500	0.22738	2,3,8,9	0.28571	0.32261	4,1,8,9	0.40	0.39486
11,9,9	0.50000	0.19766	2,3,9,9	0.14286	0.30838	4,1,9,9	0.20	0.38713
11,10,9	0.37500	0.15468	2,3,10,9	0.00000	0.28966	4,1,10,9	0.00	0.38297
1,2,4,9	1.00000	0.29167	2,4,4,9	0.71429	0.34960	4,2,4,9	1.00	0.46667
1,2,5,9	0.87500	0.28877	2,4,5,9	0.57143	0.35496	4,2,5,9	0.80	0.46053
1,2,6,9	0.75000	0.28144	2,4,6,9	0.42857	0.35400	4,2,6,9	0.60	0.45743
1,2,7,9	0.62500	0.26933	2,4,7,9	0.28571	0.34960	4,2,7,9	0.40	0.45743
1,2,8,9	0.50000	0.25173	2,4,8,9	0.14286	0.34318	4,2,8,9	0.20	0.46053
1,2,9,9	0.37500	0.22738	2,4,9,9	0.00000	0.33333	4,2,9,9	0.00	0.46667
1,2,10,9	0.25000	0.19376	2,5,5,9	0.42857	0.36034	4,3,3,9	1.00	0.47610
1,3,3,9	1.00000	0.29756	2,5,6,9	0.28571	0.36234	4,3,4,9	0.80	0.47944
1,3,4,9	0.87500	0.30055	2,5,7,9	0.14286	0.36246	4,3,5,9	0.60	0.48571
1,3,5,9	0.75000	0.29938	2,5,8,9	0.00000	0.35952	4,3,6,9	0.40	0.49477
1,3,6,9	0.62500	0.29398	2,6,6,9	0.14286	0.36867	4,3,7,9	0.20	0.50649
1,3,7,9	0.50000	0.28413	2,6,7,9	0.00000	0.37192	4,3,8,9	0.00	0.52068
1,3,8,9	0.37500	0.26933	3,0,6,9	1.00000	0.31914	4,4,4,9	0.60	0.49477

TABLE I (Continued)
TABLE FOR CALCULATION OF MEDIAN-EFFECTIVE DOSE BY MOVING AVERAGE

r-values	n = 10, K = 3 f	σf	r-values	n = 10, K = 3 f	σf	r-values	n = 10, K = 3 f	σf
1,3,9,9	0.25000	0.24869	3,0,7,9	0.83333	0.29310	4,4,5,9	0.40	0.51242
1,3,10,9	0.12500	0.22060	3,0,8,9	0.66667	0.26254	4,4,6,9	0.20	0.53216
1,4,4,9	0.75000	0.30512	3,0,9,9	0.50000	0.22567	4,4,7,9	0.00	0.55377
1,4,5,9	0.62500	0.30557	3,0,10,9	0.33333	0.18703	4,5,5,9	0.20	0.54045
1,4,6,9	0.50000	0.30190	3,1,5,9	1.00000	0.36340	4,5,6,9	0.00	0.56960
1,4,7,9	0.37500	0.29398	3,1,6,9	0.83333	0.35000	5,0,6,9	1.00	0.47871
1,4,8,9	0.25000	0.28144	3,1,7,9	0.66667	0.33487	5,0,7,9	0.75	0.43800
1,4,9,9	0.12500	0.26363	3,1,8,9	0.50000	0.31672	5,0,8,9	0.50	0.41248
1,4,10,9	0.00000	0.23936	3,1,9,9	0.33333	0.30089	5,0,9,9	0.25	0.40505
1,5,5,9	0.50000	0.30760	3,1,10,9	0.16667	0.26692	5,0,10,9	0.00	0.41667
1,5,6,9	0.37500	0.30557	3,2,4,9	1.00000	0.38889	5,1,5,9	1.00	0.54645
1,5,7,9	0.25000	0.29938	3,2,5,9	0.83333	0.38423	5,1,6,9	0.75	0.52457
1,5,8,9	0.12500	0.28887	3,2,6,9	0.66667	0.37816	5,1,7,9	0.50	0.51707
1,5,9,9	0.00000	0.27323	3,2,7,9	0.50000	0.37060	5,1,8,9	0.25000	0.52457
1,6,6,9	0.25000	0.30512	3,2,8,9	0.33333	0.36571	5,1,9,9	0.00000	0.54645
1,6,7,9	0.12500	0.30055	3,2,9,9	0.16667	0.34731	5,2,4,9	1.00000	0.58333
1,6,8,9	0.00000	0.29167	3,2,10,9	0.00000	0.33793	5,2,5,9	0.75000	0.57509
1,7,7,9	0.00000	0.29756	3,3,3,9	1.00000	0.39674	5,2,6,9	0.50000	0.58035
2,0,6,9	1.00000	0.27355	3,3,4,9	0.83333	0.39997	5,2,7,9	0.25000	0.59875

n = 10, K = 3			n = 10, K = 3			n = 10, K = 3		
r-values	f	σf	r-values	f	σf	r-values	f	σf
2,0,7,9	0.85714	0.25170	3,3,5,9	0.66667	0.40190	5,2,8,9	0.00000	0.62915
2,0,8,9	0.71429	0.22283	3,3,6,9	0.50000	0.40254	5,3,3,9	1.00000	0.59512
2,0,9,9	0.57143	0.18786	3,3,7,9	0.33333	0.40572	5,3,4,9	0.75000	0.59875
2,0,10,9	0.42857	0.12834	3,3,8,9	0.16667	0.39707	5,3,5,9	0.50000	0.61520
2,1,5,9	1.00000	0.31226	3,3,9,9	0.00000	0.35573	5,3,6,9	0.25000	0.64348
2,1,6,9	0.85714	0.30094	3,4,4,9	0.66667	0.40965	5,3,7,9	0.00000	0.68211
2,1,7,9	0.71429	0.28531	3,4,5,9	0.50000	0.41759	5,4,4,9	0.50000	0.62639
2,1,8,9	0.57143	0.26753	3,4,6,9	0.33333	0.42793	5,4,5,9	0.25000	0.66471
2,1,9,9	0.42857	0.23934	3,4,7,9	0.16667	0.42703	5,4,6,9	0.00000	0.71200
2,1,10,9	0.28571	0.20146	3,4,8,9	0.00000	0.39674	5,5,5,9	0.00000	0.72169
2,2,4,9	1.00000	0.33333	3,5,5,9	0.33333	0.43509	6,0,6,9	1.00000	0.63828
2,2,5,9	0.85714	0.32970	3,5,6,9	0.16667	0.44125	6,0,7,9	0.66667	0.58443
2,2,6,9	0.71429	0.32261	3,5,7,9	0.00000	0.41944	6,0,8,9	0.33333	0.58443
2,2,7,9	0.57143	0.31430	3,6,6,9	0.00000	0.42673	6,0,9,9	0.00000	0.63828
2,2,8,9	0.42857	0.29838	4,0,6,9	1.00	0.38297	6,1,5,9	1.00000	0.72860
2,2,9,9	0.28571	0.27725	4,0,7,9	0.80	0.35100	6,1,6,9	0.66667	0.69979
2,2,10,9	0.14286	0.25170	4,0,8,9	0.60	0.32028	6,1,7,9	0.33333	0.71722
2,3,3,9	1.00000	0.34007	4,0,9,9	0.40	0.29120	6,1,8,9	0.00000	0.77778
2,3,4,9	0.85714	0.34318	4,0,10,9	0.20	0.26432	6,2,4,9	1.00000	0.77778
2,3,5,9	0.71429	0.34305	4,1,5,9	1.00	0.43716	6,2,5,9	0.66667	0.7672
6,2,6,9	0.33333	0.79866	0,4,10,8	0.125	0.20465	2,1,8,8	0.66667	0.32341
6,2,7,9	0.00000	0.79349	0,5,5,8	0.625	0.30369	2,1,9,9	0.50000	0.28328
6,3,3,9	1.00000	0.79349	0,5,6,8	0.500	0.29756	2,1,10,8	0.33333	0.23497

r-values	$n = 10, K = 3$ f	σf
6,3,4,9	0.66667	0.79866
6,3,5,9	0.33333	0.84376
6,3,6,9	0.00000	0.85346
6,4,4,9	0.33333	0.85827
6,4,5,9	0.00000	0.88192
7,0,6,9	1.00000	0.95743
7,0,6,9	1.00000	0.95743
7,0,7,9	0.50000	0.88976
7,0,8,9	0.00000	1.01379
7,1,5,9	1.00	1.09291
7,1,6,9	0.50	1.06066
7,1,7,9	0.00	1.10924
7,2,4,9	1.00	1.16667
7,2,5,9	0.50	1.16070
7,2,6,9	0.00	1.30171
7,3,3,9	1.00	1.19024
7,3,4,9	0.50	1.20761
7,3,5,9	0.00	1.36422
7,4,4,9	0.00	1.38444

r-values	$n = 10, K = 3$ f	σf
0,5,7,8	0.375	0.28603
0,5,8,8	0.250	0.26842
0,5,9,8	0.125	0.22902
0,5,10,8	0.000	0.20833
0,6,6,8	0.375	0.29204
0,6,7,8	0.250	0.28106
0,6,7,8	0.250	0.28106
0,6,8,8	0.125	0.26393
0,6,9,8	0.000	0.23936
0,7,7,8	0.125	0.27043
0,7,8,8	0.000	0.25345
1,0,7,8	1.00000	0.28966
1,0,8,8	0.85714	0.25170
1,0,9,8	0.71429	0.20146
1,0,10,8	0.57143	0.12834
1,1,6,8	1.00000	0.33333
1,1,7,8	0.58714	0.30838
1,1,8,8	0.71429	0.27725
1,1,9,8	0.57143	0.23934

r-values	$n = 10, K = 3$ f	σf
2,2,5,8	1.00000	0.41944
2,2,6,8	0.83333	0.39890
2,2,7,8	0.66667	0.37634
2,2,8,8	0.50000	0.35136
2,2,9,8	0.33333	0.32341
2,2,10,8	0.16667	0.29163
2,2,10,8	0.16667	0.29163
2,3,4,8	1.00000	0.43390
2,3,5,8	0.83333	0.42174
2,3,6,8	0.66667	0.40783
2,3,7,8	0.50000	0.40062
2,3,8,8	0.33333	0.37634
2,3,9,8	0.16667	0.35813
2,3,10,8	0.00000	0.33793
2,4,4,8	0.83333	0.42783
2,4,5,8	0.66667	0.42269
2,4,6,8	0.50000	0.43033
2,4,7,8	0.33333	0.40783
2,4,8,8	0.16667	0.39890

r-values	n = 10, K = 3 f	σf	r-values	n = 10, K = 3 f	σf	r-values	n = 10, K = 3 f	σf
8,0,6,9	1.00	1.77951	1,1,10,8	0.42857	0.18786	2,4,9,8	0.00000	0.38888
8,0,7,9	0.00	2.02759	1,2,5,8	1.00000	0.35952	2,5,5,8	0.50000	0.44445
8,1,5,9	1.00	2.18581	1,2,6,8	0.58714	0.34318	2,5,6,8	0.33333	0.42269
8,1,6,9	0.00	2.33333	1,2,7,8	0.71429	0.32261	2,5,7,8	0.16667	0.42147
8,2,4,9	1.00	2.33333	1,2,8,8	0.57143	0.29839	2,5,8,8	0.00000	0.41944
8,2,5,9	0.00	2.51661	1,2,9,8	0.42857	0.26753	2,6,6,8	0.16667	0.42873
8,3,3,9	1.00	2.38048	1,2,10,8	0.28571	0.22283	2,6,7,8	0.00000	0.43390
8,3,4,9	0.00	2.60342	1,3,4,8	1.00000	0.37192	3,0,7,8	1.00000	0.40552
0,0,7,8	1.000	0.25345	1,3,5,8	0.58	0.36246	3,0,8,8	0.80000	0.34692
0,0,8,8	0.875	0.22140	1,3,6,8	0.71429	0.34960	3,0,9,8	0.60000	0.28378
0,0,9,0	0.750	0.17678	1,3,7,8	0.57143	0.33423	3,0,10,8	0.40000	0.21208
0,0,10,8	0.625	0.07365	1,3,8,8	0.42857	0.31430	3,1,6,8	1.00000	0.46667
0,1,6,8	1.000	0.29166	1,3,9,8	0.28571	0.28531	3,1,7,8	0.80000	0.42729
0,1,7,8	0.875	0.27081	1,3,10,8	0.14286	0.25170	3,1,8,8	0.60000	0.38941
0,1,8,8	0.750	0.24296	1,4,4,8	0.85714	0.36867	3,1,9,8	0.40000	0.35352
0,1,9,8	0.625	0.19151	1,4,5,8	0.71429	0.36234	3,1,10,8	0.20000	0.32028
0,1,10,8	0.500	0.10534	1,4,6,8	0.57143	0.35400	3,2,5,8	1.00000	0.50332
0,2,5,8	1.000	0.31458	1,4,7,8	0.42857	0.34194	3,2,6,8	0.80000	0.47647
0,2,6,8	0.875	0.30117	1,4,8,8	0.28571	0.32261	3,2,7,8	0.60000	0.45274
0,2,7,8	0.750	0.28260	1,4,9,8	0.14286	0.30094	3,2,8,8	0.40000	0.43267
0,2,8,8	0.625	0.24694	1,4,10,8	0.00000	0.27355	3,2,10,8	0.20000	0.41676
0,2,9,8	0.500	0.21651	1,5,5,8	0.57143	0.26034	3,2,10,8	0.00000	0.40552

TABLE I (Continued)
TABLE FOR CALCULATION OF MEDIAN-EFFECTIVE DOSE BY
MOVING AVERAGE

r-values	n = 10, K = 3 f	r-values	n = 10, K = 3 f	f	r-values	n = 10, K = 3 f	f
0,2,10,8	0.375	1,5,6,8	0.42857	0.35496	3,3,4,8	1.00000	0.52068
0,3,4,8	1.000	1,5,7,8	0.28571	0.34305	3,3,5,8	0.80000	0.50368
0,3,5,8	0.875	1,5,8,8	0.14286	0.32970	3,3,6,8	0.60000	0.49044
0,3,6,8	0.750	1,5,9,8	0.00000	0.31226	3,3,7,8	0.40000	0.48129
0,3,7,8	0.625	1,6,6,8	0.28571	0.34960	3,3,8,8	0.20000	0.47647
0,3,8,8	0.500	1,6,7,8	0.14286	0.34318	3,3,9,8	0.00000	0.47610
0,3,9,8	0.375	1,6,8,8	0.00000	0.33333	3,4,4,8	0.80000	0.51242
0,3,10,8	0.250	1,7,7,8	0.00000	0.34007	3,4,5,8	0.60000	0.50824
0,4,4,8	0.875	2,0,7,8	1.00000	0.33793	3,4,6,8	0.40000	0.50824
0,4,5,8	0.750	2,0,8,8	0.83333	0.29163	3,4,7,8	0.20000	0.51242
0,4,6,8	0.625	2,0,9,8	0.66667	0.23497	3,4,8,8	0.00000	0.52068
0,4,7,8	0.500	2,0,10,8	0.50000	0.15713	3,5,5,8	0.40000	0.51691
0,4,8,8	0.375	2,1,6,8	1.00000	0.38888	3,5,6,8	0.20000	0.52949
0,4,9,8	0.250	2,1,7,8	0.83333	0.35813	3,5,7,8	0.00000	0.54569
3,6,6,8	0.00000	6,3,6,8	0.00000	1.38444	1,2,7,7	0.83333	0.39707
4,0,7,8	1.00000	6,4,4,8	0.50000	1.26930	1,2,8,7	0.66667	0.36571
4,0,8,8	0.75000	6,4,5,8	0.00000	1.42400	1,2,9,7	0.50000	0.31672
4,0,9,8	0.50000	7,0,7,8	1.00000	2.02759	1,2,10,7	0.33333	0.26254
4,0,10,8	0.25000	7,0,8,8	0.00000	2.02759	1,3,5,7	1.00000	0.41944

n = 10, K = 3		
r-values	f	f
4,1,6,8	1.00000	0.58333
4,1,7,8	0.75000	0.53033
4,1,8,8	0.50000	0.49301
4,1,9,8	0.25000	0.47507
4,1,10,8	0.00000	0.47871
4,2,5,8	1.00000	0.62915
4,2,6,8	0.75000	0.59219
4,2,7,8	0.50000	0.57130
4,2,8,8	0.25000	0.56826
4,2,9,8	0.00000	0.58333
4,3,4,8	1.00000	0.65085
4,3,5,8	0.75000	0.62639
4,3,6,8	0.50000	0.61802
4,3,7,8	0.25000	0.62639
4,3,8,8	0.00000	0.65085
4,4,4,8	0.75000	0.63191
4,4,5,8	0.50000	0.64010
4,4,6,8	0.25000	0.66926
4,4,7,8	0.00000	0.69222
4,5,5,8	0.25000	0.68971
4,5,6,8	0.00000	0.71200
5,0,7,8	1.00000	0.67586
5,0,8,8	0.66667	0.56534

n = 10, K = 3		
r-values	f	f
7,1,6,8	1.00000	2.33333
7,1,7,8	0.00000	2.38048
7,2,5,8	1.00000	2.51661
7,2,6,8	0.00000	2.60342
7,3,4,8	1.00000	2.60342
7,3,5,8	0.00000	2.72845
7,4,4,8	0.00000	2.76887
0,0,8,7	1.00000	0.28965
0,0,9,7	0.85714	0.23536
0,0,10,7	0.71429	0.15587
0,1,7,7	1.00000	0.34007
0,1,8,7	0.85714	0.30278
0,1,9,7	0.71429	0.25517
0,1,10,7	0.57143	0.18962
0,2,6,7	1.00000	0.37192
0,2,7,7	0.85714	0.34480
0,2,8,7	0.71429	0.31122
0,2,9,7	0.57143	0.26877
0,2,10,7	0.42857	0.21695
0,3,5,7	1.00000	0.38978
0,3,6,7	0.85714	0.37017
0,3,7,7	0.71429	0.34574
0,3,8,7	0.57143	0.31536

n = 10, K = 3		
r-values	f	f
1,3,6,7	0.83333	0.42703
1,3,7,7	0.66667	0.40572
1,3,8,7	0.50000	0.37060
1,3,9,7	0.33333	0.33487
1,3,10,7	0.16667	0.29310
1,4,4,7	1.00000	0.42673
1,4,5,7	0.83333	0.44125
1,4,6,7	0.66667	0.42793
1,4,7,7	0.50000	0.40254
1,4,8,7	0.33333	0.37816
1,4,9,7	0.16667	0.35000
1,4,10,7	0.00000	0.31914
1,5,5,7	0.66667	0.43509
1,5,6,7	0.50000	0.41759
1,5,7,7	0.33333	0.40190
1,5,8,7	0.16667	0.38423
1,5,9,7	0.00000	0.36430
1,6,6,7	0.33333	0.40965
1,6,7,7	0.16667	0.39997
1,6,8,7	0.00000	0.38889
1,7,7,7	0.00000	0.39674
2,0,8,7	1.00000	0.40552
2,0,9,7	0.80000	0.32028

TABLE I (Continued)
TABLE FOR CALCULATION OF MEDIAN-EFFECTIVE DOSE BY MOVING AVERAGE

n = 10, K = 3			n = 10, K = 3			n = 10, K = 3		
r-values	f	f	r-values	f	f	r-values	f	f
5,0,9,8	0.33333	0.51984	0,3,9,7	0.42857	0.28074	2,0,10,7	0.60000	0.21208
5,0,10,8	0.00000	0.55556	0,3,10,7	0.28571	0.22695	2,1,7,7	1.00000	0.47610
5,1,6,8	1.00000	0.77778	0,4,4,7	1.00000	0.39555	2,1,8,7	0.80000	0.41676
5,1,7,8	0.66667	0.70175	0,4,5,7	0.85714	0.38223	2,1,9,7	0.60000	0.35352
5,1,8,8	0.33333	0.68393	0,4,6,7	0.71429	0.36488	2,1,10,7	0.40000	0.28378
5,1,9,8	0.00000	0.72860	0,4,7,7	0.57143	0.34291	2,2,6,7	1.00000	0.52068
5,2,5,8	1.00000	0.83887	0,4,8,7	0.42857	0.31857	2,2,7,7	0.80000	0.47647
5,2,6,8	0.66667	0.78480	0,4,9,7	0.28571	0.28057	2,2,8,7	0.60000	0.43267
5,2,7,8	0.33333	0.78480	0,4,10,7	0.14286	0.23536	2,2,9,7	0.40000	0.48941
5,2,8,8	0.00000	0.83887	0,5,5,7	0.71429	0.37104	2,2,10,7	0.20000	0.34692
5,3,4,8	1.00000	0.86780	0,5,6,7	0.57143	0.35589	2,3,5,7	1.00000	0.54569
5,3,5,8	0.66667	0.83065	0,5,7,7	0.42857	0.33927	2,3,6,7	0.80000	0.51242
5,3,6,8	0.33333	0.84539	0,5,8,7	0.28571	0.31122	2,3,7,7	0.60000	0.48129
5,3,7,8	0.00000	0.90948	0,5,9,7	0.14286	0.37941	2,3,8,7	0.40000	0.45274
5,4,4,8	0.66667	0.84539	0,5,10,7	0.00000	0.23809	2,3,9,7	0.20000	0.42729
5,4,5,8	0.33333	0.87410	0,6,6,7	0.42857	0.34588	2,3,10,7	0.00000	0.40552
5,4,6,8	0.00000	0.94933	0,6,7,7	0.28571	0.32546	2,4,4,7	1.00000	0.55377
5,5,5,8	0.00000	0.96225	0,6,8,7	0.14286	0.30278	2,4,5,7	0.80000	0.52949
6,0,7,8	1.00000	1.01379	0,6,9,7	0.00000	0.27355	2,4,6,7	0.60000	0.50824

n = 10, K = 3

r-values	f	f
6,0,8,8	0.50000	0.84984
6,0,9,8	0.00000	0.95743
6,1,6,8	1.00000	1.16667
6,1,7,8	0.50000	1.05409
6,1,8,8	0.00000	1.16667
6,2,5,8	1.00000	1.25830
6,2,6,8	0.50000	1.17851
6,3,7,8	0.00000	1.30171
6,3,4,8	1.00000	1.30171
6,3,5,8	0.50000	1.24722
3,0,9,7	0.75000	0.39198
3,0,10,7	0.50000	0.27003
3,1,7,7	1.00000	0.59512
3,1,8,7	0.75000	0.51454
3,1,9,7	0.50000	0.44488
3,1,10,7	0.25000	0.39198
3,2,6,7	1.00000	0.65085
3,2,7,7	0.75000	0.58999
3,2,8,7	0.50000	0.54327
3,2,9,7	0.25000	0.51454
3,2,10,7	0.00000	0.50690
3,3,5,7	1.00000	0.68211
3,3,6,7	0.75000	0.63533

n = 10, K = 3

r-values	f	f
0,7,7,7	0.14286	0.31018
0,7,8,7	0.00000	0.28965
1,0,8,7	1.00000	0.33793
1,0,9,7	0.83333	0.26692
1,0,10,7	0.66667	0.18793
1,1,7,7	1.00000	0.35573
1,1,8,7	0.83333	0.34731
1,1,9,7	0.66667	0.30089
1,1,10,7	0.50000	0.22567
1,2,6,7	1.00000	0.39674
5,3,7,7	0.00000	1.36422
5,4,4,7	1.00000	1.38444
5,4,5,7	0.50000	1.29636
5,4,6,7	0.00000	1.42400
5,5,5,7	0.00000	1.44338
6,0,8,7	1.00000	2.10818
6,0,9,7	0.00000	1.77951
6,1,7,7	1.00000	2.44949
6,1,8,7	0.00000	2.33333
6,2,6,7	1.00000	2.66667
6,2,7,7	0.00000	2.60342
6,3,5,7	1.00000	2.78887
6,3,6,7	0.00000	2.76887

n = 10, K = 3

r-values	f	f
2,4,7,7	0.40000	0.49044
2,4,8,7	0.20000	0.47647
2,4,9,7	0.00000	0.46667
2,5,5,7	0.60000	0.51691
2,5,6,7	0.40000	0.50824
2,5,7,7	0.20000	0.50368
2,5,8,7	0.00000	0.50332
2,6,6,7	0.20000	0.51242
2,6,7,7	0.00000	0.52068
3,0,8,7	1.00000	0.50690
1,3,7,6	0.80000	0.50649
1,3,8,6	0.60000	0.45743
1,3,9,6	0.40000	0.40596
1,3,10,6	0.20000	0.35100
1,4,5,6	1.00000	0.56960
1,4,6,6	0.80000	0.53216
1,4,7,6	0.60000	0.49477
1,4,8,6	0.40000	0.45743
1,4,9,6	0.20000	0.42016
1,4,10,6	0.00000	0.38297
1,5,5,6	0.80000	0.54045
1,5,6,6	0.60000	0.51242
1,5,7,6	0.40000	0.48571

TABLE I (Continued)
TABLE FOR CALCULATION OF MEDIAN-EFFECTIVE DOSE BY MOVING AVERAGE

r-values	n = 10, K = 3 f	f	r-values	n = 10, K = 3 f	f	r-values	n = 10, K = 3 f	f
3,3,7,7	0.50000	0.60403	6,4,4,7	1.00000	2.82427	1,5,8,6	0.20000	0.46053
3,3,8,7	0.25000	0.58999	6,4,5,7	0.00000	2.84800	1,5,9,6	0.00000	0.43716
3,3,9,7	0.00000	0.59512	0,0,9,6	1.00000	0.31914	1,6,6,6	0.40000	0.49477
3,4,4,7	1.00000	0.69222	0,0,10,6	0.83333	0.22680	1,6,7,6	0.20000	0.47944
3,4,5,7	0.75000	0.65683	0,1,8,6	1.00000	0.38889	1,6,8,6	0.00000	0.46667
3,4,6,7	0.50000	0.63191	0,1,9,6	0.83333	0.32710	1,7,7,6	0.00000	0.47610
3,4,7,7	0.25000	0.63533	0,1,10,6	0.66667	0.24637	2,0,9,6	1.00000	0.47871
3,4,8,7	0.00000	0.65085	0,2,7,6	1.00000	0.43390	3,0,10,6	0.75000	0.31732
3,5,5,7	0.50000	0.64818	0,2,8,6	0.83333	0.38756	2,1,8,6	1.00000	0.58333
3,5,6,7	0.25000	0.65683	0,2,9,6	0.66667	0.33178	2,1,9,6	0.75000	0.47507
3,5,7,7	0.00000	0.68211	0,2,10,6	0.50000	0.26058	2,1,10,6	0.50000	0.36324
3,6,6,7	0.00000	0.69222	0,3,6,6	1.00000	0.46148	2,2,7,6	1.00000	0.65085
4,0,8,7	1.00000	0.67586	0,3,7,6	0.83333	0.42552	2,2,8,6	0.75000	0.56826
4,0,9,7	0.66667	0.50917	0,3,8,6	0.66667	0.38356	2,2,9,6	0.50000	0.49301
4,0,10,7	0.33333	0.40062	0,3,9,6	0.50000	0.33333	2,2,10,6	0.25000	0.42998
4,1,7,7	1.00000	0.79349	0,3,10,6	0.33333	0.27027	2,3,6,6	1.00000	0.69222
4,1,8,7	0.66667	0.67586	0,4,5,6	1.00000	0.47466	2,3,7,6	0.75000	0.62639
4,1,9,7	0.33333	0.61864	0,4,6,6	0.83333	0.44675	2,3,8,6	0.50000	0.57130
4,1,10,7	0.00000	0.63828	0,4,7,6	0.66667	0.41450	2,3,9,6	0.25000	0.53033

n = 10, K = 3			n = 10, K = 3			n = 10, K = 3		
r-values	f	f	r-values	f	f	r-values	f	f
4,2,6,7	1.00000	0.86780	0,4,8,6	0.50000	0.37679	2,3,10,6	0.00000	0.50690
4,2,7,7	0.66667	0.77778	0,4,9,6	0.33333	0.33178	2,4,5,6	1.00000	0.71200
4,2,8,7	0.33333	0.74536	0,4,10,6	0.16667	0.27592	2,4,6,6	0.75000	0.66926
4,2,9,7	0.00000	0.77778	0,5,5,6	0.83333	0.45361	2,4,7,6	0.50000	0.61802
4,3,5,7	1.00000	0.90948	0,5,6,6	0.66667	0.42913	2,4,8,6	0.25000	0.59219
4,3,6,7	0.66667	0.83887	0,5,7,6	0.50000	0.40062	2,4,9,6	0.00000	0.58333
4,3,7,7	0.33333	0.82402	0,5,8,6	0.33333	0.36711	2,5,5,6	0.75000	0.68971
4,2,8,7	0.00000	0.86780	0,5,9,6	0.16667	0.32710	2,5,6,6	0.50000	0.64010
4,4,4,7	1.00000	0.92296	0,5,10,6	0.00000	0.27778	2,5,7,6	0.25000	0.62639
4,4,5,7	0.66667	0.86780	0,6,6,6	0.50000	0.40825	2,5,8,6	0.00000	0.62915
4,4,6,7	0.33333	0.86780	0,6,7,6	0.33333	0.38356	2,6,6,6	0.25000	0.63191
4,4,7,7	0.00000	0.92296	0,6,8,6	0.16667	0.35428	2,6,7,6	0.00000	0.65085
4,5,5,7	0.33333	0.88192	0,6,9,2	0.00000	0.31914	3,0,9,6	1.00000	0.63828
4,5,6,7	0.00000	0.94933	0,7,7,6	0.16667	0.36289	3,0,10,6	0.66667	0.40062
5,0,8,7	1.00000	1.01379	0,7,8,6	0.00000	0.33793	3,1,8,6	1.00000	0.77778
5,0,9,7	0.50000	0.75462	1,0,9,6	1.00000	0.38297	3,1,9,6	0.66667	0.61864
5,0,10,7	0.00000	0.83333	1,0,10,6	0.80000	0.26432	3,1,10,6	0.33333	0.50917
5,1,7,7	1.00000	1.19024	1,1,8,6	1.00000	0.46667	3,2,7,6	1.00000	0.86780
5,1,8,7	0.50000	1.00692	1,1,9,6	0.80000	0.38713	3,2,8,6	0.66667	0.74536
5,1,9,7	0.00000	1.09291	1,1,10,6	0.60000	0.29120	3,2,9,6	0.33333	0.67586
5,2,6,7	1.00000	1.30171	1,2,7,6	1.00000	0.52068	3,2,10,6	0.00000	0.67586
5,2,7,7	0.50000	1.16070	1,2,8,6	0.80000	0.46053	3,3,6,6	1.00000	0.92296
5,2,8,7	0.00000	1.25830	1,2,9,6	0.60000	0.39486	3,3,7,6	0.66667	0.82402

TABLE I (Continued)
TABLE FOR CALCULATION OF MEDIAN-EFFECTIVE DOSE BY MOVING AVERAGE

r-values	n = 10, K = 3 f	f	r-values	n = 10, K = 3 f	f	r-values	n = 10, K = 3 f	f
5,3,5,7	1.00000	1.36422	1,2,10,6	0.40000	0.32028	3,3,8,6	0.33333	0.77778
5,3,6,7	0.50000	1.25277	1,3,6,6	1.00000	0.55377	3,3,9,6	0.00000	0.79349
3,4,5,6	1.00000	0.94933	0,6,7,5	0.40000	0.46667	3,3,9,5	0.00000	1.19024
3,4,6,6	0.66667	0.86780	0,6,8,5	0.20000	0.42688	3,4,6,5	1.00000	1.42400
3,4,7,6	0.33333	0.83887	0,6,9,5	0.00000	0.38297	3,4,7,5	0.50000	1.25277
3,4,8,6	0.00000	0.86780	0,7,7,5	0.20000	0.43716	3,4,8,5	0.00000	1.30171
3,5,5,6	0.66667	0.88192	0,7,8,5	0.00000	0.40552	3,5,5,5	1.00000	1.44388
3,5,6,6	0.33333	0.86780	1,0,10,5	1.00000	0.41667	3,5,6,5	0.50000	1.29636
3,5,7,6	0.00000	0.90948	1,1,9,5	1.00000	0.54645	3,5,7,5	0.00000	1.36422
3,6,6,6	0.00000	0.92296	1,1,10,5	0.75000	0.40505	3,6,6,5	0.00000	1.38444
4,0,9,6	1.00000	0.95743	1,2,8,5	1.00000	0.62915	4,0,10,5	1.00000	1.66667
4,0,10,6	0.50000	0.57735	1,2,9,5	0.75000	0.52457	4,1,9,5	1.00000	2.18581
4,1,8,6	1.00000	0.16667	1,2,10,5	0.50000	0.41248	4,1,10,5	0.00000	2.23607
4,1,9,6	0.50000	0.91287	1,3,7,5	1.00000	0.68211	4,2,8,5	1.00000	2.51661
4,1,10,6	0.00000	0.95743	1,3,8,5	0.75000	0.59875	4,2,9,5	0.00000	2.60342
4,2,7,6	1.00000	1.19024	1,3,9,5	0.50000	0.51707	4,3,7,5	1.00000	2.72845
4,2,8,6	0.50000	1.10554	1,3,10,5	0.25000	0.43800	4,3,8,5	0.00000	2.84800
4,2,9,6	0.00000	1.16667	1,4,6,5	1.00000	0.71200	4,4,6,5	1.00000	2.84800
4,3,6,6	1.0	1.28019	1,4,7,5	0.75000	0.64348	4,4,7,5	0.00000	3.00000
4,3,7,6	0.5	1.22474	1,4,8,5	0.50000	0.58035	4,5,5,5	1.00000	2.88675
4,3,8,6	0.0	1.19024	1,4,9,5	0.25000	0.52457	4,5,6,5	0.00000	3.07318

r-values	n = 10, K = 3 f	f	r-values	n = 10, K = 3 f	f	r-values	n = 10, K = 3 f	f
4,4,5,6	1.0	1.32288	1,4,10,5	0.00000	0.47871	0,1,10,4	1.00000	0.47871
4,4,6,6	0.5	1.29099	1,5,5,5	1.00000	0.72169	0,2,9,4	1.00000	0.58333
4,4,7,6	0.0	1.28019	1,5,6,5	0.75000	0.66471	0,2,10,4	0.75000	0.45262
4,5,5,6	0.5	1.31233	1,5,7,5	0.50000	0.61520	0,3,8,4	1.00000	0.65085
4,5,6,6	0.0	1.32288	1,5,8,5	0.25000	0.57509	0,3,9,4	0.75000	0.54962
5,0,9,6	1.0	2.23607	1,5,9,5	0.00000	0.54645	0,3,10,4	0.50000	0.53301
5,0,10,6	0.0	1.66667	1,6,6,5	0.50000	0.62639	0,4,7,4	1.00000	0.69222
5,1,8,6	1.0	2.60342	1,6,7,5	0.25000	0.59875	0,4,8,4	0.75000	0.60953
5,1,9,6	0.0	2.18581	1,6,8,5	0.00000	0.58333	0,4,9,4	0.50000	0.52042
5,2,7,6	1.0	2.84800	1,7,7,5	0.00000	0.59512	0,4,10,4	0.25000	0.45644
5,2,8,6	0.0	2.51661	2,1,9,5	1.00000	0.72860	0,5,7,4	0.75000	0.64280
5,3,7,6	0.0	2.72845	2,1,10,5	0.66667	0.51985	0,5,8,4	0.50000	0.57130
5,4,5,6	1.0	3.07318	2,2,8,5	1.00000	0.83887	0,5,9,4	0.25000	0.52705
5,4,6,6	0.0	2.84800	2,2,9,5	0.66667	0.68393	0,5,10,4	0.00000	0.41667
5,5,5,6	0.0	2.88675	2,2,10,5	0.33333	0.56534	0,6,6,4	0.75000	0.65352
0,0,10,5	1.0	0.33333	2,3,7,5	1.00000	0.90948	0,6,7,4	0.50000	0.59512
0,1,9,5	1.0	0.43716	2,3,8,5	0.66667	0.78480	0,6,8,4	0.25000	0.56519
0,1,10,5	0.8	0.33333	2,3,9,5	0.33333	0.70175	0,6,9,4	0.00000	0.47871
0,2,8,5	1.0	0.50332	2,3,10,5	0.00000	0.67586	0,7,7,4	0.25000	0.57735
0,2,9,5	0.8	0.42687	2,4,6,5	1.00000	0.94933	0,7,8,4	0.00000	0.50690
0,2,10,5	0.6	0.33333	2,4,7,5	0.66667	0.84539	1,1,10,4	1.00000	0.63828
0,3,7,5	1.0	0.54569	2,4,8,5	0.33333	0.78480	1,2,9,4	1.00000	0.77778
0,3,8,5	0.8	0.48534	2,4,9,5	0.00000	0.77778	1,2,10,4	0.66667	0.58443

TABLE I (Continued)
TABLE FOR CALCULATION OF MEDIAN-EFFECTIVE DOSE BY MOVING AVERAGE

r-values	n = 10, K = 3 f	r-values	n = 10, K = 3 f	f	r-values	n = 10, K = 3 f	f
0,3,9,5	0.6	2,5,5,5	1.00000	0.96225	1,3,8,4	1.00000	0.79349
0,3,10,5	0.4	2,5,6,5	0.66667	0.87410	1,3,9,4	0.66667	0.71722
0,4,6,5	1.0	2,5,7,5	0.33333	0.83065	1,3,10,4	0.33333	0.58443
0,4,7,5	0.8	2,5,8,5	0.00000	0.83887	1,4,7,4	1.00000	0.85346
0,4,8,5	0.6	2,6,6,5	0.33333	0.84539	1,4,8,4	0.66667	0.79866
0,4,9,5	0.4	2,6,7,5	0.00000	0.86780	1,4,9,4	0.33333	0.69979
0,4,10,5	0.2	3,0,10,5	1.00000	0.83333	1,4,10,4	0.00000	0.63828
0,5,5,5	1.0	3,1,9,5	1.00000	1.09291	1,5,6,4	1.00000	0.88192
0,5,6,5	0.8	3,1,10,5	0.50000	0.75462	1,5,7,4	0.66667	0.84376
0,5,7,5	0.6	3,2,8,5	1.00000	1.25830	1,5,8,4	0.33333	0.7672
0,5,8,5	0.40000	3,2,9,5	0.50000	1.00692	1,5,9,4	0.00000	0.72860
0,5,9,5	0.20000	3,2,10,5	0.00000	1.01379	1,6,6,4	0.66667	0.85827
0,5,10,5	0.00000	3,3,7,5	1.00000	1.36422	1,6,7,4	0.33333	0.79866
0,6,6,5	0.60000	3,3,8,5	0.50000	1.16070	1,6,8,4	0.00000	0.77778
1,7,7,4	0.00000	0,4,10,3	0.33333	0.57013	2,5,8,3	0.0	2.51661
2,1,10,4	1.00000	0,5,7,3	1.00000	0.90948	2,6,6,3	1.0	2.76887
2,2,9,4	1.00000	0,5,8,3	0.66667	0.78829	2,6,7,3	0.0	2.60342
2,2,10,4	0.50000	0,5,9,3	0.33333	0.66975	0,3,10,2	1.0	1.01379
2,3,8,4	1.00000	0,5,10,3	0.00000	0.55556	0,4,9,2	1.0	1.16667
2,3,9,4	0.50000	0,6,6,3	1.00000	0.92296	0,4,10,2	0.5	0.88192
2,3,10,4	0.00000	0,6,7,3	0.66667	0.81901	0,5,8,2	1.0	1.25830

n = 10, K = 3

r-values	f	f
2,4,7,4	1.00000	1.38444
2,4,8,4	0.50000	1.17851
2,4,9,4	0.00000	1.16667
2,5,6,4	1.00000	1.42400
2,5,7,4	0.50000	1.24722
2,5,8,4	0.00000	1.25830
2,6,6,4	0.50000	1.26930
2,6,7,4	0.00000	1.30171
3,10,4	1.00000	1.79951
3,2,9,4	1.00000	2.33333
3,2,10,4	0.00000	2.10818
3,3,8,4	1.00000	2.60342
3,3,9,4	0.00000	2.44949
3,4,7,4	1.00000	2.76887
3,4,8,4	0.00000	2.66667
3,5,6,4	1.00000	2.84800
3,5,7,4	0.00000	2.78887
3,6,6,4	0.00000	2.82427
0,2,10,3	1.00000	0.67586
0,3,9,3	1.00000	0.79349
0,3,10,3	0.66667	0.61195
0,4,8,3	1.00000	0.86780
0,4,9,3	0.66667	0.72293

n = 10, K = 3

r-values	f	f
0,6,8,3	0.33333	0.72293
0,6,9,3	0.00000	0.63828
0,7,7,3	0.33333	0.73981
0,7,8,3	0.00000	0.67586
1,2,10,3	1.0	1.01379
1,3,9,3	1.0	1.19024
1,3,10,3	0.5	0.88976
1,4,8,3	1.0	1.30171
1,49,3	0.5	1.06066
1,4,10,3	0.0	0.95743
1,5,7,3	1.0	1.36422
1,5,8,3	0.5	1.16070
1,5,9,3	0.0	1.09291
1,6,6,3	1.0	1.38444
1,6,7,3	0.5	1.20761
1,6,8,3	0.0	1.16667
1,7,7,3	0.0	1.19024
2,2,10,3	1.0	2.02759
2,3,9,3	1.0	2.38048
2,3,10,3	0.0	2.02759
2,4,8,3	1.0	2.60342
2,4,9,3	0.0	2.33333
2,5,7,3	1.0	2.72845

n = 10, K = 3

r-values	f	f
0,5,9,2	0.5	1.02740
0,5,10,2	0.0	0.83333
0,6,7,2	1.0	1.30171
0,6,8,2	0.5	1.10554
0,6,9,2	0.0	0.95743
0,7,7,2	0.5	1.13039
0,7,8,2	0.0	1.01379
1,3,10,2	1.0	2.02759
1,4,9,2	1.0	2.33333
1,4,10,2	0.0	1.77951
1,5,8,2	1.0	2.51661
1,5,9,2	0.0	2.18581
1,6,7,2	1.0	2.60342
1,6,8,2	0.0	2.33333
1,7,7,2	0.0	2.38048
0,4,10,1	1.0	.77951
0,5,9,1	1.0	2.18581
0,5,10,1	0.0	1.66667
0,6,8,1	1.0	2.33333
0,6,9,1	0.0	1.77951
0,7,7,1	1.0	2.38048
0,7,8,1	0.0	2.02759

TABLE I (continued)†
Table for calculation of median - effective dose

r-values	f	σf	d(f + 0.5)	2.306 d σf
			d = 0.30103	
0,0,5	1.0	(0)	0.45154	(0)
0,1,5	0.8	0.20000	0.39134	0.13884
0,2,5	0.6	0.24495	0.33113	0.17004
0,3,5	0.4	0.24495	0.27093	0.17004
0,4,5	0.2	0.20000	0.21072	0.13884
0,5,5	0.0	(0)	0.15052	(0)
1,0,5	1.0	(0)	0.45154	(0)
1,1,5	0.75	0.25769	0.37629	0.17888
1,2,5	0.5	0.33072	0.30103	0.22958
1,3,5	0.25	0.35904	0.22577	0.24924
1,4,5	0.0	0.35355	0.15052	0.24543
2,0,5	1.0	(0)	0.45154	(0)
2,1,5	0.66667	0.36004	0.35120	0.24993
2,2,5	0.33333	0.49065	0.25086	0.34060
2,3,5	0.0	0.57735	0.15052	0.40078
3,0,5	1.0	(0)	0.45154	(0)
3,1,5	0.5	0.58630	0.30103	0.40700
3,2,5	0.0	0.86603	0.15052	0.60118
4,0,5	1.0	(0)	0.45154	(0)
4,1,5	0.0	1.41421	0.15052	0.98171

r-values	f	σf	d(f + 0.5)	d = 0.30103 2.306 d σf
0,1,4	1.0	0.35355	0.45154	0.24543
0,2,4	0.75	0.35904	0.37629	0.24924
0,3,4	0.5	0.33072	0.30103	0.22958
0,4,4	0.25	0.25769	0.22577	0.17888
0,5,4	0.0	(0)	0.15052	(0)
1,1,4	1.0	0.47140	0.45154	0.32723
1,2,4	0.6667	0.47791	0.35120	0.33175
1,3,4	0.3333	0.47791	0.25086	0.33175
1,4,4	0.0	0.47140	0.15052	0.32723
2,1,4	1.0	0.70711	0.45154	0.49086
2,2,4	0.5	0.72887	0.30103	0.50596
2,3,4	0.0	0.86603	0.15052	0.60118
3,1,4	1.0	1.41421	0.45154	0.98171
3,2,4	0.0	1.73205	0.15052	1.20235
0,2,3	1.0	0.57735	0.45154	0.40078
0,3,3	0.66667	0.49065	0.35120	0.35060
0,4,3	0.33333	0.36004	0.25086	0.24993
0,5,3	0.0	(0)	0.15052	(0)
1,2,3	1.0	0.86603	0.45154	1.20235

†Calculation by moving average interpolation for $N = 5$, $K = 2$, $d = 0.30103$ from the formula: $\text{Log } m = \log D_a + d(f + 0.5) = \log D_a + \frac{d(K - 1)}{2} + df =$ $\log D_a + d(f + 0.5)$ in this case. $2.306 \, \sigma_{\log m} = 2.306 \, d\sigma_f$.

TABLE I (continued)†
Table for calculation of median - effective dose

r-values	f	σ_f	d = 0.30103	
			d(f + 0.5)	2.306 d σ_f
1,3,3	0.5	0.72887	0.30103	0.50596
1,4,3	0.0	0.70711	0.15052	0.49806
2,2,3	1.0	1.73205	0.45154	1.20235
2,3,3	0.0	1.73205	0.15052	1.20235
0,3,2	1.0	0.86603	0.45154	0.60118
0,4,2	0.5	0.58630	0.30103	0.40700
0,5,2	0.0	(0)	0.15052	(0)
1,3,2	1.0	1.73205	0.45154	1.20235
1,4,2	0.0	1.41421	0.15052	0.98171
0,4,1	1.0	1.41421	0.45154	0.98171
0,5,1	0.0	(0)	0.15052	(0)

†Calculation by moving average interpolation for N = 4, K = 2, d = 0.30103 from the formula: Log m = log D_a + d(f + 0.5). 2.447 σ = 2.447 σ_f(d).

$$\log m = \log D_a + \frac{d(K - 1)}{2} + df = \log D_a + d(f + 0.5)$$

TABLE I (continued)†

Table for calculation of median-effective dose

r-values	f	σf	d = 0.30103 d(f+1)	2.179 d σf	r-values	f	σf	d = 0.30103 d(f+1)	2.179 d σf
0,0,3,5	0.9	0.24495	0.57196	0.16067	0,2,4,4	0.375	0.40625	0.41392	0.26648
0,0,4,5	0.7	0.20000	0.51175	0.13119	0,2,5,4	0.125	0.30778	0.33866	0.20189
0,0,5,5	0.5	0.0	0.45154	0.0	0,3,3,4	0.375	0.44304	0.41392	0.29061
0,1,2,5	0.9	0.31623	0.57196	0.20743	0,3,4,4	0.125	0.39652	0.33866	0.26010
0,1,3,5	0.7	0.31623	0.51175	0.20743	1,0,4,4	0.83333	0.43744	0.55189	0.28694
0,1,4,5	0.5	0.28284	0.45154	0.18553	1,0,5,4	0.50	0.23570	0.45154	0.15461
0,1,5,5	0.3	0.20000	0.39134	0.13119	1,1,3,4	0.83333	0.59835	0.55189	0.39248
0,2,2,5	0.7	0.34641	0.51175	0.22723	1,1,4,4	0.50	0.52705	0.45154	0.34572
0,2,3,5	0.5	0.34641	0.45154	0.22723	1,1,5,4	0.16667	0.43744	0.35120	0.28694
0,2,4,5	0.3	0.31623	0.39134	0.20743	1,2,2,4	0.83333	0.64310	0.55189	0.42184
0,2,5,5	0.1	0.24495	0.33113	0.16067	1,2,3,4	0.50	0.62361	0.45154	0.40905
03,3,5	0.3	0.34641	0.39134	0.22723	1,2,4,4	1.16667	0.59835	0.35120	0.39248
0,3,4,5	0.1	0.31623	0.33113	0.20743	1,3,3,4	0.16667	0.64310	0.35120	0.42184
1,0,3,5	0.875	0.30778	0.56443	0.20189	2,0,4,4	0.75	0.64348	0.52680	0.42209
1,0,4,5	0.625	0.26700	0.48917	0.17514	2,0,5,4	0.25	0.47598	0.37629	0.31222
1,0,5,5	0.375	0.15625	0.41392	0.10249	2,1,3,4	0.75	0.88829	0.52680	0.58267
1,1,2,5	0.875	0.39652	0.56443	0.26010	2,1,4,4	0.25	0.85239	0.37629	0.55912
1,1,3,5	0.625	0.40625	0.48917	0.26648	2,2,2,4	0.75	0.95607	0.52680	0.62713
1,1,4,5	0.375	0.38654	0.41392	0.25355	2,2,3,4	0.25	0.98821	0.37629	0.64821

†Calculation by moving average interpolation. for N = 5, K = 3, d = 0.30103 from the formula: Log m = log D_a + d(K − 1)/2 + df = log D_a + d(f + 1) in this case. 2.179$\sigma_{\log m}$ = 2.179 σ_f (d)

TABLE I (continued)†
Table for calculation of median-effective dose

r-values	f	σf	d = 0.30103 d(f+1)	d = 0.30103 2.179 d_σf
1,1,5,5	0.125	0.33219	0.33866	0.21790
1,2,2,5	0.625	0.44304	0.48917	0.29061
1,2,3,5	0.375	0.46034	0.41392	0.30196
1,2,4,5	0.125	0.45178	0.33866	0.29634
1,3,3,5	0.125	0.48513	0.33866	0.31822
2,0,3,5	0.83333	0.41388	0.55189	0.27148
2,0,4,5	0.50000	0.39087	0.45154	0.25639
2,0,5,5	0.16667	0.34021	0.35120	0.22316
2,1,2,5	0.83333	0.53142	0.55189	0.34858
2,1,3,5	0.50	0.56519	0.45154	0.37073
2,1,4,5	0.16667	0.58134	0.35120	0.38133
2,2,2,5	0.50	0.61237	0.45154	0.40168
2,2,3,5	0.16667	0.67013	0.35120	0.43957
3,0,3,5	0.75	0.63122	0.52680	0.41404
3,0,4,5	0.25	0.67892	0.37629	0.44533
3,1,2,5	0.75	0.80526	0.52680	0.52820
3,1,3,5	0.25	0.91430	0.37629	0.59973
3,2,2,5	0.25	0.98028	0.37629	0.64301
4,0,3,5	0.5	1,32288	0.45154	0.86774
4,1,2,5	0.5	1.64831	0.45154	1.08776
0,0,4,4	0.875	0.33219	0.56443	0.21790

r-values	f	σf	d = 0.30103 d(f+1)	d = 0.30103 2.179 d_σf
3,0,4,4	0.5	1.27475	0.45154	0.83616
3,1,3,4	0.5	1.76777	0.45154	1.15956
3,2,2,4	0.5	1.90394	0.45154	1.24888
0,0,5,3	0.83333	0.34021	0.55189	0.22316
0,1,4,3	0.83333	0.58134	0.55134	0.38133
0,1,5,3	0.50000	0.39087	0.45154	0.25639
0,2,3,3	0.83333	0.67013	0.55189	0.43957
0,2,4,3	0.50000	0.56519	0.45154	0.37073
0,2,5,3	0.16667	0.41388	0.35120	0.27148
0,3,3,3	0.50000	0.61237	0.45154	0.40168
0,3,4,3	0.16667	0.53142	0.35120	0.34858
1,0,5,3	0.75	0.47598	0.52680	0.31222
1,1,4,3	0.75	0.85239	0.52680	0.55912
1,1,5,3	0.25	0.64348	0.37629	0.42209
1,2,3,3	0.75	0.98821	0.52680	0.64821
1,2,4,3	0.25	0.88829	0.37629	0.58267
1,3,3,3	0.25	0.95607	0.37629	0.62713
2,0,5,3	0.5	0.86602	0.45154	0.56806
0,1,5,2	0.75	0.67892	0.52680	0.44533
0,2,4,2	0.25	0.91430	0.37629	0.59973
0,2,5,2	0.25	0.63122	0.37629	0.41404

r-values	f	σf	d = 0.30103	
			d(f + 1)	2.179 d$_{\sigma f}$
0,0,5,4	0.625	0.15625	0.48917	0.10249
0,1,3,4	0.875	0.45178	0.56443	0.29634
0,1,4,4	0.625	0.38654	0.48917	0.25355
0,1,5,4	0.375	0.26700	0.41392	0.17514
0,2,2,4	0.875	0.48513	0.56443	0.31822
0,2,3,4	0.625	0.46034	0.48917	0.30196

r-values	f	σf	d = 0.30103	
			d(f + 1)	2.179 d$_{\sigma f}$
0,3,3,2	0.75	0.98028	0.52680	0.64301
0,3,4,2	0.25	0.80526	0.37625	0.52820
1,1,5,2	0.5	1.27475	0.45154	0.83616
1,2,4,2	0.5	1.76777	0.45154	1.15956
1,3,3,2	0.5	1.90394	0.45154	1.24888
0,2,5,1	0.5	1.32288	0.45154	0.86774
0,3,4,1	0.5	1.65831	0.45154	1.08776

†Calculation by moving average interpolation for N = 5, K = 3, d = 0.30103 from the formula: Log m = log D_a + d(k − 1)/2 + df = log D_a + d(f + 1) in this case. 2.179σ log m = 2.179 σ$_r$(d)

TABLE I (continued)†
Table for calculation of median - effective dose

r-values	f	σf	d = 0.30103 d(f + 0.5)	2.447 d σf
0,0,4	1.0	(0)	0.45154	(0)
0,1,4	0.75	0.25000	0.37629	0.18416
0,2,4	0.5	0.28868	0.30103	0.21265
0,3,4	0.25	0.25000	0.22577	0.18416
0,4,4	0.0	(0)	0.15052	(0)
1,0,4	1.0	(0)	0.45154	(0)
1,1,4	0.66667	0.35138	0.35120	0.25883
1,2,4	0.33333	0.44444	0.25086	0.32738
1,3,4	0.0	0.47140	0.15052	0.34724
2,0,4	1.0	(0)	0.45154	(0)
2,1,4	0.5	0.57735	0.30103	0.42529
2,2,4	0.0	0.81650	0.15052	0.60145
3,0,4	1.0	(0)	0.45154	(0)
3,1,4	0.0	1.41421	0.15052	1.04174
0,1,3	1.0	0.47140	0.45154	0.34724
0,2,3	0.66667	0.44444	0.35120	0.32738
0,3,3	0.33333	0.35138	0.25086	0.25883
0,4,3	0.0	(0)	0.15052	(0)
1,1,3	1.0	0.70711	0.45154	0.52087
1,2,3	0.5	0.6770	0.30103	0.49869

r-values	f	σf	d = 0.30103	
			d(f + 0.5)	2.447 d σ$_f$
1,3,3	0.0	0.70711	0.15052	0.52087
2,1,3	1.0	1.41421	0.45154	1.04174
2,2,3	0.0	1.63299	0.15052	1.20289
0,2,2	1.0	0.81650	0.45154	0.60145
0,3,2	0.5	0.57735	0.30103	0.42529
0,4,2	0.0	(0)	0.15052	(0)
1,2,2	1.0	1.63299	0.45154	1.20289
1,3,2	0.0	1.41421	0.15052	1.04174
0,3,1	1.0	1.41421	0.45154	1.04174
0,4,1	0.0	(0)	0.15052	(0)

†Calculation by moving average interpolation for N = 4, K = 2, d = 0.30103 from the formula: $\text{Log } m = \log D_a + \frac{d(K - 1)}{2} + df = \log D_a + d(f + 0.5)$. 2.447 σ = 2.447 σ_f(d).

TABLE I (continued)†

r-values	f	σf	d = 0.30103 df	d = 0.30103 3.182 dσf
0,4	0.5	(0)	0.15052	(0)
1,4	0.33333	0.22222	0.10034	0.21286
2,4	0.0	0.57735	0.0	0.55303
0,3	0.66667	0.22222	0.20069	0.21286
1,3	0.5	0.34355	0.15052	0.33866
2,3	0.0	1,15470	0.0	1.10606
0,2	1.0	0.57735	0.30103	0.55303
1,2	1.0	1.15470	0.30103	1.1060
				2.776 dσf
0,5	0.5	(0)	0.1505	(0)
1,5	0.375	0.15625	0.11289	0.13057
2,5	0.16667	0.34021	0.05017	0.28430
0,4	0.625	0.15625	0.18814	0.13057
1,4	0.5	0.23570	0.15052	0.19696
2,4	0.25	0.47599	0.07526	0.39776
0,3	0.83333	0.34021	0.25086	0.28430
1,3	0.75	0.47599	0.22577	0.39776
2,3	0.5	0.86603	0.15052	0.72371

†Calculation by moving average interpolation for N = 4 or 5, K = 1, d = 0.30103 from the formula: $\text{Log } m = \log D_a + \frac{d(K-1)}{2} + df = \log D_a + df$ in this case.

N = 4; upper section
N = 5; lower section

TABLE I (continued)†

Table for calculation of median-effective dose

| r-values | | d = 0.30103 | | | r-values | | d = 0.30103 | | |
	f	σf	d(f+1)	2.262 dσf		f	σf	d(f+1)	2.262 dσf
0,0,2,4	1.00000	0.28868	0.60206	0.19657	0,1,4,3	0.33333	0.35136	0.40137	0.23925
0,0,3,4	0.7500	0.2500	0.52680	0.17023	0,2,2,3,	0.66667	0.58794	0.50172	0.40035
0,0,4,4	0.50000	0.0	0.45154	0.0	0,2,3,3	0.33333	0.52116	0.40137	0.35487
0,1,1,4	1.00000	0.35355	0.60206	0.24074	0,2,4,3	0.00000	0.38490	0.30103	0.26209
0,1,2,4	0.75000	0.38188	0.52680	0.26003	0,3,3,3	0.00000	0.47140	0.30103	0.26209
0,1,3,4	0.50000	0.35355	0.45154	0.24074	1,0,3,3	1.00000	0.70711	0.60206	0.48149
0,1,4,4	0.25000	0.25000	0.37629	0.17023	1,0,4,3	0.50000	0.35355	0.45154	0.24074
0,2,2,4	0.50000	0.40825	0.45154	0.27799	1,1,2,3	1.00000	0.91287	0.60206	0.62160
0,2,3,4	0.25000	0.38188	0.37629	0.26003	1,1,3,3	0.50000	0.79057	0.45154	0.53832
0,2,4,4	0.00000	0.28868	0.30103	0.19657	1,1,4,3	0.00000	0.70711	0.30103	0.48149
0,3,3,4	0.00000	0.35355	0.30103	0.24074	1,2,2,3	0.50000	0.88976	0.45154	0.60586
1,0,2,4	1.00000	0.38490	0.60206	0.26209	1,2,3,3	0.00000	0.91287	0.30103	0.62160
1,0,3,4	0.66667	0.35136	0.50172	0.23925	2,0,3,3	1.00000	1.41421	0.60206	0.96298
1,0,4,4	0.33333	0.22222	0.40137	0.15132	2,0,4,3	0.00000	1.15470	0.30103	0.78627
1,1,1,4	1.00000	0.47140	0.60206	0.32099	2,1,2,3	1.00000	1.82574	0.60206	1.24320
1,1,2,4	0.66667	0.52116	0.50172	0.35487	2,1,3,3	0.00000	1.82574	0.30103	1.24320
1,1,3,4	0.33333	0.52116	0.40137	0.35487	2,2,2,3	0.00000	2.00000	0.30103	1.36186
1,1,4,4	0.00000	0.47140	0.30103	0.32099	0,0,4,2	1.00000	0.57735	0.60206	0.39313
1,2,2,4	0.33333	0.58794	0.40137	0.40035	0,1,3,2	1.00000	0.91287	0.60206	0.62160

†Calculation by moving average interpolation for N = 4, K = 3, d = 0.30103, from the formula: $\log m = \log D_a = \dfrac{d\,(k-1)}{2+\delta f}$

TABLE I (continued)†
Table for calculation of median-effective dose

r-values	f		d = 0.30103	
		σf	d(f+1)	2.179 d_σf
1,2,3,4	0.00000	0.60858	0.30103	0.41440
2,0,2,4	1.00000	0.57735	0.60206	0.39313
2,0,3,4	0.50000	0.57735	0.45154	0.39313
2,0,4,4	0.00000	0.57735	0.30103	0.39313
2,1,1,4	1.00000	0.70711	0.60206	0.48149
2,1,2,4	0.50000	0.81650	0.45154	0.55598
2,1,3,4	0.00000	0.91287	0.60206	0.62160
2,2,2,4	0.00000	1.00000	0.30103	0.68093
3,0,2,4	1.00000	1.15470	0.60206	0.78627
3,0,3,4	0.00000	1.41421	0.30103	0.96298
3,1,1,4	1.00000	1.41421	0.60206	0.96298
3,1,2,4	0.00000	1.82574	0.30103	1.24320
0,0,3,3	1.00000	0.47140	0.60206	0.32099
0,0,4,3	0.66667	0.22222	0.50172	0.15132
0,1,2,3	1.00000	0.60858	0.60206	0.41440
0,1,3,3	0.66667	0.52116	0.50172	0.35487

r-values	f		d = 0.30103	
		σf	d(f+1)	2.179 d_σf
0,1,4,2	0.50000	0.57735	0.45154	0.39313
0,2,2,2	1.00000	1.00000	0.60206	0.68093
0,2,3,2	0.50000	0.81650	0.45154	0.55598
0,2,4,2	0.00000	0.57735	0.30103	0.39313
0,3,3,2	0.00000	0.70711	0.30103	0.48149
1,0,4,2	1.00000	1.15470	0.60206	0.78627
1,1,3,2	1.00000	1.82574	0.60206	1.24320
1,1,4,2	0.00000	1.41421	0.30103	0.96298
1,2,2,2	1.00000	2.00000	0.60206	1.36186
1,2,3,2	0.00000	1.82574	0.30103	1.24320
0,2,3,1	1.00000	1.82574	0.60206	1.24320
0,2,4,1	0.00000	1.15470	0.80103	0.78627
0,3,3,1	1.00000	1.41421	0.30103	0.96298
0,1,4,1	0.66667	1.41421	0.60206	0.96298

†Calculation by moving average interpolation for N = 4, K = 3, d = 0.30103, from the formula: $\log m = \log D_a = d\frac{(k-1)}{2+\delta f}$

TABLE J: CRITICAL VALUES FOR THE WILCOXON RANK SUM TEST

(N_1 = larger group)

P = .05 one sided; P = .10 two-sided

N_1	$N_2=3$	$N_2=4$	$N_2=5$	$N_2=6$	$N_2=7$	$N_2=8$	$N_2=9$	$N_1=10$	$N_2=11$	$N_2=12$	$N_2=13$	$N_2=14$
$N_1=N_2$	6,15	12,24	19,36	28,50	39,66	52,84	66,105	83,127	101,152	121,179	143,208	167,239
$N_1=N_2+1$	7,17	13,27	20,40	30,54	41,71	54,90	69,111	86,134	105,159	125,187	148,216	172,248
$N_1=N_2+2$	7,20	14,30	22,43	32,58	43,76	57,95	72,117	89,141	109,166	129,195	152,225	177,257
$N_1=N_2+3$	8,22	15,33	24,46	33,63	46,80	60,100	75,123	93,147	112,174	134,202	157,233	182,266
$N_1=N_2+4$	9,24	16,36	25,50	35,67	48,85	62,106	78,129	96,154	116,181	138,210	162,241	187,275
$N_1=N_2+5$	9,27	17,39	26,54	37,71	50,90	65,111	81,135	100,160	120,188	142,218	166,250	192,284
$N_1=N_2+6$	10,29	18,42	27,58	39,75	52,95	67,117	84,141	103,167	124,195	147,225	171,258	197,293
$N_1=N_2+7$	11,31	19,45	29,61	41,79	54,100	70,122	87,147	107,173	128,202	151,233	176,266	203,301
$N_1=N_2+8$	11,34	20,48	30,65	42,84	57,104	73,127	90,153	110,180	132,209	155,241	181,274	208,310
$N_1=N_2+9$	12,36	21,51	32,68	44,88	59,109	75,133	93,159	114,186	136,216	159,249	185,283	213,319
$N_1=N_2+10$	13,38	22,54	33,72	46,92	61,114	78,138	96,165	117,193	139,224	164,256	190,291	218,328
$N_1=N_2+11$	13,41	23,57	34,76	48,96	63,119	80,144	100,170	120,200	143,231	168,264	195,299	223,337
$N_1=N_2+12$	14,43	24,60	36,79	50,100	65,124	83,149	103,176	124,206	147,238	172,272	199,308	228,346
$N_1=N_2+13$	15,45	25,63	37,83	52,104	68,128	86,154	106,182	127,213	151,245	177,279	204,316	234,354
$N_1=N_2+14$	15,48	26,66	39,86	53,109	70,133	88,160	109,188	131,219	155,252	181,287	209,324	239,363
$N_1=N_2+15$	16,50	27,69	40,90	55,113	72,138	91,165	112,194	134,226	159,259	185,295	214,332	244,372
$N_1=N_2+16$	17,52	28,72	42,93	57,117	74,143	94,170	115,200	138,232	163,266	190,302	218,341	249,381
$N_1=N_2+17$	17,55	29,75	43,97	59,121	77,147	96,176	118,206	141,239	167,273	194,310	223,349	254,390
$N_1=N_2+18$	18,57	30,78	44,101	61,125	79,152	99,181	121,212	145,245	171,280	198,318	228,357	260,398
$N_1=N_2+19$	19,59	31,81	46,104	62,130	81,157	102,186	124,218	148,252	175,287	203,325	233,365	265,407
$N_1=N_2+20$	19,62	32,84	47,108	64,134	83,162	104,192	127,224	152,258	178,295	207,333	237,374	270,416
$N_1=N_2+21$	20,64	33,87	49,111	66,138	86,166	107,197	130,230	155,265	182,302	211,341	242,382	275,425
$N_1=N_2+22$	21,66	34,90	50,115	68,142	88,171	109,203	133,236	159,271	186,309	216,348	247,390	280,434
$N_1=N_2+23$	21,69	35,93	52,118	70,146	90,176	112,208	136,242	162,278	190,316	220,356	252,398	285,443
$N_1=N_2+24$	22,71	37,95	53,122	72,150	92,181	115,213	139,248	166,284	194,323	224,364	257,406	291,451
$N_1=N_2+25$	23,73	38,98	54,126	73,155	94,186	117,219	142,254	169,291	198,330	229,371	261,415	296,460

TABLE J: Continued

P = .05 one sided; P = .10 two-sided

N_1	$N_2=15$	$N_2=16$	$N_2=17$	$N_2=18$	$N_2=19$	$N_2=20$	$N_2=21$	$N_1=22$	$N_2=23$	$N_2=24$	$N_2=25$
$N_1 = N_2$	192,273	220,308	249,346	280,386	314,427	349,471	386,517	424,566	465,616	508,668	552,723
$N_1 = N_2+1$	198,282	226,318	256,356	287,397	321,439	356,484	394,530	433,579	474,630	517,683	562,738
$N_1 = N_2+2$	203,292	232,328	262,367	294,408	328,451	364,496	402,543	442,592	483,644	527,697	572,753
$N_1 = N_2+3$	209,301	238,338	268,378	301,419	336,462	372,508	410,556	450,606	492,658	536,712	582,768
$N_1 = N_2+4$	215,310	244,348	275,388	308,430	343,474	380,520	418,569	459,619	501,672	546,726	592,783
$N_1 = N_2+5$	220,320	250,358	281,399	315,441	350,486	387,533	427,581	468,632	511,685	555,741	602,798
$N_1 = N_2+6$	226,329	256,368	288,409	322,452	358,497	395,545	435,594	476,646	520,699	565,755	612,813
$N_1 = N_2+7$	231,339	262,378	294,420	329,463	365,509	403,557	443,607	485,659	529,713	574,770	622,828
$N_1 = N_2+8$	237,348	268,388	301,430	336,474	372,521	411,569	451,620	494,672	538,727	584,784	632,843
$N_1 = N_2+9$	242,358	274,398	307,441	342,486	380,532	419,581	459,633	502,686	547,741	594,798	642,858
$N_1 = N_2+10$	248,367	280,408	314,451	349,497	387,544	426,594	468,645	511,699	556,755	603,813	652,873
$N_1 = N_2+11$	254,376	286,418	320,462	356,508	394,556	434,606	476,658	520,712	565,769	613,827	662,888
$N_1 = N_2+12$	259,386	292,428	327,472	363,519	402,567	442,618	484,671	528,726	574,783	622,842	672,903
$N_1 = N_2+13$	265,395	298,438	333,483	370,530	409,579	450,630	492,684	537,739	584,796	632,856	682,918
$N_1 = N_2+14$	270,405	304,448	340,493	377,541	416,591	458,642	501,696	546,752	593,810	642,870	692,933
$N_1 = N_2+15$	276,414	310,458	346,504	384,552	424,602	465,655	509,709	554,766	602,824	651,885	702,948
$N_1 = N_2+16$	282,423	316,468	353,514	391,563	431,614	473,667	517,722	563,779	611,838	661,899	712,963
$N_1 = N_2+17$	287,433	322,478	359,525	398,574	438,626	481,679	526,734	572,792	620,852	670,914	723,977
$N_1 = N_2+18$	293,442	328,488	366,535	405,585	446,637	489,691	534,747	581,805	629,866	680,928	733,992
$N_1 = N_2+19$	299,451	334,498	372,546	412,596	453,649	497,703	542,760	589,819	639,879	690,942	473,1007
$N_1 = N_2+20$	304,461	340,508	379,556	419,607	461,660	505,715	550,773	598,832	648,893	699,957	753,1022
$N_1 = N_2+21$	310,470	347,517	385,568	426,618	468,672	512,728	559,785	607,845	657,907	709,971	763,1037
$N_1 = N_2+22$	315,480	353,527	392,577	433,629	475,684	520,740	567,798	615,859	666,921	718,986	773,1052
$N_1 = N_2+23$	321,489	359,537	398,588	439,641	483,695	528,752	575,811	624,872	675,935	728,1000	783,1067
$N_1 = N_2+24$	327,498	365,547	405,598	446,652	490,707	536,764	583,824	633,885	684,949	738,1014	793,1082
$N_1 = N_2+25$	332,508	371,557	411,609	453,663	498,718	544,776	592,836	642,898	694,962	747,1029	803,1097

TABLE J: Continued

P = .025 one sided; P = .05 two-sided

N_1	$N_2=3$	$N_2=4$	$N_2=5$	$N_2=6$	$N_2=7$	$N_2=8$	$N_2=9$	$N_1=10$	$N_2=11$	$N_2=12$	$N_2=13$	$N_2=14$
$N_1=N_2$	5,16	11,25	18,37	26,52	37,68	49,87	63,108	79,131	96,157	116,184	137,214	160,246
$N_1=N_2+1$	6,18	12,28	19,41	28,56	39,73	51,93	66,114	82,138	100,164	120,192	141,223	165,255
$N_1=N_2+2$	6,21	12,32	20,45	29,61	41,78	54,98	69,121	85,145	103,172	124,200	146,231	170,264
$N_1=N_2+3$	7,23	13,35	21,49	31,65	43,83	56,104	71,127	88,152	107,179	128,208	150,240	174,274
$N_1=N_2+4$	7,26	14,38	22,53	32,70	45,88	58,110	74,133	91,159	110,187	131,217	154,249	179,283
$N_1=N_2+5$	8,28	15,41	24,56	34,74	46,94	61,115	77,139	94,166	114,194	135,225	159,257	184,292
$N_1=N_2+6$	8,31	16,44	25,60	36,78	48,99	63,121	79,146	97,173	118,201	139,233	163,266	189,301
$N_1=N_2+7$	9,33	17,47	26,64	37,83	50,104	65,127	82,152	101,179	121,209	143,241	168,274	194,310
$N_1=N_2+8$	10,35	17,51	27,68	39,87	52,109	68,132	85,158	104,186	125,216	147,249	172,283	198,320
$N_1=N_2+9$	10,38	18,54	29,71	41,91	54,114	70,138	88,164	107,193	128,224	151,257	176,292	203,329
$N_1=N_2+10$	11,40	19,57	30,75	42,96	56,119	72,144	90,171	110,200	132,231	155,265	181,300	208,338
$N_1=N_2+11$	11,43	20,60	31,79	44,100	58,124	75,149	93,177	113,207	135,239	159,273	185,309	213,347
$N_1=N_2+12$	12,45	21,63	32,83	45,105	60,129	77,155	96,183	117,213	139,246	163,281	190,317	218,356
$N_1=N_2+13$	12,48	22,66	33,87	47,109	62,134	80,160	99,189	120,220	143,253	167,289	194,326	222,366
$N_1=N_2+14$	13,50	23,69	35,90	49,113	64,139	82,166	101,196	123,227	146,261	171,297	198,335	227,375
$N_1=N_2+15$	13,53	24,72	36,94	50,118	66,144	84,172	104,202	126,234	150,268	175,305	203,343	232,384
$N_1=N_2+16$	14,55	24,76	37,98	52,122	68,149	87,177	107,208	129,241	153,276	179,313	207,352	237,393
$N_1=N_2+17$	14,58	25,79	38,102	53,127	70,154	89,183	110,214	132,248	157,283	183,321	212,360	242,402
$N_1=N_2+18$	15,60	26,82	40,105	55,131	72,159	92,188	113,220	136,254	161,290	187,329	216,369	247,411
$N_1=N_2+19$	15,63	27,85	41,109	57,135	74,164	94,194	115,227	139,261	164,298	191,337	221,377	252,420
$N_1=N_2+20$	16,65	28,88	42,113	58,140	76,169	96,200	118,233	142,268	168,305	195,345	225,386	256,430
$N_1=N_2+21$	16,68	29,91	43,117	60,144	78,174	99,205	121,239	145,275	171,313	199,353	229,395	261,739
$N_1=N_2+22$	17,70	30,94	45,120	61,149	80,179	101,211	124,245	148,282	175,320	203,361	234,403	266,448
$N_1=N_2+23$	17,73	31,97	46,124	63,153	82,184	103,217	127,251	152,288	179,327	207,369	238,412	271,457
$N_1=N_2+24$	18,75	31,101	47,128	65,157	84,189	106,222	129,258	155,295	182,335	211,377	243,420	276,466
$N_1=N_2+25$	18,78	32,104	48,132	66,162	86,194	108,228	132,264	158,302	186,342	216,384	247,429	281,475

TABLE J: Continued

P = .025 one sided; P = .05 two-sided

N_1	$N_2=15$	$N_2=16$	$N_2=17$	$N_2=18$	$N_2=19$	$N_2=20$	$N_2=21$	$N_1=22$	$N_2=23$	$N_2=24$	$N_2=25$
$N_1 = N_2$	185,280	212,316	240,355	271,395	303,438	337,483	373,530	411,579	451,630	493,683	536,739
$N_1 = N_2 + 1$	190,290	217,327	246,366	277,407	310,450	345,495	381,543	419,593	460,644	502,698	546,754
$N_1 = N_2 + 2$	195,300	223,337	252,377	284,418	317,462	352,508	389,556	428,606	468,659	511,713	555,770
$N_1 = N_2 + 3$	201,309	229,347	258,388	290,430	324,474	359,521	397,569	436,620	477,673	520,728	565,785
$N_1 = N_2 + 4$	206,319	234,358	264,399	297,441	331,486	367,533	404,583	444,634	486,687	529,743	574,801
$N_1 = N_2 + 5$	211,329	240,368	271,409	303,453	338,498	374,546	412,596	452,648	494,702	538,758	584,816
$N_1 = N_2 + 6$	216,339	245,379	277,420	310,464	345,510	381,559	420,609	460,662	503,716	547,773	593,832
$N_1 = N_2 + 7$	221,349	251,389	283,431	316,476	351,523	389,571	428,622	469,675	512,730	556,788	603,847
$N_1 = N_2 + 8$	227,358	257,399	289,442	323,487	358,535	396,584	436,635	477,689	520,745	565,803	612,863
$N_1 = N_2 + 9$	232,368	262,410	295,453	329,499	365,547	403,597	443,649	485,703	529,759	575,817	622,878
$N_1 = N_2 + 10$	237,378	268,420	301,464	336,510	372,559	411,609	451,662	493,717	538,773	584,832	632,893
$N_1 = N_2 + 11$	242,388	274,430	307,475	342,522	379,571	418,622	459,675	502,730	546,788	593,847	641,909
$N_1 = N_2 + 12$	248,397	279,441	313,486	349,533	386,583	426,634	467,688	510,744	555,802	602,862	651,924
$N_1 = N_2 + 13$	253,407	285,451	319,497	355,545	393,595	433,647	475,701	518,758	564,816	611,877	660,940
$N_1 = N_2 + 14$	258,417	291,461	325,508	362,556	400,607	440,660	482,715	526,772	572,831	620,892	670,955
$N_1 = N_2 + 15$	263,427	296,472	331,519	368,568	407,619	448,672	490,728	535,785	581,845	629,907	679,971
$N_1 = N_2 + 16$	269,436	302,482	338,529	375,579	414,631	455,685	498,741	543,799	590,859	638,922	689,986
$N_1 = N_2 + 17$	274,446	308,492	344,540	381,591	421,643	463,697	506,754	551,813	599,873	648,936	699,1001
$N_1 = N_2 + 18$	279,456	314,502	350,551	388,602	428,655	470,710	514,767	560,826	607,888	657,951	708,1017
$N_1 = N_2 + 19$	284,466	319,513	356,562	395,613	435,667	477,723	522,780	568,840	616,902	666,966	718,1032
$N_1 = N_2 + 20$	290,475	325,523	362,573	401,625	442,679	485,735	530,793	576,854	625,916	675,981	727,1048
$N_1 = N_2 + 21$	295,485	331,533	368,584	408,636	449,691	492,748	537,807	584,868	633,931	684,996	737,1063
$N_1 = N_2 + 22$	300,495	336,544	374,595	414,648	456,703	500,760	545,820	593,881	642,945	693,1011	747,1078
$N_1 = N_2 + 23$	306,504	342,554	374,595	414,648	456,703	500,760	545,820	593,881	642,945	693,1011	747,1078
$N_1 = N_2 + 24$	311,514	348,564	387,616	427,671	470,727	515,785	561,846	609,909	660,973	712,1040	766,1109
$N_1 = N_2 + 25$	316,524	353,575	393,627	434,682	477,739	522,798	569,859	618,922	668,988	721,1055	775,1125

TABLE J: Continued

$P = .005$ one sided; $P = .01$ two-sided

N_1	$N_2=3$	$N_2=4$	$N_2=5$	$N_2=6$	$N_2=7$	$N_2=8$	$N_2=9$	$N_1=10$	$N_2=11$	$N_2=12$	$N_2=13$	$N_2=14$
$N_1 = N_2$	5,16	9,27	15,40	23,55	33,72	44,92	57,114	71,139	88,165	106,194	126,225	148,258
$N_1 = N_2 + 1$	5,19	10,30	16,44	24,60	34,78	46,98	59,121	74,146	91,173	109,203	130,234	152,268
$N_1 = N_2 + 2$	5,22	10,34	17,48	25,65	36,83	47,105	61,128	76,154	94,181	113,211	133,244	156,278
$N_1 = N_2 + 3$	5,25	11,37	18,52	27,69	37,89	49,111	63,135	79,161	97,189	116,220	137,253	160,288
$N_1 = N_2 + 4$	6,27	11,41	19,56	28,74	39,94	51,117	65,142	82,168	100,197	119,229	141,262	164,298
$N_1 = N_2 + 5$	6,30	12,44	19,61	29,79	40,100	53,123	68,148	84,176	102,206	123,237	144,272	168,308
$N_1 = N_2 + 6$	6,33	12,48	20,65	30,84	42,105	55,129	70,155	87,183	105,214	126,246	148,281	172,318
$N_1 = N_2 + 7$	6,36	13,51	21,69	31,89	43,111	57,135	72,162	89,191	108,222	129,255	152,290	176,328
$N_1 = N_2 + 8$	7,38	13,55	22,73	32,94	45,116	59,141	75,168	92,198	111,230	133,263	155,300	181,337
$N_1 = N_2 + 9$	7,41	14,58	23,77	34,98	46,122	61,147	77,175	95,205	114,238	136,272	159,309	185,347
$N_1 = N_2 + 10$	7,44	15,61	24,81	35,103	48,127	62,154	79,182	97,213	117,246	139,281	163,318	189,357
$N_1 = N_2 + 11$	8,46	15,65	25,85	36,108	49,133	64,160	81,189	100,220	120,254	143,289	167,327	193,367
$N_1 = N_2 + 12$	8,49	16,68	26,89	37,113	51,138	66,166	83,196	103,227	123,262	146,298	171,336	197,377
$N_1 = N_2 + 13$	8,52	16,72	26,94	38,118	52,144	68,172	86,202	105,235	126,270	150,306	175,345	201,387
$N_1 = N_2 + 14$	9,54	17,75	27,98	40,122	54,149	70,178	88,209	108,242	129,278	153,315	178,355	205,397
$N_1 = N_2 + 15$	9,57	17,79	28,102	41,127	55,155	72,184	90,216	110,250	132,286	156,324	182,364	210,406
$N_1 = N_2 + 16$	9,60	18,82	29,106	42,132	57,160	74,190	93,222	113,257	136,293	160,332	186,373	214,416
$N_1 = N_2 + 17$	9,63	19,85	30,110	43,137	59,165	76,196	95,229	116,264	139,301	163,341	190,382	218,426
$N_1 = N_2 + 18$	10,65	19,89	31,114	45,141	60,171	78,202	97,236	118,272	142,309	167,349	194,391	222,436
$N_1 = N_2 + 19$	10,68	20,92	32,118	46,146	62,176	80,208	99,243	121,279	145,317	170,358	197,401	226,446
$N_1 = N_2 + 20$	10,71	20,96	33,122	47,151	63,182	82,214	102,249	124,286	148,325	173,367	201,410	231,455
$N_1 = N_2 + 21$	11,73	21,99	33,127	48,156	65,187	83,221	104,256	126,294	151,333	177,375	205,419	235,465
$N_1 = N_2 + 22$	11,76	21,103	34,131	49,161	66,193	85,227	106,263	129,301	154,341	180,384	209,428	239,475
$N_1 = N_2 + 23$	11,79	22,106	35,135	51,165	68,198	87,233	109,269	132,308	157,349	184,392	213,437	243,485
$N_1 = N_2 + 24$	12,81	23,109	36,139	52,170	70,203	89,239	111,276	134,316	160,357	187,401	216,447	247,495
$N_1 = N_2 + 25$	12,84	23,113	37,143	53,175	71,209	91,245	113,283	137,323	163,365	191,409	220,456	252,504

TABLE J: Continued

P = .005 one sided; P = .01 two-sided

N_1	$N_2=15$	$N_2=16$	$N_2=17$	$N_2=18$	$N_2=19$	$N_2=20$	$N_2=21$	$N_1=22$	$N_2=23$	$N_2=24$	$N_2=25$
$N_1 = N_2$	171,294	196,332	223,372	252,414	283,458	316,504	250,553	386,604	424,657	464,712	506,679
$N_1 = N_2 + 1$	176,304	201,343	229,383	258,426	289,471	322,518	357,567	393,619	432,672	472,728	514,786
$N_1 = N_2 + 2$	180,315	206,354	234,395	264,438	295,484	329,531	364,581	401,633	440,687	480,744	532,802
$N_1 = N_2 + 3$	184,326	211,365	239,407	269,451	301,497	335,545	371,595	408,648	447,703	489,759	531,819
$N_1 = N_2 + 4$	189,336	216,376	245,418	275,463	307,510	342,558	378,609	415,663	455,718	497,775	540,835
$N_1 = N_2 + 5$	194,346	221,387	250,430	281,475	314,522	348,572	385,623	423,677	463,733	505,791	549,851
$N_1 = N_2 + 6$	198,357	226,398	255,442	287,487	320,535	355,585	392,637	430,692	471,748	513,807	557,868
$N_1 = N_2 + 7$	203,367	231,409	261,453	292,500	326,548	361,599	399,651	438,706	479,763	521,823	566,884
$N_1 = N_2 + 8$	207,378	236,420	266,465	298,512	332,561	368,612	405,666	445,721	486,779	530,838	575,900
$N_1 = N_2 + 9$	212,388	241,431	271,477	304,524	338,574	374,626	412,680	452,736	494,794	538,854	583,917
$N_1 = N_2 + 10$	216,399	245,443	277,488	310,536	344,587	381,639	419,694	460,750	502,809	546,870	592,933
$N_1 = N_2 + 11$	221,409	250,454	282,500	315,549	351,599	388,652	426,708	467,765	510,824	554,886	601,949
$N_1 = N_2 + 12$	225,420	255,465	287,512	321,561	357,612	394,666	433,722	475,779	518,839	563,901	609,966
$N_1 = N_2 + 13$	230,430	260,476	293,523	327,573	363,625	401,679	440,736	482,794	526,854	571,917	618,982
$N_1 = N_2 + 14$	235,440	265,487	298,535	333,585	369,638	407,693	447,750	490,808	533,870	579,933	627,998
$N_1 = N_2 + 15$	239,451	270,498	303,547	338,598	375,651	414,706	454,764	497,823	541,885	587,949	635,1015
$N_1 = N_2 + 16$	244,461	275,509	309,558	344,610	381,664	421,719	462,777	504,838	549,900	596,964	644,1031
$N_1 = N_2 + 17$	248,472	280,520	314,570	350,622	388,676	427,733	469,791	512,852	557,915	604,980	653,1047
$N_1 = N_2 + 18$	253,482	285,531	320,581	356,634	394,689	434,746	476,805	519,867	565,930	612,996	661,1064
$N_1 = N_2 + 19$	257,493	290,542	325,593	362,646	400,702	440,760	483,819	527,881	573,945	620,1012	670,1080
$N_1 = N_2 + 20$	262,503	295,553	330,605	367,659	406,715	447,773	490,833	534,896	580,961	629,1027	679,1096
$N_1 = N_2 + 21$	267,513	300,564	336,616	373,671	413,727	454,786	497,847	542,910	588,976	637,1043	687,1113
$N_1 = N_2 + 22$	271,524	305,575	341,628	379,683	419,740	460,800	504,861	549,925	596,991	645,1059	696,1129
$N_1 = N_2 + 23$	276,534	310,586	347,639	385,695	425,753	467,813	511,875	556,940	604,1006	654,1074.	705,1145
$N_1 = N_2 + 24$	280,545	315,597	352,651	391,707	431,766	474,826	518,889	564,954	612,1021	662,1090	714,1161
$N_1 = N_2 + 25$	285,555	320,608	357,663	397,719	438,778	480,840	525,903	571,969	620,1106	670,1106	722,1178

TABLE J: Continued

P = .01 one sided; P = .012 two-sided

N_1	$N_2=3$	$N_2=4$	$N_2=5$	$N_2=6$	$N_2=7$	$N_2=8$	$N_2=9$	$N_1=10$	$N_2=11$	$N_2=12$	$N_2=13$	$N_2=14$
$N_1 = N_2$	5,16	10,26	16,39	24,54	34,71	46,90	59,112	74,136	91,162	110,190	130,221	153,253
$N_1 = N_2 + 1$	5,19	10,30	17,43	26,58	36,76	48,96	62,118	77,143	94,170	113,199	134,230	157,263
$N_1 = N_2 + 2$	6,21	11,33	18,47	27,63	38,81	50,102	64,125	80,150	97,178	117,207	138,239	161,273
$N_1 = N_2 + 3$	6,24	12,36	19,51	28,68	39,87	52,108	66,132	83,157	101,185	120,216	142,248	166,282
$N_1 = N_2 + 4$	6,27	12,40	20,55	30,72	41,92	54,114	69,138	85,165	104,193	124,224	146,257	170,292
$N_1 = N_2 + 5$	7,29	13,43	21,59	31,77	43,97	56,120	71,145	88,172	107,201	128,232	150,266	174,302
$N_1 = N_2 + 6$	7,32	14,46	22,63	32,82	44,103	58,126	74,151	91,179	110,209	131,241	154,275	179,311
$N_1 = N_2 + 7$	7,35	14,50	23,67	34,86	46,108	60,132	76,158	94,186	113,217	135,249	158,284	183,321
$N_1 = N_2 + 8$	8,37	15,53	24,71	35,91	48,113	62,138	79,164	97,193	117,224	138,258	162,293	188,330
$N_1 = N_2 + 9$	8,40	16,56	25,75	36,96	49,119	64,144	81,171	100,200	120,232	142,266	166,302	192,340
$N_1 = N_2 + 10$	9,42	16,60	26,79	38,100	51,124	66,150	83,178	102,208	123,240	146,274	170,311	196,350
$N_1 = N_2 + 11$	9,45	17,63	27,83	39,105	53,129	68,156	86,184	105,215	126,248	149,283	174,320	201,359
$N_1 = N_2 + 12$	9,48	18,66	28,87	40,110	55,134	71,161	88,191	108,222	130,255	153,291	178,329	205,369
$N_1 = N_2 + 13$	10,50	18,70	29,91	42,114	56,140	73,167	91,197	111,229	133,263	157,299	182,338	210,378
$N_1 = N_2 + 14$	10,53	19,73	30,95	43,119	58,145	75,173	93,204	114,236	136,271	160,308	186,347	214,388
$N_1 = N_2 + 15$	10,56	20,76	31,99	45,123	60,150	77,179	96,210	117,243	139,279	164,316	190,356	219,397
$N_1 = N_2 + 16$	11,58	20,80	32,103	46,128	61,156	79,185	98,217	120,250	143,286	168,324	194,365	223,407
$N_1 = N_2 + 17$	11,61	21,83	33,107	47,133	63,161	81,191	101,223	122,258	146,294	171,333	198,374	228,416
$N_1 = N_2 + 18$	12,63	22,86	34,111	49,137	65,166	83,197	103,230	125,265	149,302	175,341	203,382	232,426
$N_1 = N_2 + 19$	12,66	23,89	35,115	50,142	67,171	85,203	106,236	128,272	152,310	179,349	207,391	236,436
$N_1 = N_2 + 20$	12,69	23,93	36,119	51,147	68,177	87,209	108,243	131,279	156,317	182,358	211,400	241,445
$N_1 = N_2 + 21$	13,71	24,96	37,123	53,151	70,182	90,214	111,249	134,286	159,325	186,366	215,409	245,455
$N_1 = N_2 + 22$	13,74	25,99	39,127	54,156	72,187	92,220	113,256	137,293	162,333	190,374	219,418	250,464
$N_1 = N_2 + 23$	14,76	25,103	39,131	56,160	74,192	94,226	116,262	140,300	165,341	193,383	223,427	254,474
$N_1 = N_2 + 24$	14,79	26,106	40,135	57,165	75,198	96,232	118,269	143,307	169,348	197,391	227,436	259,483
$N_1 = N_2 + 25$	14,82	27,109	41,139	58,170	77,203	98,238	121,275	145,315	172,356	201,399	231,445	263,493

TABLE J: Continued

P = .01 one sided; P = .02 two-sided

N_1	$N_2=15$	$N_2=16$	$N_2=17$	$N_2=18$	$N_2=19$	$N_2=20$	$N_2=21$	$N_1=22$	$N_2=23$	$N_2=24$	$N_2=25$
$N_1 = N_2$	177,288	202,326	230,365	260,406	291,450	324,496	359,544	396,594	435,646	476,700	518,757
$N_1 = N_2 + 1$	181,299	208,336	236,376	266,418	297,463	331,509	367,557	404,608	443,661	484,716	527,773
$N_1 = N_2 + 2$	186,309	213,347	241,388	272,430	304,475	338,522	374,571	412,622	451,676	493,731	536,789
$N_1 = N_2 + 3$	191,319	218,358	247,399	278,442	310,488	345,535	381,585	419,637	459,691	501,747	545,805
$N_1 = N_2 + 4$	196,329	223,369	253,410	284,454	317,500	352,548	388,599	427,651	467,706	510,762	554,821
$N_1 = N_2 + 5$	200,340	228,380	258,422	290,466	323,513	359,561	396,612	435,665	476,720	518,778	563,837
$N_1 = N_2 + 6$	205,350	234,390	264,433	296,478	330,525	365,575	403,626	442,680	484,735	527,793	572,853
$N_1 = N_2 + 7$	210,360	239,401	269,445	302,490	336,538	372,588	410,640	450,694	492,750	535,809	581,869
$N_1 = N_2 + 8$	215,370	244,412	275,456	308,502	343,550	379,601	418,653	458,708	500,765	544,824	590,885
$N_1 = N_2 + 9$	220,380	249,423	281,467	314,514	349,563	386,614	425,667	466,722	508,780	553,839	599,901
$N_1 = N_2 + 10$	225,390	255,433	286,479	320,526	356,575	393,627	432,681	473,737	516,795	561,855	608,917
$N_1 = N_2 + 11$	229,401	260,444	292,490	326,538	362,588	400,640	440,694	481,751	524,810	570,870	617,933
$N_1 = N_2 + 12$	234,411	265,455	298,501	332,550	369,600	407,653	447,708	489,765	533,824	578,886	626,949
$N_1 = N_2 + 13$	239,421	270,466	303,513	338,562	375,613	414,666	454,722	497,779	541,839	587,901	635,965
$N_1 = N_2 + 14$	244,431	276,476	309,524	344,574	382,625	421,679	462,735	504,794	549,854	596,916	644,981
$N_1 = N_2 + 15$	249,441	281,487	315,535	350,586	388,638	428,692	469,749	512,808	557,869	604,932	653,997
$N_1 = N_2 + 16$	254,451	286,498	320,547	357,597	395,650	434,706	476,763	520,822	565,884	613,947	662,1013
$N_1 = N_2 + 17$	259,461	291,509	326,558	363,609	401,663	441,719	484,776	528,836	574,898	621,963	671,1029
$N_1 = N_2 + 18$	264,472	297,519	332,569	369,621	408,675	448,732	491,790	535,851	582,913	630,978	680,1045
$N_1 = N_2 + 19$	268,482	302,530	337,581	375,633	414,688	455,745	498,804	543,865	590,928	639,993	689,1061
$N_1 = N_2 + 20$	273,492	307,541	343,592	381,645	421,700	462,758	506,817	551,879	598,943	647,1009	689,1077
$N_1 = N_2 + 21$	278,502	312,552	349,603	387,657	427,713	469,771	513,831	559,893	606,958	656,1024	707,1093
$N_1 = N_2 + 22$	283,512	318,562	355,614	393,669	434,725	476,784	520,845	567,907	615,972	665,1039	716,1109
$N_1 = N_2 + 23$	288,522	323,573	361,626	399,681	440,738	483,797	528,858	574,922	623,987	673,1055	726,1124
$N_1 = N_2 + 24$	293,532	328,584	366,637	405,693	447,750	490,810	535,872	582,936	631,1002	682,1070	735,1140
$N_1 = N_2 + 25$	298,542	334,594	372,648	412,704	453,763	497,823	543,885	590,950	639,1017	691,1085	744,1156

APPENDIX 2: DEFINITION OF TERMS

Accuracy - The degree to which a measurement reflects the true value of a variable.

Assumptions - Accepted properties of populations, samples, or of the variables that make them up. Every test or technique has a set of underlying assumptions without which it is not completely valid. Robust tests suffer less from violations of assumptions.

Continuous - Data that can be considered as points on an unbroken line. Meters, minutes, and kilograms are generally measured so that they are examples of continuous data.

Degree of Freedom (df) - Choices or freedom to vary. If testing one group, the dfs are N-1. If two groups, it is N-2. Each additional group "costs" another df.

Dependent Variable - Response or predicted value (such as the number of animals dying given a certain dose).

Discontinuous - Data based on measurements which can only be expressed as whole numbers or units, such as numbers of animals. Also called discrete data.

False Negative - When there is an actual effect (difference between groups) but it is statistically judged not to be significant. See type II error.

False Positive - When a statistical test detects a significant difference where, in fact, there is none. See type I error.

Frequency Distribution - The manner in which data points are distributed in accordance with their values. A histogram is a plot of a frequency distribution. The Gaussian curve is a plot of the frequency distribution of a normal distribution.

Homoscedasticity - The condition when variability of the data of two or more groups, expressed as standard deviations, is equivalent.

Hypothesis - A statement of the proposed relationship between two sets of variables. Usually presented as the null hypothesis, H_0, which states that there is no relationship.

Independence - An assumption basic to many statistical techniques and to experimental design: that the measurement of any one datum (or collection of any sample) does not affect or is not affected by that of another sample.

Independent Variable - Treatment or predictor variables.

Kurtosis - Peakedness. A leptokurtic curve is very thin and pointed. A normal curve is mesokurtic. A platykurtic curve is flattened.

Mean - Usually refers to the arithmetic mean. The average computed as the sum of values divided by the total number of values.

Measurement Scales - Quantal/Nominal - Classified as one sort or another such as dead or alive. Ordinal - Numbers reflect the rank order of the values but not the distance between values. Numerical/Interval - Each value is by definition a precise degree greater or lesser than every other value.

Median - The middle value in a sample or population. Exactly half the values are greater and half are less.

Mode - The most common value in a sample or population - the value that occurs the most often.

Multivariate - The study of one or more independent and one or more dependent variables, and the relationships between them.

N - The number of cases in a sample, such as the number of animals in a treatment group.

Normal - The most common frequency distribution, which describes such variables as heights, body weights, and red blood cell counts. The distribution is such that 68% of the population is within ± 1.0 standard deviation of the mean and 95% of the population is within ± 1.96 standard deviation of the mean.

Outlier - An extreme value which seemingly is not part of the data set (in comparison to the other data).

Parameters - Values which describe characteristics of a population - Mean, Standard Deviation, Variance, Proportion, Number of Cases.

Power - The probability of rejecting the null hypothesis when it is actually false. This is equal to 1.0 minus the probability of making a type II error, or $1-\alpha$.

Precision - The reproducibility of measurement of a variable.

Population - All the possible values in a set, such as all second graders in the United States.

Quartile - A portion of a sample or population which contains one quarter of all values.

Range - The entire expanse of values in a sample or population, the interval that includes all possible values.

Rank - To arrange all the values in a data set from lowest to highest (or from highest to lowest). Once a data set is so arranged, then the order in which values occur in the set (first, second, third, etc.) is the value's assigned rank (1,2,3, etc.).

Residuals - What remain after a summary or fitted model has been subtracted out of the data according to the equation.

$$residual = data - fit.$$

Resistance - Insensitivity to localized "misbehavior" in data. Resistant methods pay much attention to the main body of the data and little to outliers. The median is a resistant statistic, whereas the sample mean is not.

Robustness - Generally implies insensitivity to departures from the assumptions underlying the use of a method.

Rounding - Reducing the number of digits in a number in such a manner that the information present in those digits that are dropped is reflected in a modification of the last digit that is retained.

Sample - A subset of a population on which data actually are collected. Usually designed so as to be randomly collected and therefore unbiased.

Semi Quartile Distance - That portion of the range which contains the middle two quarters of all values.

Sensitivity - Ability to detect relationships between variables. Must strike a balance between the levels of different types of errors it will accept.

Significance - A measure of the probability (p) that an occurrence is due to random chance. An acceptable level of significance is usually $P \geqslant 0.05$ - that is, by random chance such a set of events would occur no more than 5% of the time.

Skewness - Tendency of a frequency distribution to be to one side or other of the mean - to the left or the right.

Standard Deviation - A measure of the dispersion of data in a normal population or sample. It is calculated as the square root of $x^{-2}/N-1$.

Type I Error - Rejecting the null hypothesis when it is in fact, true. Probability of this is called the alpha level. Also called a false positive.

Type II Error - Not rejecting the null hypothesis when it is false. The probability of this is called the beta level. Also called a false negative.

Univariate - The study of one independent and one dependent variable and the relationship between these.

APPENDIX 3: GREEK ALPHABET, ABBREVIATIONS AND SYMBOLS

A. GREEK ALPHABET

Greek character		Greek name	Use in Statistics
A α	*A α*	alpha	Type I error; False negative rate
B β	*B β*	beta	Type II error; False positive rate
Γ γ	*Γ γ*	gamma	Number of "hits" in risk assessment needed rate of change
Δ δ	*Δ δ*	delta	
E ε	*E ε*	epsilon	
Z ζ	*Z ζ*	seta	
H η	*H η*	eta	
Θ θ	*Θ θ*	theta	
I ι	*I ι*	iota	
K κ	*K κ*	kappa	
Λ λ	*Λ λ*	lambda	
M μ	*M μ*	mu	Lower case letter - arithmetic mean of population; also micro or 1×10^{-6}
N ν	*N ν*	nu	
Ξ ξ	*Ξ ξ*	xi	
O o	*O o*	omicron	
Π π	*Π π*	pi	Constant = 3.14159...
P ρ	*P ρ*	rho	
Σ σ	*Σ σ*	sigma	Capital letter-summation; lower case - standard deviation
T τ	*T τ*	tau	
Υ υ	*Υ υ*	upsilon	
Φ φ	*Φ φ*	phi	
X χ	*X χ*	chi	
Ψ ψ	*Ψ ψ*	psi	
Ω ω	*Ω ω*	omega	

B. MATHEMATICAL SYMBOLS

Symbol	Meaning
∞	Infinity
lim	Limiting value
$a \sim b$	a approximately equal to b
$a > b$	a greater than b
$a < b$	a smaller than b
$a \neq b$	a not equal to b
$\lvert a \rvert$	Absolute value of a; this is always positive
$\sum_{i}^{k} x_i$	Sum of all values $x_1, x_2, x_3, \ldots$, of all values x_1 from $i = 1$ to $i = k$ inclusive, or $$\sum_{1}^{k} x_i = x_1 + x_2 + x_3 + \ldots + x_k$$
$\int$	indefinite integral
$\int_{a}^{b}$	Definite integral, or integral between $x = a$ and $x = b$.
$a^b = c$	a^b, read as "a to the power b", known as involution, a is the base, b the exponent; a^b, or c, is the bth power of a.
$\sqrt[b]{a} = c$	$\sqrt[b]{}$ a, is the bth root of a, b being known as the root exponent. In the special case of $\sqrt[2]{a} = c$ $\sqrt[2]{a}$ or c is known as the square root of a, and the root exponent is omitted.
log	Base ten logarithm
ln	Natural logarithm
$x!$	x factorial, equal to $x\,(x-1)\,(x-2)\ldots(3)\,(2)\,(1)$
$\bar{x}$	Arithmetic mean of sample
$\bar{x}_g$	Geometric mean of sample

C. ABBREVIATIONS

ANCOVA	Analysis of Covariance
ANOVA	Analysis of Variance
CV	Coefficient of variation
df	Degree of freedom
EDA	Exploratory data analysis
N	Number of data in group
Q	Quartile
QD	Semiquartile distance (also called quartile deviation)
SAR	Structure Activity Relationship
SD	Standard deviation
SEM	Standard error of measurement

CONTENTS

I. TECHNIQUE   PROBLEM SETS NUMBER

Problem 1:

Body weights were collected from the five groups of male rats in a acute oral toxicity study. These weights are given below.

Group:	A	B	C	D	E
	204.7	196.7	208.9	206.5	205.9
	198.6	207.9	204.7	202.3	187.6
	210.3	204.5	204.1	208.7	182.4
	207.4	210.2	192.3	191.1	192.5
	202.9	203.9	206.7	189.6	203.7

Calculate the mean and standard deviation for each of these groups and for the entire set of male rats in this experiment.

Problem 2:

During the course of a chronic study, a portion of the female animals from four dose groups were necropsied and their spleens weighed. These weights are presented below.

Group A	Group B	Group C	Group D
2.14	1.97	1.92	1.87
2.12	2.14	2.14	1.74
2.21	2.16	1.85	1.98
2.11	1.87	1.92	1.89
1.99	2.17	2.17	2.01
2.05	2.04	1.97	2.03
2.04	2.01	1.89	1.95
2.00	2.06	2.05	1.86
1.97	2.19		
2.08	2.03		

Calculate the mean and standard deviation for each of these groups and for the entire set of spleens.

Problem 3:

In a cytotoxicity asaay, the number of viable cells in samples from each of three treatment groups were counted. These cell counts are presented below.

Control	Treatment A	Treatment B
362	318	312
258	247	287
347	219	317
319	308	321
297	251	374
278	293	285
321	286	326

Calculate the mean and standard deviation for each group and for the combined 21 samples.

Problem 4:

As part of a metabolism study, urine samples were collected from a group of animals at different times and the concentration of metabolite present in each sample determined. These data are presented below.

Animal	Hour 1	Hour 2	Hour 3	Hour 4
1	18	47	104	59
2	30	59	98	48
3	19	46	105	64
4	34	55	118	84
5	12	31	107	51
6	26	56	121	69
7	21	38	111	67
8	29	61	83	63
9	28	63	116	56
10	23	64	112	72

Calculate the mean and standard deviation for each of the intervals, and for each animal across the entire sampling period.

Problem 5:

Using the data presented in problem number 2, calculate the standard error of the mean for each group and for the entire data set.

Problem 6:

Using the data set from problem 4, calculate the standard error of the mean for each interval and each animal. Compare these SEM's with the SD's for the same sets of data.

Problem 7:

For each of the following three sets of data, determine the median and the semiquartile distance.

Set A: 1, 13, 47, 26, 63, 34, 3, 18, 29, 9, 31, and 39.
Set B: 53, 9, 4, 18, 25, 30, 29, 15, 41, 23, 33, 15, and 31.
Set C: 16, 43, 51, 86, 24, 26, 31, 91, 59, 68, 53, 47, 29, 46, 5, and 55.
Set D: 4, 11, 17, 19, 13, 27, 15, 6, 22, 7, 18, 23, and 15.

Problem 8:

In performing an evaluation of the neurobehavioral effects of a series of solvents, righting reflex scores were obtained and recorded for three separate groups of animals. These values are presented below.

Control	Low Dose	High Dose
0	3	3
0	1	7
1	0	4
0	3	5
0	2	8
2	1	3
1	3	4
0	2	5
0	0	8
0	1	4

Determine the median righting reflex scores and semiquartile distances for each test group.

Problem 9:
Using the data presented in problem 7, calculate both the arithmetic and geometric means for each of the four data sets.

Problem 10:
As part of an inhalation study, samples of dust particles were collected from three different generation systems. The aerodynamic diameter of portions of each sample were determined and are presented below.

Generator A	Generator B	Generator C
18	4	1
250	1	7
164	29	6
142	19	9
187	16	9
129	23	1
178	26	5
225	11	8
153	18	12
46	37	39

Calculate the arithmetic and geometric means of particle diameters for each of the three generation systems.

Problem 11:
Using the data presented in problem one, calculate coefficients of variation for the five groups of animal weights.

Problem 12:
Using the data presented in problem 10, calculate the coefficients of variation for the particle size measurements from each of the three generators.

Problem 13:
During an acute oral study, several technicians weighed members of groups of animals. Use Chauvenet's criterion to identify outliers (from the data sets presented below) which may represent operator errors.

Group A	Group B	Group C
164.08	177.58	209.84
163.32	168.28	223.46
162.98	172.78	214.46
167.80	180.94	213.14
165.16	110.44	204.46

Problem 14:
During the course of a dermal study, blood samples were collected and analyzed for methemoglobin levels. The cooximeter which was used for these measurements jammed with blood clots several times during the measurements, and it is suspected that this may have interferred with the proper evaluation of some samples. Using Chauvenet's criterion, identify outlier values from the following three data sets.

Control	Low Dose	High Dose
0.16	0.94	5.64
0.14	0.86	4.97
0.21	0.65	4.85
0.23	0.42	0.01
0.19	0.47	6.12
0.11	0.54	5.89
0.12	0.02	5.94
0.26	0.46	3.87
0.20	0.75	5.61
0.17	0.01	1.04

Problem 15:
Using the rule and procedures presented in the text, present the following ten values as both rounded and truncated to three digits.

A.	163.32	F.	165.49
B.	14.51	G.	0.0953
C.	10.50	H.	1.0953
D.	165.42	I.	14.18
E.	0.0987	J.	11.56

Problem 16:
Using the rule and procedures presented in the text, present the following six values as both rounded and truncated to four digits.

A.	1053.26	D.	19.9850
B.	0.5326	E.	162.49
C.	19.9950	F.	162.51

Problem 17:

Using the data presented in problem 1 to estimate sample standard deviation, calculate the group sample sizes necessary to have a p level of 0.05. The acceptable range of variations in weights is five grams.

Problem 18:

Using the data presented in problem 2 to estimate sample standard deviation, calculate the group sample sizes necessary to have a p level of 0.05. The acceptable range of variations in spleen weights is 0.10 grams.

Problem 19:

Using the same procedure and data as detailed in problems 17 and 18, calculate the sample sizes necessary to have a p level of 0.01 for both these sets of controls and experimental groups.

Problem 20:

Prepare scattergrams of the following data sets such that the nature of the distribution and occurrence of outliers can be evaluated.

Group A: 1.6, 2.4, 3.3, 3.5, 4.1, 4.3, 4.4, 4.7, 5.2, 5.3, 5.5, 5.6, 5.7, 6.3, 6.4, 6.6, 6.8, 7.2, 7.5, 8.3, 9.2

Group B: 1.0, 2.1, 3.2, 4.1, 5.2, 6.3, 7.0, 7.6, 7.7, 7.8, 8.2, 8.3, 8.4, 8.5, 8.6, 8.7, 8.9, 9.1, 9.2, 9.5, 10.0

Problem 21:

Calculate Bartletts homogenicity of variance for the body weights of the male and female rats body weights presented below, and state whether (at a $p \leq 0.05$ level) the variances are such that an analysis of variance should be employed in further analyses.

	Group A	Group B	Group C	Group D
Males:	194.4	201.8	216.0	235.4
	189.3	230.8	225.5	207.8
	195.1	190.4	219.2	221.5
	212.5	201.7	218.0	210.1
	223.3	218.8	208.5	204.2
	195.5	216.7	214.4	213.5
	203.2	178.9	222.2	191.4
	187.5	225.3	213.5	214.1
	186.1	231.7	195.6	204.5
	220.4	223.8	243.2	225.9

	Group A	Group B	Group C	Group D
Females:	152.4	142.3	129.7	141.6
	154.8	145.8	134.8	124.4
	140.9	140.9	146.8	134.7
	137.7	138.6	152.9	148.8
	135.6	139.2	168.5	135.9
	136.6	138.0	154.0	132.8
	148.2	140.8	144.1	136.9
	141.5	142.2	147.3	145.2
	143.1	153.9	149.8	144.5
	141.4	141.8	146.2	140.6

Problem 22:

Calculate the Bartlett's homogenicity of variance for the male and female brain weights presented below.

	Group A	Group B	Group C	Group D
Males:	1.70	1.66	1.82	1.79
	1.70	1.78	1.81	1.72
	1.70	1.69	1.80	1.81
	1.77	1.74	1.89	1.72
	1.81	1.73	1.60	1.73
	1.71	1.81	1.73	1.71
	1.70	1.72	1.80	1.74
	1.70	1.81	1.77	1.87
	1.71	1.80	1.80	1.82
	1.72	1.86	1.79	1.88

	Group A	Group B	Group C	Group D
Females:	1.63	1.65	1.60	1.63
	1.63	1.50	1.62	1.66
	1.66	1.55	1.66	1.65
	1.58	1.58	1.71	1.64
	1.57	1.56	1.70	1.62
	1.66	1.64	1.68	1.58
	1.65	1.72	1.69	1.63
	1.67	1.62	1.63	1.69
	1.65	0.58	1.68	1.60
	1.61	1.70	1.67	1.68

Problem 23:

In reviewing a study conducted in another laboratory, you want to ensure that animals were randomly assigned to each of the five test groups. Using a sign test, evaluate the validity of randomization of the five groups of animals presented as below.

Group I	Group II	Group III	Group IV	Group V
17	19	20	22	36
21	27	26	23	38
24	37	34	25	44
30	50	45	29	49
31	52	54	32	51
40	53	57	33	69
41	68	60	35	71
43	73	67	39	79
55	81	75	42	83
59	82	85	47	88

Problem 24:

While reviewing acute studies on a series of related compounds, you notice that the incidence of clinical observations by some technicians seems higher than others. Given the number of times in each study that each of four technicians have recorded seeing effects during clinical tests, and using a sign test as a quick and easy assessment, evaluate the possibility that the different technicans are not equivalent in their performance of clinical observations.

Technician A	Technician B	Technician C	Technician D
12	4	31	7
15	25	27	9
10	32	13	6
26	6	29	5
15	16	24	14
16	26	28	21
10	15	30	11
4	36	9	19
8	21	8	0
18	7	10	15

Problem 25:

Determine the arcsin transformed values of the following ten incidence rates.

A. 13/50
B. 3/10
C. 4/25
D. 7/49
E. 3/21
F. 5/50
G. 10/18
H. 12/100
I. 12/50
J. 7/50

Problem 26:
Determine the probit transformation values associated with the ten incidences presented below:

    A. 7/10
    B. 2/100
    C. 3/9
    D. 8/30
    E. 49/50
    F. 7/29
    G. 5/12
    H. 7/28
    I. 34/46
    J. 99/100

Problem 27:
Using Fisher's Exact test, determine if any of the tumor incidences presented below are statistically higher in test group animals.

Site	Control		Test Group	
	Males	**Females**	**Males**	**Females**
Liver	2/50	4/50	17/50	8/50
Pituitary	4/50	6/49	7/50	5/50
Lung	2/50	1/50	7/50	6/50
Kidney	4/50	1/50	15/50	14/50
Mammary	NA	12/50	NA	19/50

Present the exact p values for each of the nine test group incidences.

Problem 28:
Calculate and present the Fishers exact values for the following incidence rates.

A.	0/10 vs. 3/10	F.	6/12 vs. 12/12
B.	0/10 vs. 4/10	G.	5/15 vs. 9/15
C.	3/10 vs. 7/10	H.	5/15 vs. 10/15
D.	3/10 vs. 8/10	I.	5/15 vs. 11/15
E.	2/10 vs. 6/8	J.	5/20 vs. 10/20

Problem 29:
Using Fisher's exact test, determine which of the five following incidence rates is significantly different from a control rate of 1/25 at $p \leq 0.05$.

    A. 3/10
    B. 4/10
    C. 7/25
    D. 10/25
    E. 20/100

What do these results suggest about the influence of differences in group sizes on test results?

Problem 30:
Using Fisher's exact test, determine which of the five following incidence rates is significantly different from a control rate of 9/100 at $p \leqslant 0.05$.

    A.   9/50
    B.   13/100
    C.   18/100
    D.   8/50
    E.   13/96

Problem 31:
Using a 2 x 2 chi square test, determine which of the following incidence rates are significantly different ($p \leqslant 0.05$) from a control rate of 6/15.

    A.   9/15
    B.   10/15
    C.   15/20
    D.   21/30
    E.   18/30

Problem 32:
Using a 2 x 2 chi square test, evaluate the incidence rates presented in Problem 28 for significance at $p \leqslant 0.05$ and $p \leqslant 0.01$.

Problem 33:
Using a 2 x 2 chi square test, evaluate the incidence rates presented in Problem 30 for significance at $p \leqslant 0.05$ and $p \leqslant 0.01$.

Problem 34:
Using a 2 x 2 chi square test, evaluate the significance of differences for each of the four following sets of data.

    A.   Control   8/13   Test   13/18
    B.   Control   7/13   Test   12/16
    C.   Control   13/49   Test   10/49
    D.   Control   7/92   Test   10/80

Problem 35:
In developing a new test method, each of three technicians used four different techniques to measure one of the endpoints. For each technician and technique we determine the number of times the accuracy of the measurements is unacceptable. These are presented in the table below.

	Technique				Total per technician
	A	B	C	D	
Technician 1	10	5	15	12	42
Technician 2	10	12	21	19	62
Technician 3	13	10	17	20	60
Total per Technique	33	27	53	51	164

Are there significant differences between techniques?

Problem 36:
In evaluating a *Drosophilla* mutagenesis test the following frequencies of eye color were recorded.

Eye Color	Treatment A	B	C	D	Row Total
Black	11	10	9	16	46
Red	9	38	52	54	153
Albino	12	24	56	57	149
Barred	16	18	34	74	142
Column Total	48	90	151	201	490

Were there any significant relationships between treatment and eye color at a level of $p \leq 0.05$?

Problem 37:
In evaluating the aquatic environmental effects of production plant effluents, we must determine if there is a relationship between the populations of fish in proximity to effluent streams in local rivers. A species capture study was performed and the data from it presented below.

Fish Species	Site Upstream	Plant 1	Plant 2	Row Total
A	54	15	17	86
B	27	25	22	74
C	14	27	36	77
D	32	16	28	76
E	73	47	53	173
F	9	12	37	58
Column Total	209	142	193	544

Is there a statistical relationship at the level of $p < 0.05$ in an R x C chi square test?

Problem 38:
Using an R x C chi square test, examine the tumor incidence presented in Problem 27 to determine if there is a relationship between treatment and the pattern of tumors in the female at a level of $p \leq 0.05$.

Problem 39:
Segmented RBC counts were determined for blood samples collected from rats. These are presented in the table below.

GROUP A	GROUP B
6	6
11	4
8	11
8	14
10	13
9	10
13	15
5	12
11	22
15	15

Using the Wilcoxon rank sum, determine if these groups are different at $p \leqslant 0.05$.

Problem 40:

Using the Wilcoxon rank sum test, compare the treatment group presented below with the control group.

CONTROL	TREATMENT
12	4
11	9
9	1
6	13
12	10
9	18
10	17
9	14
6	12
8	16

Are these groups different at $p \leqslant 0.05$?

Problem 41:

Using the Wilcoxon rank sum test, evaluate the difference between the following two sets of lymphocyte counts at a level of $p \leqslant 0.01$.

GROUP A	GROUP B
92	93
84	87
84	95
80	94
89	88
83	84
85	89
86	91
82	97
85	87
81	92

Problem 42:
Compare the following two sets of implantation site counts at levels of $p \leq 0.05$ and $p \leq 0.01$ using the Wilcoxon rank sum test.

Control: 13, 15, 12, 9, 12, 13, 14, 14, 10, 14, 13, 14, 12, 11, 8, 16, 12, 13, 13, 14 and 12.

Test: 11, 13, 12, 12, 11, 14, 7, 10, 11, 13, 12, 13, 9, 12, 12, 11, 10, 8, 10, 13 and 11.

Problem 43:
Use the Mann-Whitney U test to compare the two groups in Problem 41.

Problem 44:
Use the Mann-Whitney U test to compare the two groups in Problem 42.

Problem 45:
Righting reflex scores were determined for each animal in a study dosing. Are there any significant differences between the scores from the four groups of animals presented below? Use the Kruskall-Wallis nonparametric ANOVA to evaluate.

CONTROL	1 mg/kg	5 mg/kg	15 mg/kg
0	1	1	2
0	1	2	2
0	1	2	3
0	2	2	3
0	2	2	3
0	2	2	4
1	3	3	8
1	3	3	8
1	3	3	8
1	3	4	8

Problem 46:
As in Problem 45 use the Kruskall-Wallis test to determine if there are any significant differences between groups in the following data.

CONTROL	LOW DOSE	MID DOSE	HIGH DOSE
0	1	2	4
0	1	3	5
0	2	3	5
0	2	3	6
0	2	4	6
0	2	4	6
0	2	4	6
1	2	4	7
1	3	5	7
1	3	5	7

How do the arithmetic means of these groups vary from those in problem 45? What is the major difference between the two sets of data?

Problem 47:
Use the Kruskall-Wallis test to compare the three sets of implantation site counts below. Are any of the groups significantly different from another group at $p \leq 0.05$?

CONTROL	LOW DOSE	HIGH DOSE
8	7	3
9	8	3
10	9	4
11	9	4
11	10	5
12	10	6
12	10	6
12	11	6
12	11	7
13	11	7
13	11	7
13	11	7
13	11	7
13	11	8
14	12	8
14	12	10
14	12	10
15	12	10
15	13	11
16	14	13

Problem 48:
Compare the following two sets of body weights using the Student's t-Test. Are they significantly different? At what level?

CONTROL	TREATMENT
148.6	154.3
154.7	149.4
151.7	153.6
144.7	151.8
155.8	154.0
160.8	155.1
151.4	151.1
152.1	152.3
148.3	147.3
150.1	156.7

Problem 49:

Compare the following two sets of body weights using the Student's t-Test at a level of $p \leq 0.05$.

CONTROL	TREATMENT
224.7	217.3
213.3	217.8
226.3	220.8
229.6	228.3
213.8	220.8
209.2	223.5
208.4	209.6
214.0	212.8
207.2	222.2
210.9	218.8

Problem 50:

Using Student's t-Test, compare the following two sets of creatinine values presented below at the level of $p \leq 0.05$.

CONTROL	TREATMENT
201.3	113.3
171.6	128.7
149.6	141.9
206.8	152.9
192.5	150.7

Problem 51:

Using Student's t-test, compare the following two sets of alkaline phosphatase data.

A	B
531	504
500	530
498	470
538	528
519	510
582	506
538	542
519	496
612	526
540	491

Problem 52:

Using the Student's t-Test, compare the following two sets of alkaline phosphotase data. How does this data set differ from that in Problem 51?

A	B
521	494
500	540
498	470
548	538
509	500
582	496
548	542
509	486
612	546
550	491
567	
508	

Problem 53:

Compare the following unequal groups of data using the Cochran t-test. Are they significantly different?

A	B
521	504
510	527
498	470
538	524
519	510
572	502
538	525
519	490
602	538
540	
557	
518	
544	
543	

Problem 54:

Using the Cochran's t-test, compare the two groups of serum glucose values presented below. Are they significantly different at a $p \leq 0.05$ level?

GROUP A	GROUP B
166	179
157	180
168	169
174	182
178	188
174	177
168	186
170	166
169	
174	
168	

Problem 55:
Using the F-test, evaluate the two data sets in Problems 53 and 54 for homogeneity of variance. Use the first 9 pairs of values in 53 and the first 8 in 54.

Problem 56:
Using the F-test, evaluate the two data sets in Problems 51 and 52 for homogeneity of variance.

Problem 57:
Using an analysis of variance, analyze the body weights from the following four groups of rats to determine if there are any statistically significant differences between groups.

GROUP A	GROUP B	GROUP C	GROUP D
148.5	146.8	148.7	148.0
153.2	157.3	154.5	144.8
148.9	143.5	152.3	148.7
141.8	156.6	139.4	150.7
149.8	148.0	146.9	146.7
152.2	151.6	151.7	146.1
147.7	150.4	149.8	146.7
145.4	155.1	144.0	151.9
144.2	144.1	150.5	142.4
146.2	145.8	151.3	152.3
145.7	149.2	144.0	150.1
152.1	151.1	148.9	146.8

Problem 58:

Using an analysis of variance, compare the body weights from five groups of rats to determine if there are any statistically significant differences between groups. Data is presented below.

GROUP A	GROUP B	GROUP C	GROUP D	GROUP E
326.2	314.5	324.9	306.2	274.0
296.1	312.5	316.2	314.6	279.2
316.9	312.2	286.4	302.5	292.2
328.2	333.7	334.7	317.8	293.9
327.8	298.3	303.88	319.3	274.2
311.1	320.7	325.5	300.1	285.5
340.9	324.4	314.4	316.6	279.5
327.2	324.4	348.4	301.3	290.9
314.8	331.1	284.1	333.4	276.7
325.5	335.1	317.8	303.5	297.7
326.6	331.6	311.5	305.3	252.8
305.1	303.4	306.2	292.9	271.0
302.2	333.9	325.1	283.8	265.7
343.6	301.1	322.4	323.9	277.9
335.5	335.7	270.2	310.4	273.2

Problem 59:

Using an analysis of variance, compare the following four sets of alkaline phosphatase data and determine if there are any significant differences between the groups.

GROUP A	GROUP B	GROUP C	GROUP D
418	437	380	272
367	413	501	334
328	348	356	368
276	307	386	357
421	416	341	448
312	388	413	390
279	426	332	376
306	401	373	314
342	384	370	517
379	359	400	340

Problem 60:

Using an analysis of variance, compare the SGPT values presented below for five groups of rats.

GROUP A	GROUP B	GROUP C	GROUP D	GROUP E
65	53	65	79	80
66	65	83	73	70
59	58	66	56	87
46	88	57	58	86
77	133	82	56	76
52	58	69	85	71
48	69	86	72	84
52	66	77	66	102
63	58	68	59	93
76	66		74	

Problem 61:
Using Duncan's Multiple range test, compare the groups in Problem 57 to determine which, if any, groups are significantly different at the $p \leq 0.05$ level.

Problem 62:
Using Duncan's Multiple range test, compare the groups in Problem 58 to determine which, if any, groups are significantly different.

Problem 63:
Using Duncan's Multiple range test, compare the groups in problem 60 to determine which, if any, are significantly different.

Problem 64:
Using Scheffe's method, compare the groups in Problem 59 to determine which, if any, are significantly different.

Problem 65:
Using Scheffe's method, compare the groups in Problem 60 to determine which, if any, are significantly different.

Problem 66:
Using Dunnet's t-Test, compare the groups in Problem 58 to determine which, if any, are significantly different. For the purposes of this problem, assume Group A is the control group while Groups B - E are successively higher dosage groups.

Problem 67:
Using Dunnet's t-Test, compare the groups in Problem 60 to determine which, if any, are significantly different. For the purposes of this problem, assume Group A is the control group while Groups B - E are groups with successively higher inhalation exposure levels.

Problem 68:

Use analysis of covariance to adjust for body weight (BW) effects and determine if there is any difference between combined kidney weights of the four groups of animals below at a $p \leq 0.05$ level.

CONTROL		LOW DOSE		MID DOSE		HIGH DOSE	
BW	KIDNEY WT	BW	KIDNEY WT	BW	KIDNEY WT	BW	KIDNEY WT
184.2	1.74	174.3	1.63	182.0	1.64	176.4	1.55
183.5	1.73	178.6	1.67	179.8	1.62	167.4	1.47
186.9	1.76	184.2	1.72	174.2	1.56	172.4	1.53
188.8	1.78	183.9	1.72	179.3	1.61	171.5	1.51
188.6	1.77	182.4	1.70	178.6	1.63	177.3	1.56
189.7	1.79	192.7	1.80	180.7	1.62	173.6	1.53
194.4	1.83	186.3	1.73	176.3	1.59	172.9	1.52
192.6	1.82	194.8	1.83	186.5	1.69	168.1	1.48

Problem 69:

Using analysis of covariance to adjust for body weight (BW) effects, determine if there is any difference between spleen weights of the four groups of animals presented below at a $p < 0.05$ level.

CONTROL		LOW DOSE		MID DOSE		HIGH DOSE	
BW	SPLEEN WT	BW	SPLEEN WT	BW	SPLEEN WT	BW	SPLEEN WT
142.2	0.40	147.5	0.45	138.6	0.45	132.2	0.49
146.9	0.42	143.6	0.43	142.9	0.46	130.2	0.47
138.7	0.39	140.4	0.43	130.3	0.42	134.6	0.50
144.3	0.41	138.2	0.41	134.6	0.43	125.4	0.46
140.5	0.40	133.9	0.40	146.7	0.47	127.8	0.47

Problem 70:

We would like to determine if a pollutant had an effect on the average height of pine trees over a period of time. We measure both the ages (in years, by counting rings) and height of two random samples of pines (one from the contaminated area and the other from a noncontaminated area). These data are presented below.

CONTROL		CONTAMINATED	
AGE (YEARS)	HEIGHT (FEET)	AGE (YEARS)	HEIGHT (FEET)
71	79.0	59	77.6
71	80.9	63	87.8
78	74.9	65	77.6
79	89.5	66	80.7
81	88.7	70	72.7
82	71.0	71	85.4
83	82.3	74	75.0

CONTROL		CONTAMINATED	
AGE (YEARS)	HEIGHT (FEET)	AGE (YEARS)	HEIGHT (FEET)
84	79.9	76	73.0
88	82.9	79	88.5
88	87.7	80	87.5
88	87.7	83	88.8
90	74.6	84	73.2
90	75.8	85	87.7
90	88.5	87	92.0

Using analysis of covariance to adjust for age, determine if there is a statistically significant effect.

Problem 71:
Using the data from the control group in Problem 70, perform a linear regression of tree age vs. height. What is the predicted height of a 75 year old tree?

Problem 72:
Use linear regression to prepare a dose response curve for the following study data.

DOSE (mg/kg)	RBC SURVIVAL (days, mean)
0	59
10	57
20	55
40	44
60	38
100	22
120	17

What dose would be predicted to produce a mean survival of 50 days?

Problem 73:
The following dose response mortality data was obtained in an oral study.

DOSE (mg/kg)	% MORTALITY
10	0
20	10
40	20
60	30
80	30
140	80
160	100

Using a probit transformation for response and log transformation for dose, perform a linear regression to estimate the LD_{50} for this compound.

Problem 74:
The following dose response mortality data was obtained in an inhalation study.

CONCENTRATION (ppm)	% MORTALITY
10	0
30	10
60	20
120	30
240	60
360	80
480	80
600	100

Using a log transformation for dose and a probit transformation for response, perform a linear regression to estimate the LC_{50} for this compound.

Problem 75:
Using the moving average method, predict the LD_{50} from the data in Problem 73. Assume ten animals per group.

Problem 76:
Using the moving average method, predict the LC_{50} from the data in Problem 74. Assume ten animals per group.

Problem 77:
Using the moving average method, estimate the ED_{50} for the following oral study data. Assume eight animals per group.

DOSE (mg/kg)	EFFECTED
2	0/8
4	1/8
8	2/8
16	3/8
20	3/8
40	4/8
60	6/8
100	8/8

Problem 78:
Using the data presented in Problem 77, calculate the correlation coefficient for a linear regression.

Problem 79:
Using the data presented in Problem 74, calculate the linear correlation coefficient.

Problem 80:
Using the data presented in Problem 71, calculate the linear correlation coefficient.

Problem 81:
Using Kendall's rank correlation, determine if the height of the polluted trees in Problem 70 is rank correlated to the age.

Problem 82:
Use Kendall's rank correlation to determine if crown-rump length is inversely correlated to test error rate in the data set below.

CROWN-RUMP LENGTH	NUMBER OF ERRORS
5	24
9	18
6	24
8	19
10	16
5	26
11	17
13	14
6	23
8	22
12	15

TREND ANALYSIS

Problem 83:
Perform a Cox-Stuart trend analysis to determine if there is dose responsive increase in tumor incidence over time associated with the compound.

		COMPOUND X		
MONTH OF		TOTAL ANIMALS WITH TUMORS		
STUDY	CONTROL	LOW DOSE	MID DOSE	HIGH DOSE
10	0	0	0	0
11	1	1	2	2
12	1	3	6	6
13	1	4	10	10
14	2	6	11	13
15	3	7	13	16

Problem 83 (continued):

MONTH OF STUDY	CONTROL	COMPOUND X TOTAL ANIMALS WITH TUMORS		
		LOW DOSE	MID DOSE	HIGH DOSE
16	4	9	15	18
17	5	10	16	20
18	5	10	20	22
19	8	12	22	24
20	11	13	24	26
21	15	14	27	28
22	18	18	29	30
23	24	23	31	33
24	32	29	33	35

Problem 84:
Perform a Cox-Stuart trend analysis to determine if there is a dose responsive increase in the incidence of malformed rat pups associated with being fed either of two synthetic diets over ten generations of animals.

GENERATION	NATURAL DIET	TOTAL MALFORMED PUPS SYNTHETIC A	SYNTHETIC B
1	2	0	1
2	4	2	3
3	6	4	5
4	7	7	8
5	9	10	9
6	11	12	11
7	14	15	13
8	17	18	16
9	19	20	18
10	21	23	22

Problem 85:
Using the data presented below, perform a life table analysis to determine if there is a time-adjusted, compound-related effect on either survival or tumor incidences

Problem 85:

Interval (Months)	CONTROL ANIMALS				TEST ANIMALS			
	Alive at Beginning of Interval	Withdrawn	Dead	Animals with Tumors	Alive at Beginning of Interval	Withdrawn	Dead	Animals with Tumors
8–9	120	0	0	0	120	0	2	0
9–10	120	0	1	0	118	0	3	1
10–11	119	0	4	1	115	0	2	0
11–12	116	10	0	2	113	10	4	2
12–13	106	0	1	0	99	0	3	1
13–14	105	0	2	2	96	1	4	2
14–15	103	0	4	2	91	0	6	3
15–16	99	2	4	2	85	0	4	2
16–17	93	0	4	2	81	2	6	2
17–18	89	0	6	3	73	1	9	3
18–19	83	20	4	4	63	20	10	3
19–20	59	0	8	4	33	2	12	3
TOTAL ANIMALS FOUND WITH TUMORS				22				22

Problem 85:

Using the data presented below, perform a life table analysis to determine if there is a time adjusted compound related effect on either survival or tumor incidences

Interval (Months)	CONTROL Alive at Start of Interval	Withdrawn	Dead	TREATMENT Alive at Start of Interval	Withdrawn	Dead
0–1	100	0	1	100	0	1
1–2	99	1	1	99	0	1
2–3	98	0	3	98	0	1
3–4	95	10	2	97	10	1
4–5	83	0	3	86	0	2
5–6	80	0	5	84	0	2
6–7	75	10	4	82	0	3
7–8	61	0	6	69	0	5
8–9	55	0	5	64	0	4
9–10	50	0	8	60	0	9
10–11	42	0	7	51	0	10
11–12	35	10	9	41	10	12
TOTAL DEAD			54			51

PROBLEM SOLUTIONS

PROBLEM 1

	MEAN	STANDARD DEVIATION
Group A	204.78	4.446
Group B	204.64	5.127
Group C	203.34	6.452
Group D	199.64	8.803
Group E	194.42	10.156
Males	201.36	7.802

PROBLEM 2

	MEAN	STANDARD DEVIATION
Group A	2.071	0.07549
Group B	2.064	0.10178
Group C	1.989	0.11850
Group D	1.916	0.09561
All Spleens	2.016	0.11284

PROBLEM 3

	MEAN	STANDARD DEVIATION
Control	311.71	36.86
Treatment A	274.57	36.23
Treatment B	317.43	29.70
All Cells	301.24	38.02

PROBLEM 4

	MEAN	STANDARD DEVIATION
Hour 1	24	6.633
Hour 2	52	11.146
Hour 3	107.5	11.088
Hour 4	63.3	10.584
Animal 1	57	35.749
Animal 2	58.75	28.768
Animal 3	58.5	36.097
Animal 4	72.75	36.473
Animal 5	50.25	41.048
Animal 6	68	39.657
Animal 7	59.25	39.382
Animal 8	59	22.331
Animal 9	65.75	36.755
Animal 10	67.75	36.482

PROBLEM 5

	STANDARD ERROR OF MEAN
Group A	0.02387
Group B	0.03219
Group C	0.04189
Group D	0.03380
All Spleens	0.01881

PROBLEM 6

	STANDARD ERROR OF MEAN
Hour 1	2.098
Hour 2	3.525
Hour 3	3.506
Hour 4	3.347
Animal 1	17.875
Animal 2	14.384
Animal 3	18.048
Animal 4	18.236
Animal 5	20.524
Animal 6	19.828
Animal 7	19.691
Animal 8	11.165
Animal 9	18.377
Animal 10	18.241

PROBLEM 7

	MEDIAN	SEMIQUARTILE DISTANCE
A:	27.5	10 - 37.75
B:	25	15 - 32
C:	46.5	29 - 55
D:	15	9 - 20.5

PROBLEM 8

	MEDIAN	SEMIQUARTILE DISTANCE
Control:	0	0 - 1
Low Dose:	1.5	0.5 - 2.5
High Dose:	4.5	3.5 - 7.5

PROBLEM 9

	ARITHMETIC MEAN	GEOMETRIC MEAN
A:	26.08	16.99
B:	25.07	21.08
C:	45.62	38.07
D:	15.15	13.35

PROBLEM 10

	ARITHMETIC MEAN	GEOMETRIC MEAN
Generator A	149.2	121.70
Generator B	18.4	13.15
Generator C	9.7	6.03

PROBLEM 11

		CV
Group A	=	2.17
Group B	=	2.51
Group C	=	3.17
Group D	=	4.41
Group E	=	5.22

PROBLEM 12

		CV
Generator A	=	48.29
Generator B	=	60.31
Generator C	=	111.99

PROBLEM 13

Group A = NONE
Group B = reject 110.44
Group C = reject 227.46

PROBLEM 14

Control = reject 0.26
Low Dose = reject 0.26
High Dose = The 0.01 value is identified as an outlier. If it is dropped, then the 1.04 value would be an outlier.

PROBLEM 15

	ROUNDED	TRUNCATED
A	163	163
B	14.5	14.5
C	10.5	10.5
D	165	165
E	0.0987	0.0987
F	165	165
G	0.0953	0.0953
H	1.10	1.09
I	14.2	14.1
J	11.6	11.5

PROBLEM 16

	ROUNDED	TRUNCATED
A	1053	1053
B	0.5326	0.5326
C	20.00	19.99
D	19.99	19.98
E	162.5	162.4
F	162.5	162.5

Sample size for a p of 0.05

PROBLEM 17

3.37 or 4 animals per group.

PROBLEM 18

12.2 or 13 animals

PROBLEM 19

Problem 17 data - 6.76 or 7 animals
Problem 18 data - 24.43 or 25 animals

PROBLEM 20

Group A:

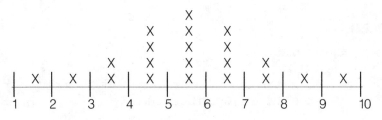

Group B:

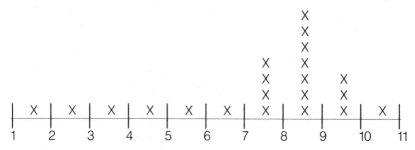

PROBLEM 21

Males: Yes p = 0.684
Females: Yes p = 0.465

PROBLEM 22

Males: Yes p = 0.235
Females: Yes p ≤ 0.01

PROBLEM 23

Group I   — 8−, 2+
Group II   — 3−, 7+
Group III   — 3−, 7+
Group IV   — 9−, 1+
Group V   — 2−, 8+
Conclusion — Assignment was not random

PROBLEM 24

Technician A — 5−, 3+, 2 midpoint
Technician B — 3−, 6+, 1 midpoint
Technician C — 4−, 6+
Technician D — 7−, 2+, 1 midpoint
Conclusion — There is no clear pattern associated with any technician

PROBLEM 25

A — 30.66
B — 33.21
C — 23.58
D — 22.21
E — 22.21
F — 18.43
G — 48.19
H — 20.27
I — 29.33
J — 21.97

PROBLEM 26

A – 5.5244
B – 2.9463
C – 4.5684
D – 4.3781
E – 7.2537
F – 4.2969
G – 4.7904
H – 4.3255
I – 5.6403
J – 7.3263

PROBLEM 27

Males   – Liver (.000098) and Kidney (0.00474)
Females – Kidney (.000194)

PROBLEM 28

A – .1052632
B – .0433436
C – .0894477
D – .0348893
E – .0306458
F – .0068650
G – .1361517
H – .0715555
I – .0327977
J – .0953963

PROBLEM 29

A – Not significant
B – Significant
C – Significant
D – Significant
E – Significant

PROBLEM 30

A – No
B – No
C – Yes : $p \leq 0.048250$
D – No
E – No

PROBLEM 31

A – NS
B – NS

C — Significant
D — Significant
E — NS

PROBLEM 32

A — $0.10 > p > 0.05$
B — $0.05 > p > 0.01$
C — $0.10 > p > 0.05$
D — $0.05 > p > 0.01$
E — $0.05 > p > 0.01$
F — $0.01 > p > 0.001$
G — $p > 0.01$
H — $0.10 > p > 0.05$
I — $0.05 > p > 0.01$
J — $0.01 > p > 0.001$

PROBLEM 33

A — $p \geqslant 0.05$
B — $p \geqslant 0.05$
C — $p \geqslant 0.05$
D — $p \geqslant 0.05$
E — $p \geqslant 0.05$

PROBLEM 34

A — $p \geqslant 0.05$
B — $p \geqslant 0.05$
C — $p > 0.05$
D — $p > 0.05$

PROBLEM 35

6 degrees of freedom. Chi square $= 2.3704$
Not significant (test statistic at $p \leqslant 0.05 = 12.592$)

PROBLEM 36

9 degrees of freedom. Chi square $= 32.1917$
$p \leqslant 0.001$ (test statistic at this level is 27.877)

PROBLEM 37

10 degrees of freedom. Chi square $= 62.1093$
$p \leqslant 0.001$ (test statistic at this level is 29.588)

PROBLEM 38

4 degrees of freedom. Chi square $= 8.7093$
Not significant (test statistic at $p \leqslant 0.05$ is 9.488)

PROBLEM 39

Group A = 86.5
Group B = 123.5
Test statistics = 79, 131 for $p \leq 0.05$
The results are not significant

PROBLEM 40

Control = 85
Treatment = 125
Test statistics = 79, 131 for $p \leq 0.05$
These results are not significant

PROBLEM 41

Group A = 81
Group B = 172
Test statistics = 96, 157 for $p \leq 0.05$
$\qquad\qquad$ = 88, 165 for $p \leq 0.01$
Groups are significantly different at $p \leq 0.01$

PROBLEM 42

Group A = 550
Group B = 353
Test statistics = 373, 530 for $p \leq 0.05$
Groups are significantly different at $p \leq 0.05$

PROBLEM 43

U_A = 106
U_B = 15
The test statistics are 35 ($p \leq 0.05$) and 26 ($p \leq 0.01$). The groups are different at $p \leq 0.05$ but not at $p \leq 0.01$.

PROBLEM 44

U_C = 122
U_T = 319
The test statistics are 146 ($p \leq 0.05$) and 122 ($p \leq 0.01$). The groups are different at $p \leq 0.05$ but not at $p \leq 0.01$.

PROBLEM 45

With three degrees of freedom, H = 25.5764. $p \leq 0.01$

PROBLEM 46

With three degrees of freedom, H = 34.7914. $p \leq 0.01$

PROBLEM 47

With two degrees of freedom, H = 31.0235. $p \leq 0.01$

PROBLEM 48

$t = 0.4425$ with eighteen degrees of freedom. Not significant at $p \leq 0.05$.

PROBLEM 49

$t = 1.1267$ with eighteen degrees of freedom. Not significant at $p \leq 0.05$.

PROBLEM 50

$t = 3.636$ with eight degrees of freedom. Not significant at $p \leq 0.05$ (and at $p \leq 0.01$).

PROBLEM 51

$t = 2.092$ with eighteen degrees of freedom. Significant at $p \leq 0.05$

PROBLEM 52

$t = 1.9447$ with twenty degrees of freedom. Not significant at $p \leq 0.05$. Though means and standard deviations are nearly equal to those of the groups in problem 51, the group sizes here are unequal.

PROBLEM 53

$t\,obs = 2.6817$
$t' = 2.2315$ (at $p \leq 0.05$), 3.180 (at $p \leq 0.0$)
Groups are significantly different at $0.05\ p > 0.01$

PROBLEM 54

$t\,obs = 2.746$
$t' = 3.401$ (at $p \leq 0.01$)
Groups are significantly different at $0.05 > p > 0.01$.

PROBLEM 55

A) For the problem 53 data set, $F = 2.38669$. The test statistic for 8 and 8df at $p \leq 0.05$ is 4.43, so the groups are suitably homogeneous.

B) For the problem 54 data set, $F = 1.43376$. The test statistic for 7 and 7df at $p \leq 0.05$ is 4.99, so the groups are suitably homogeneous.

PROBLEM 56

A) For the problem 51 data set, $F = 2.666$. The test statistic for 9 and 9df at $p \leq 0.05$ is 4.03, so the groups are suitably homogeneous.

B) For the problem 52 data set, $F = 1.6740$. The test statistic for 9 and 9df at $p \leq 0.05$ is 4.03, so the groups are suitably homogeneous.

PROBLEM 57

$F = 0.71025$, making consultation of a table unnecessary. There is no significant difference between groups.

PROBLEM 58

$F = 21.2951$, making the groups significantly different at a level of $p \leqslant 0.001$

PROBLEM 59

$F = 1.4936$, making the groups not significantly different at an .05 level (that is, $p \geqslant 0.05$)

PROBLEM 60

$F = 3.1928$, making the groups significantly different at a level of $p \leqslant 0.05$

PROBLEM 61

None of the groups are different from the others at $p \leqslant 0.05$

PROBLEM 62

Using Duncan's multiple range, group E is significantly different from all other groups at $p \leqslant 0.001$. Group D is significantly different from groups A and B at $p \leqslant 0.05$.

PROBLEM 63

Using Duncan's multipole range, group E is significantly different from group A at $p \leqslant 0.01$.

PROBLEM 64

Using Scheffe's procedure, no groups are significantly different from any others at $p \leqslant 0.05$.

PROBLEM 65

Using Scheffe's procedure, group E is significantly different from group A at $p \leqslant 0.05$.

PROBLEM 66

Using Dunnet's t-test, the only comparison is versus group A, which is designated the control. Group E is significantly different from group A at $p \leqslant 0.01$.

PROBLEM 67

Using Dunnet's t-test, the only comparison is versus gropup A, which is designated the control. Group E is significantly different from group A at $p \leqslant 0.01$.

PROBLEM 68

Using analysis of covariance, there was a significant difference between groups of kidney weights (adjusted for body weight) at $p \leqslant 0.001$. (F = 163.2)

PROBLEM 69

Using analysis of covariance, there was a significant difference between groups of spleen weights (adjusted for body weight) at $p \leqslant 0.001$. (F = 296.6)How would you determine which groups are significantly different?

PROBLEM 70

Using analysis of covariance to adjust for age, there is no significant difference between tree heights in the two samples. (F = 0.617)

PROBLEM 71

A 75 year old tree would be predicted to have a height of 80.77 feet. The correlation, however, is not particulary good ($p = 0.1197$).

PROBLEM 72

The regression should predict that a dose of 27.55 will produce a survival time of 50 days.

PROBLEM 73

The LD_{50} is predicted to be 66.67 mg/kg.

PROBLEM 74

The LC_{50} is predicted to be 153.60 ppm.

PROBLEM 75

$LD_{50} = 80.0$ mg/kg with a 95% confidence interval of 58.1 − 110.3 mg/kg. Note that you must use only the 20, 40, 80 and 160 mg/kg dose groups in the computation.

PROBLEM 76

$LC_{50} = 190.5$ ppm with a 95% confidence interval of 106.6 − 340.2 ppm. Note that you may use either the 60, 120, 240 and 480 exposure groups (which were used for these values) or the 30, 60, 120 and 240 groups (which are less desirable as they do not cover the entire range of doses).

PROBLEM 77

Cannot be calculated from the data set by this method.

PROBLEM 78

r = 0.96869

PROBLEM 79

r = 0.973

PROBLEM 80

r = 0.1197

PROBLEM 81

Kendall's rank correlation tau = 0.2857

PROBLEM 82

Kendall's rank correlation tau = 0.8727

PROBLEM 83

Cumulative scores and their probabilities under the sign test are:

low dose 6+, 9− : Sum = 3- (p ⁓0.30)
mid dose 16+, 14− : Sum = 2+ (p ⁓0.40)
high dose 18+, 14− : Sum = 4+ (p ⁓0.25)

There is a nonsignificant trend across the doses.

PROBLEM 84

Cumulative scores and their probabilities under the sign test are (compared to the natural diet)

synthetic diet A 4+ (p = 0.09)
synthetic diet B 4+, 2- (p = 0.38)